Madam Awesome

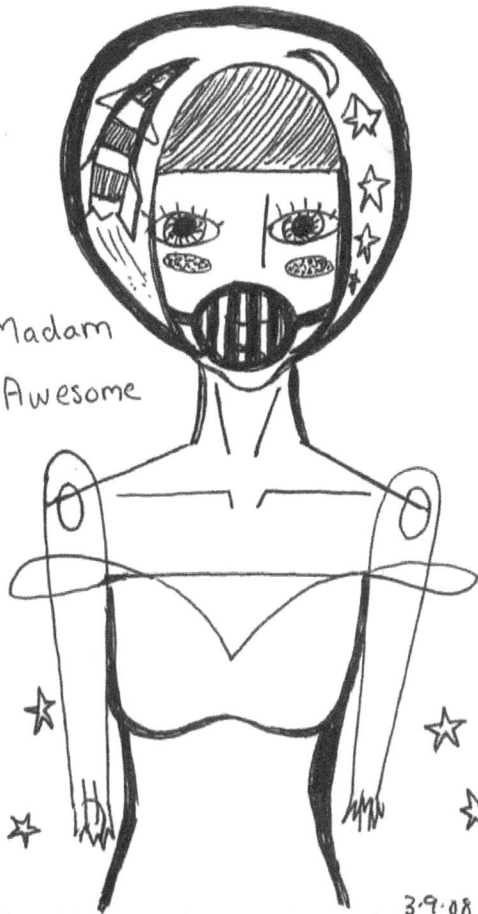

3·9·08 VG

The Delusion
The Imposter
and
The Reality

By VG. Deneen

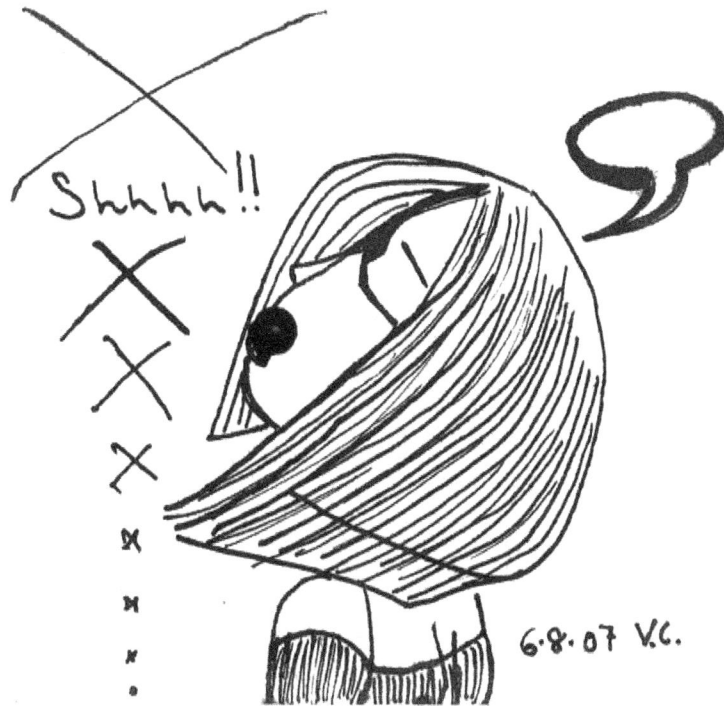

This book is
Redicated

to Every
Single Person

who thinks
This Book

is About You,
in any way.

Because
it
is.
♡ VCD

Shhhh!!

6.8.07 V.C.

Chapters

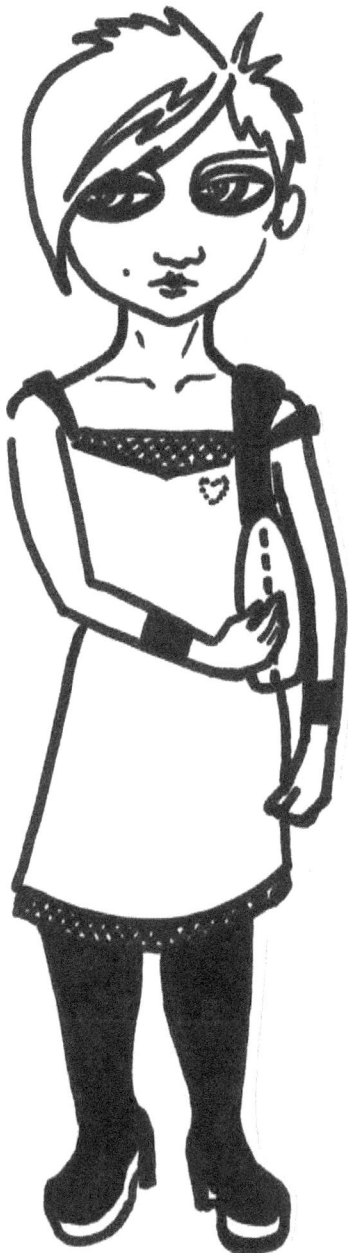

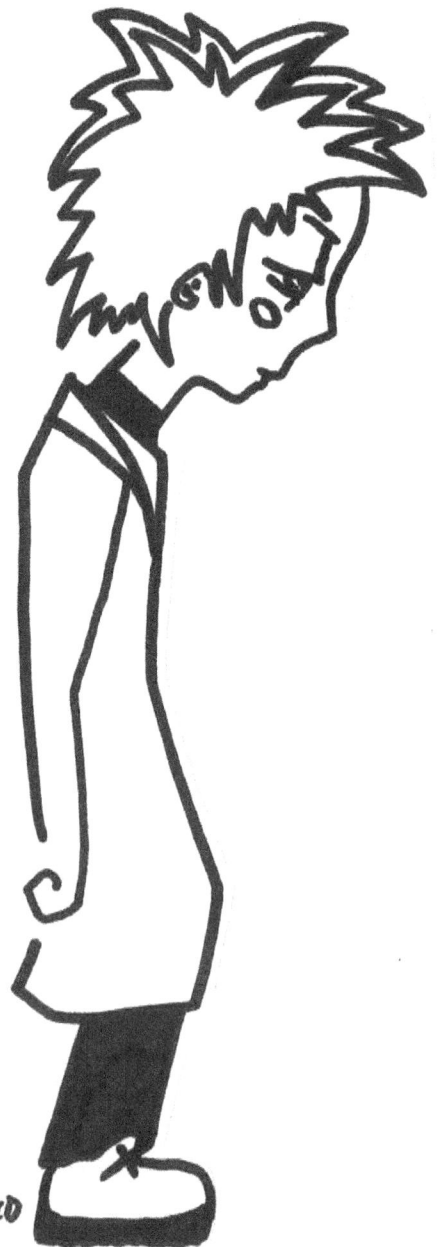

m.awesomedirofficial
IG
449·11 VCD

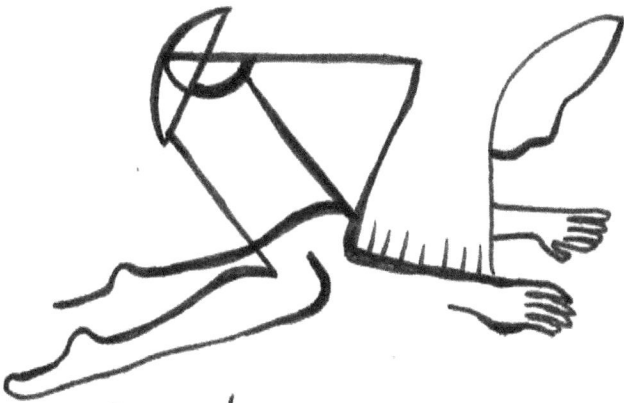

Prologue

What is Real.
Addiction.
Depression.
Anxiety.
Post Traumatic stress Disorder (PTSD).
Mental health is real.
Others like you are real.

You are real, your thoughts are not.
People in Your World are real.
Your World, not The World.
Mean people are real, what they say is not real.
Suicide is real.

Physical, mental, and emotional abuse and neglect is real.
Sexual abuse and rape is real.
These crimes are real.
Children and young suffer the most.
Many beome addicts, a lot commit suicide.
Your body is real, media bodies are not.
Babies are real, sex creates babies.
Sex trafficking and predators are real.
Human rights are real.
Racism is real.
Law corruption is real.
Good people are real, love is real.
Family of Choice is real.
Suffering is real.
You are not alone.
Really.

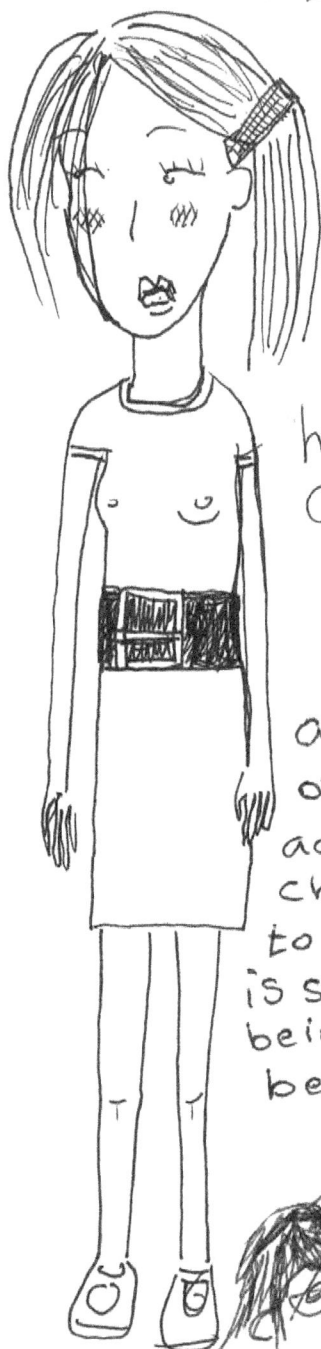

This book is for you, young adults. You are societys invisible age group. My life sucked and it messed me up. I am writing for you what I know and learned from mine and others experiences, perspective, and science.

hi. I'm clueless

Your age group should be called young adults **instead** of teens.

If elders can be called senior citizens instead, why be called teens? Adults can be bullies to young adults. Once you are adults, you can treat each other like adults. When you are legal adults, nobody gives a crap what choices you make. Young adults have to make the same choices, but the information is stupid, boring, and secritive. What are you being protected from? Young adults all become legal adults, they just do.

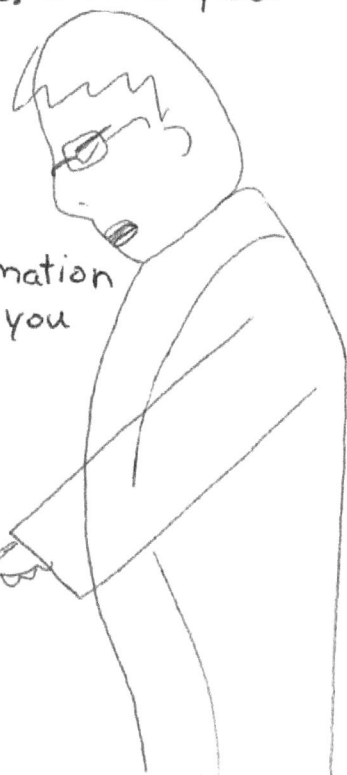

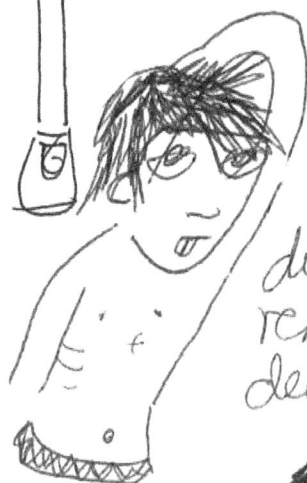

dig real deep

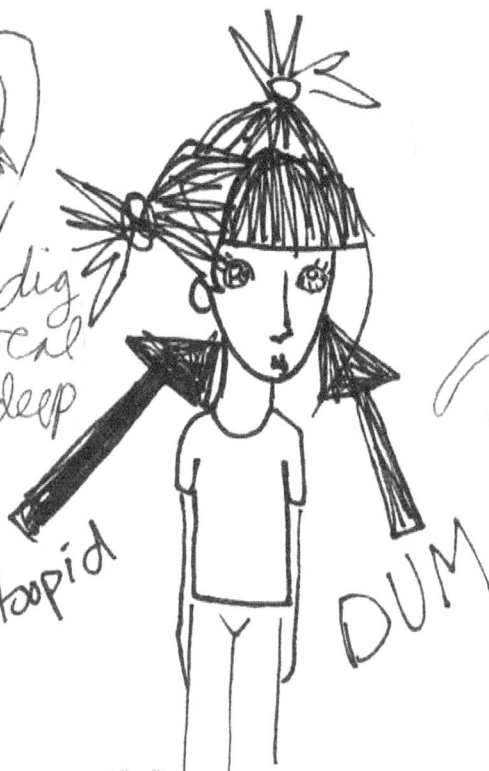

Stoopid

DUM

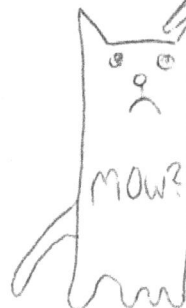

mow?

6/17/09

I don't think I am an older know-it-all.

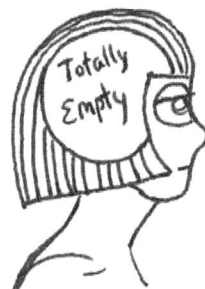

Totally Empty

There are no "did you knows?" in here. Nothing is sugar-coated or meant to scare you like children.

i know you are smart and taken for granted.

Information for young adults is condecending patronizing and dumbed-down to the point of being offensive.

There are no wrong directions in life. I was lost, but it was not my fault. Why do I care? Because life can really suck and I wish I was informed about certain things before they took a part in almost ruining my life. Young adults can grow up alone and confused, not knowing why they always feel like crap. Adults struggle with the same issues. They either "fake-it-till-they-make-it" or they make, or try to make people around them miserable like they are. I grew up with identity, image, and cultural problems. I thought I had to fit in and be successful, beautiful, smart, and rich. When I was 30, I figured out how fake all of that was. I can't change my past, it is what it was. The difference is that I am getting treated for my mental health now. Yay!

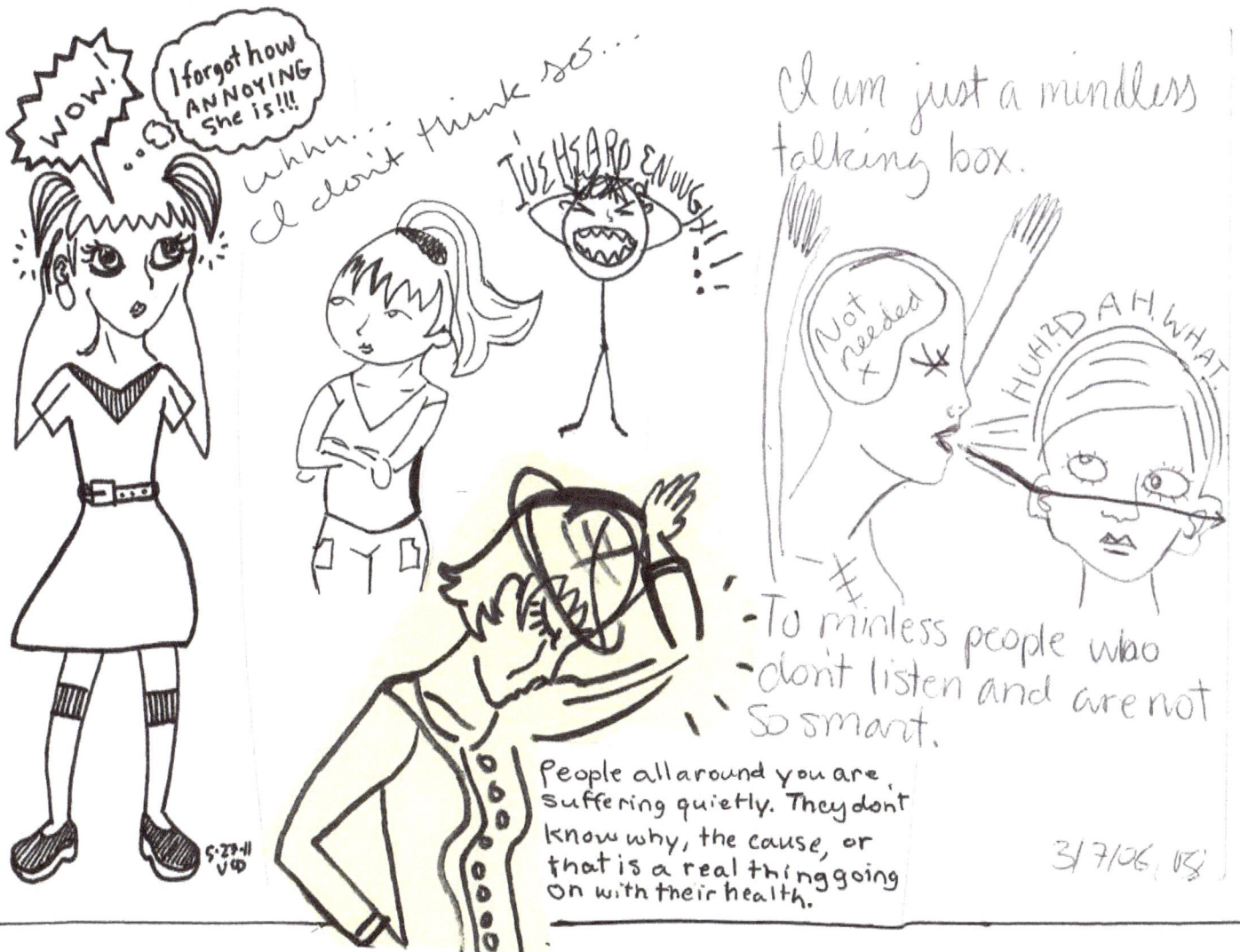

WOW.

I forgot how ANNOYING she is!!!

uhhu... I don't think so...

I'VE HEARD ENOUGH!!!

I am just a mindless talking box.

Not needed ✗

HUH? AH. WHAT.

-To mindless people who don't listen and are not so smart.

People all around you are suffering quietly. They don't know why, the cause, or that is a real thing going on with their health.

5·29·11 VO

3/7/06, 08

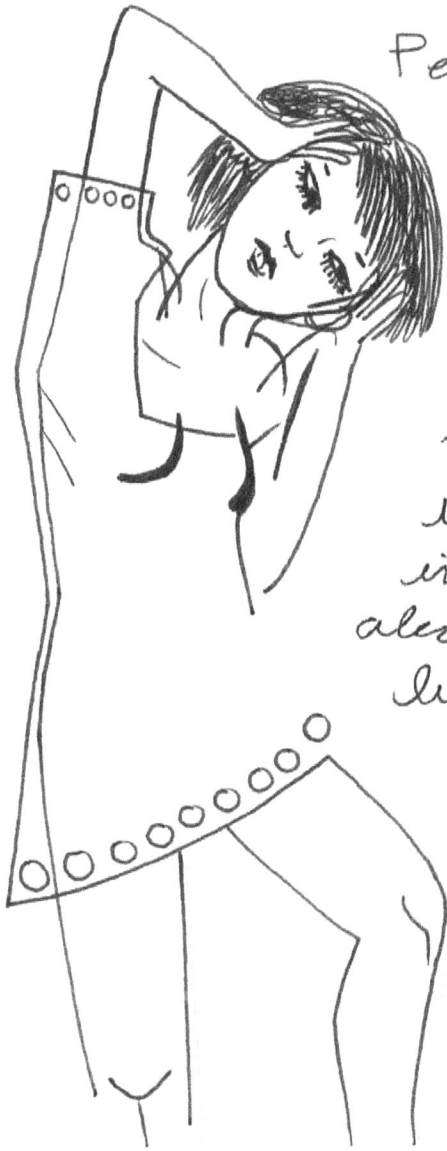

People suffer in life, they usually don't know why or what causes/caused it. Information and knowledge are powers. It can help you understand either your own behavior or the behavior of others. When life is painful, why it is easier to get so sad? into drugs and I don't know! alcohol. When you can't see the lights on your path, you can get lost like I was, I have known addicts and recovering addicts, homeless, the friend and familyless, the suicidal, depressed, anxious and untreated people. The least you can do for anyone, is see them

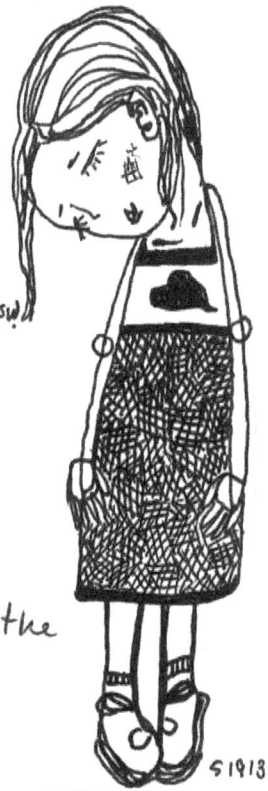

as a person. In those situations, it becomes easy for a person to expect other people to only see a worthless piece of garbage. When others see beyond The Addict, THE ALCOHOLIC, and The Crazy Person, it can mean the world to them.

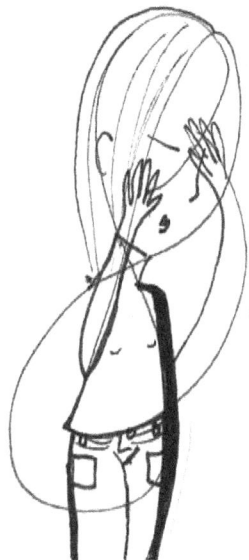

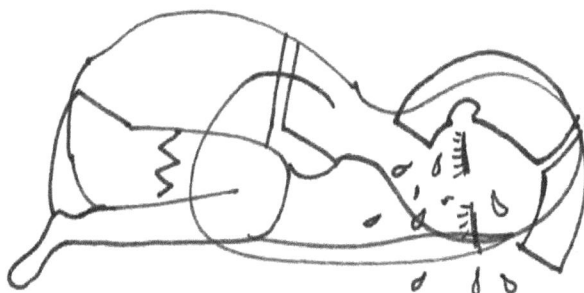

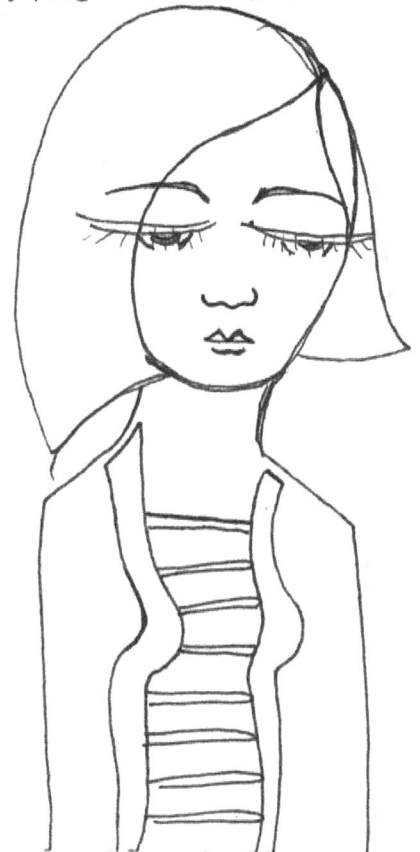

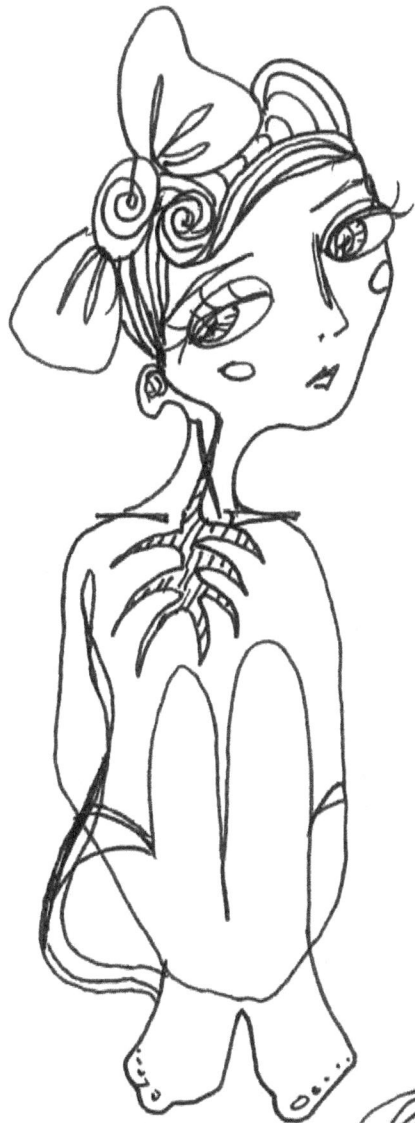

My husband is a recovering opiate addict; I am a recovering depressive. We didn't ask or expect for these things to happen, but we adapted. Our brains function differently than a "normal" brain. We can't change our pasts, but we can move forward with more knowledge and skills. You never know when addiction, depression, or anxiety will develop.

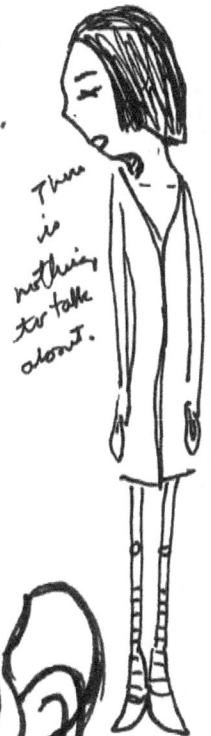

When you suffer, you may not know why at the time. It is not easy to tell others what is going on with you in your reality. I wish I had known these things instead of feeling like crap all the time and wanting to kill myself. How I felt had become who I THOUGHT I was.

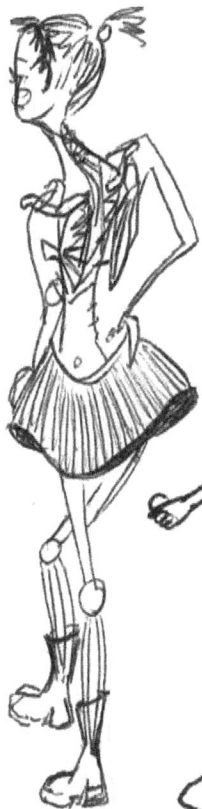

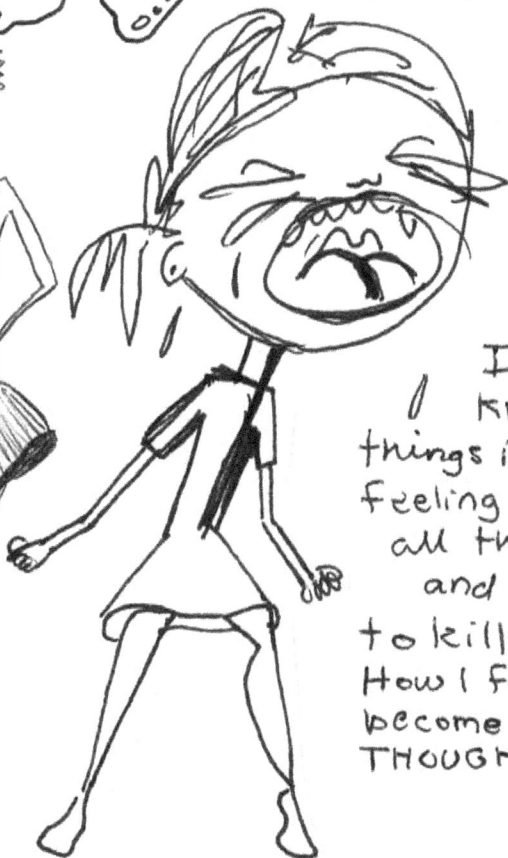

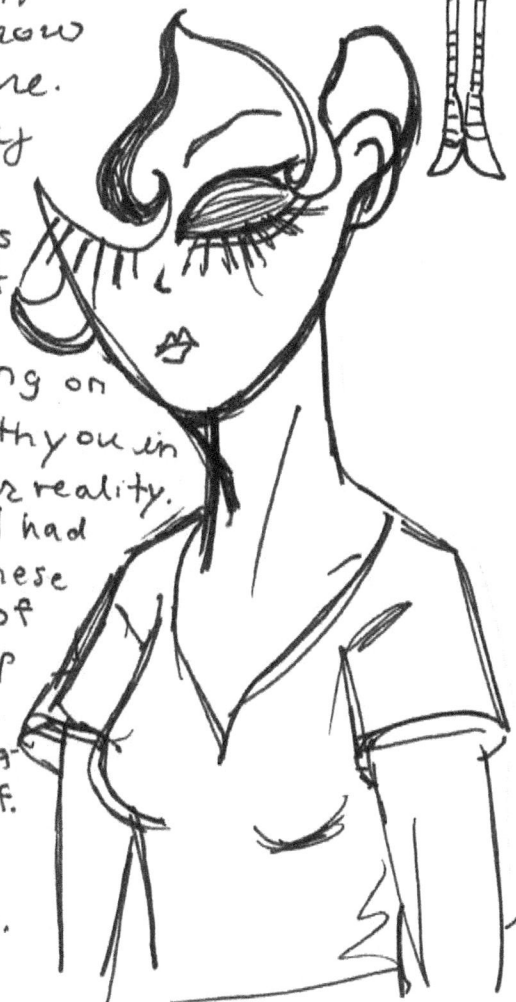

So, You Found me again.

There is nothing to talk about.

7502

The only power I had was my anger. I hurt other people and myself. I developed maladaptive behaviors like cutting and getting in trouble. I didn't care, and nobody stopped me. I was only protecting myself from getting hurt again. I have few people in my life, but they are all people I want in it, in my world. My life, not Anyone elses.

3/20/06

It is hard enough when life is bad and it always gets worse when you add alcohol or drugs. If you are already into these things, the least you can do is hold on to the tiniest HOPE that good will come.

I can feel the sadness coming back. Go away. Leave me alone.

Does your head poison your life?

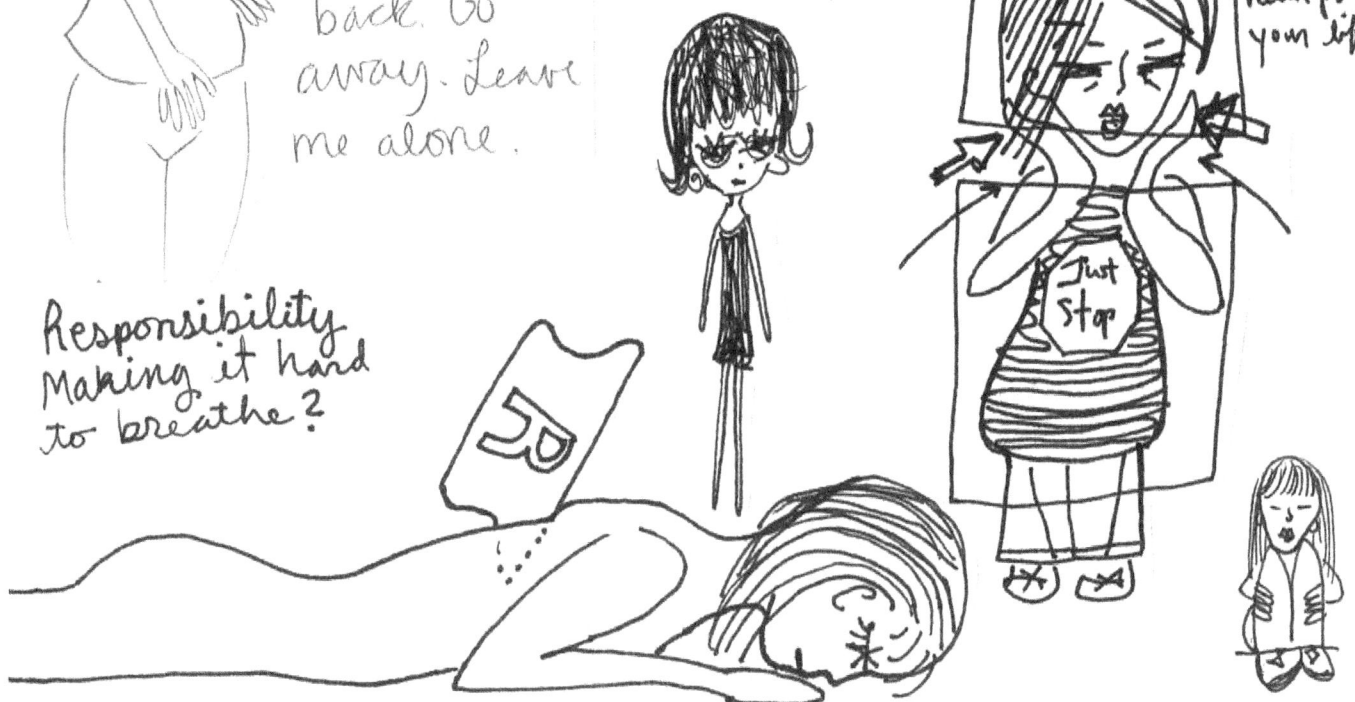

Just Stop

Responsibility Making it hard to breathe?

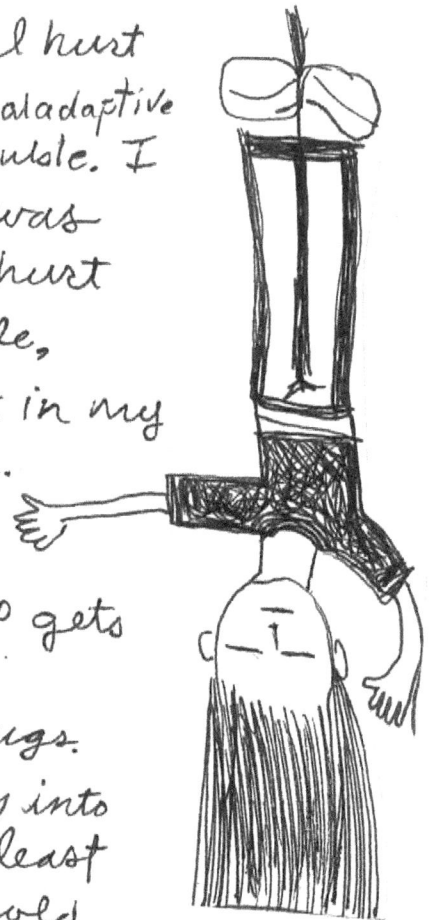

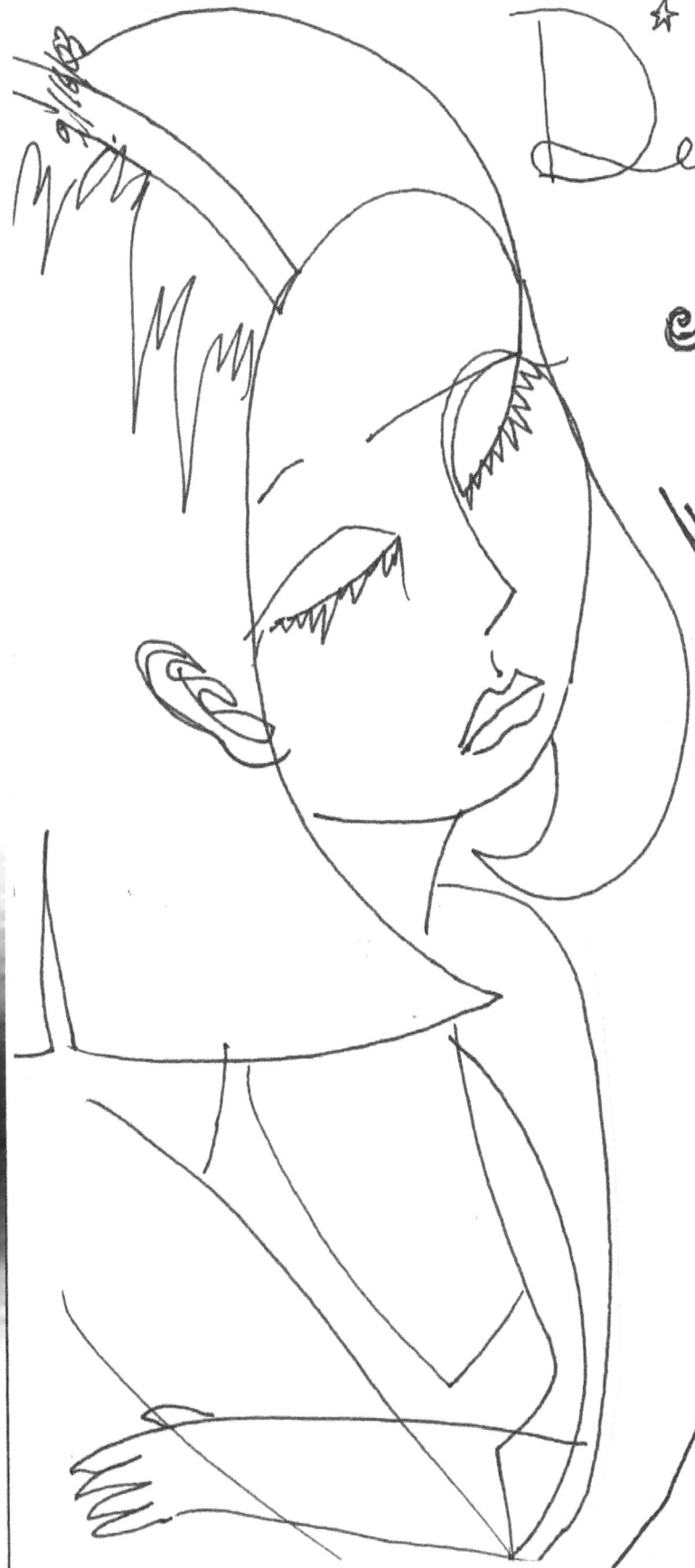

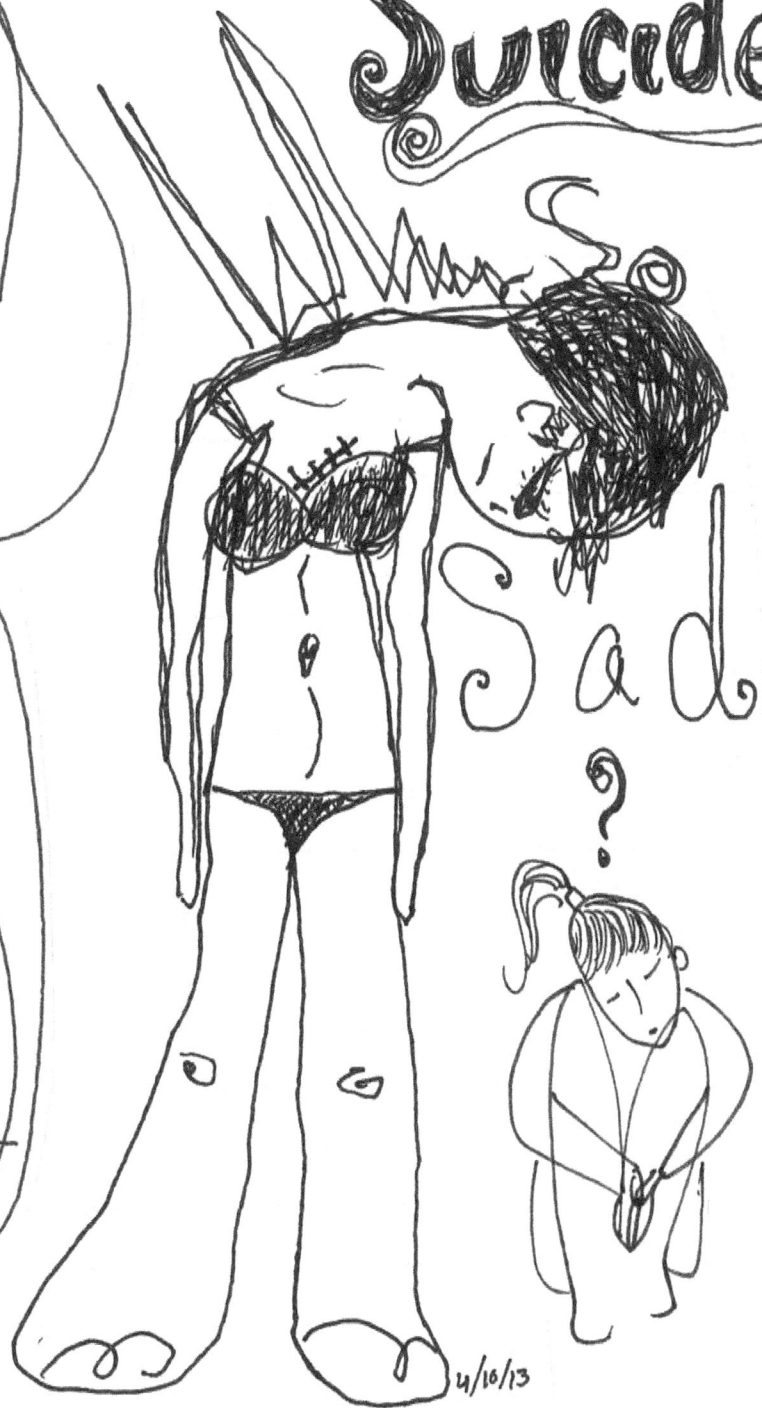

Suicide   Su = self cide = to kill

People commit suicide for many reasons. It affects everyone in that persons life. Suicide ideology usually starts when a person learns to make choices as a young adult. Children don't know any better. They do not have enough life experience to see how they are growing up and being raised is WRONG, or NOTRIGHT. Who do you turn to when your own parents are the abusers? Turn to anyone, if you can't, turn to God. He never wants you to kill yourself. If you want Him on your team, He is IN. He was with me, on the outside to the door of my heart. When my son was 2, I opened that door and it was after spending 5 days in the hospital and a couple months later.

Suicide victims are often victims of their own emotions.
They are diseases and disorders like addiction depression and anxiety. They go undiagnosed and untreated. It can get to a point where everything is not right in their perspective.

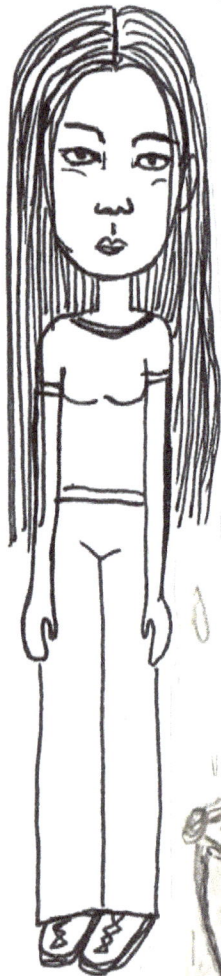

Death scratching my head and infecting.

Why now?

I AM UNPLEASANT

Catch IT Before it has a chance to turn your brain against itself.

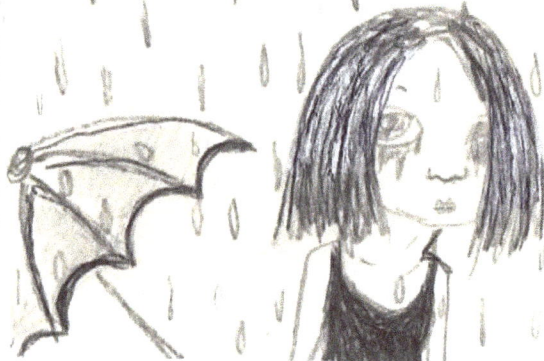

*Just because you FEEL bad does NOT mean you ARE a bad person.*Sigh* like me.

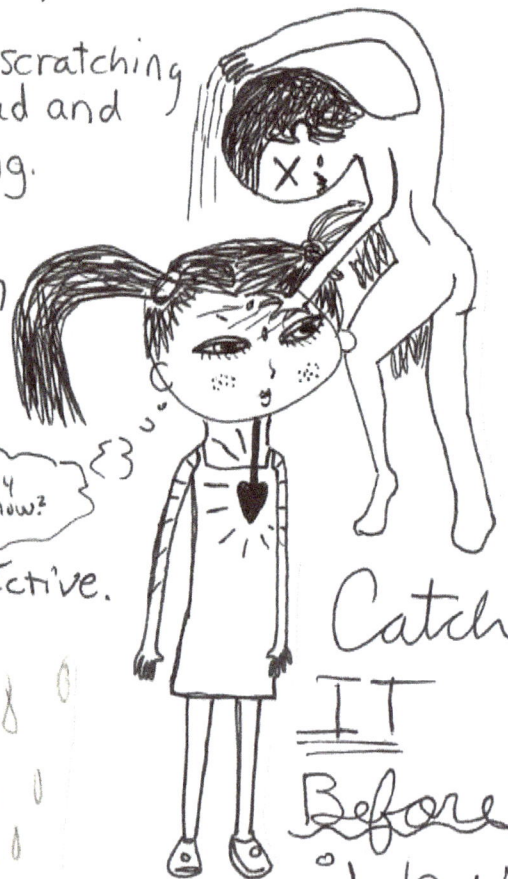

I feel fortunate to have survived my life. When I was 30 years old, I almost committed suicide. I had a Plan. With many holes in it because I wanted to be saved. I didn't do it, I just cried myself to sleep. The next day was not the same. I was an empty shell. I had an emotional circuit meltdown, everything seemed like nothing and didn't matter. Anhedonia I was broken and close to dying. I chose to go to the hospital. I stayed there for 5 days with others like myself. There were addicts, mentally ill, mentally disordered (like me) and people who just didn't feel like they could be good enough. I met with my parents and a mediator before I left. I poured my heart out for them, all they could do was accuse me of having a drug problem, which I do not.

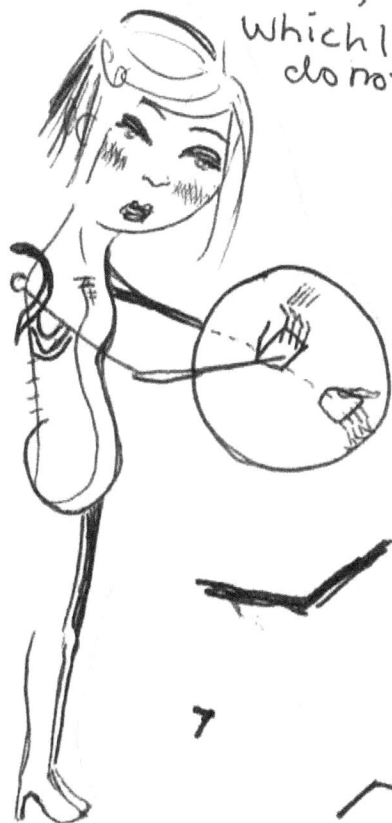

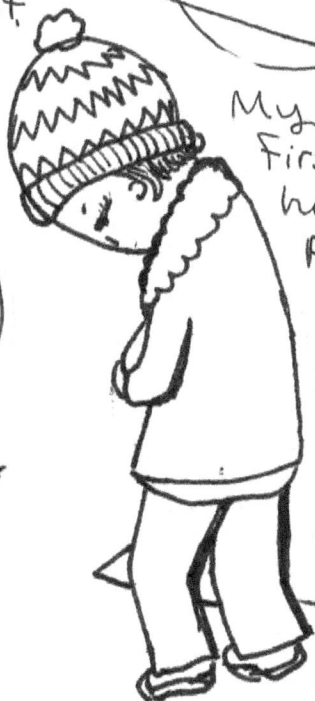

My first night home, they sent the police to my home to check on my son, who was fine and sleeping. I had learned new coping skills but this was uncalled for and I could not turn down my anxiety dial. I went back to the hospital.

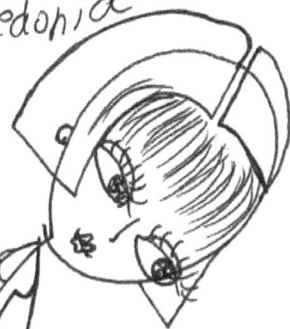

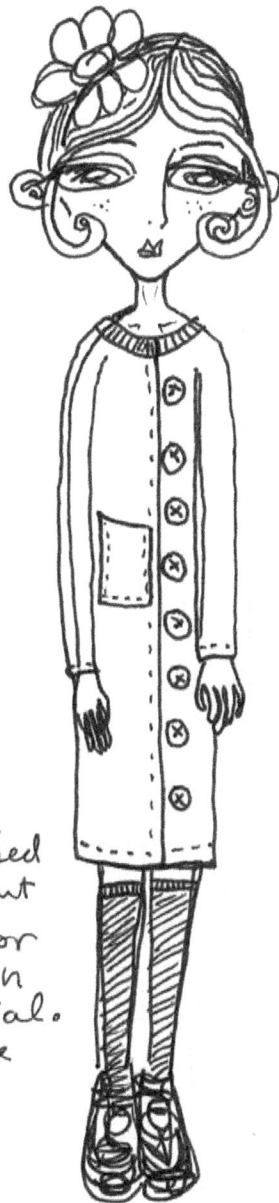

I have anxiety, depression, and Post-Traumatic Stress Disorder (PTSD). I don't like having these, but I have learned to live with it. Bad feelings come to me when something reminds me of growing up; they also come randomly. Basicly, everything in my life is ok, and I KNOW that, but I FEEL like everything is wrong or I am not doing something right. It makes me angry and sad. It used to get REALLY bad, but I have learned to identify my feelings and remind myself that they have no basis ("old feelings") in the present. *Once you find out that a shadow that looks like a bear, is not actually a bear, the fear of it goes away. Same thing with overpowering

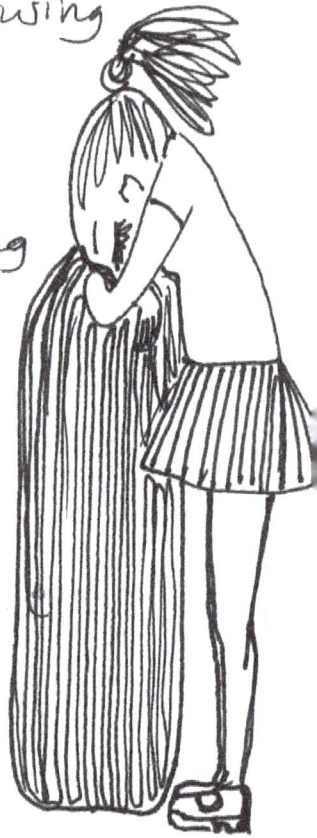

emotions* My horrible feelings that make me feel like shit come and go. Now, they don't come as often and are not as bad. They are still bad and really sucks

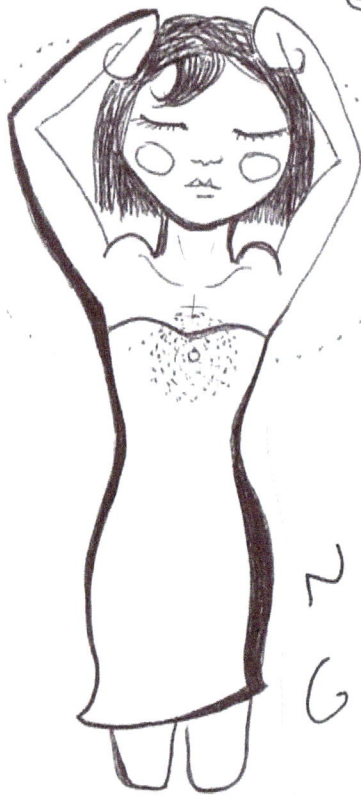

NO!
GO!
AWAY!! *
Bad
feelings
always always
ALWAYS
5/25/06 ☆go away.☆

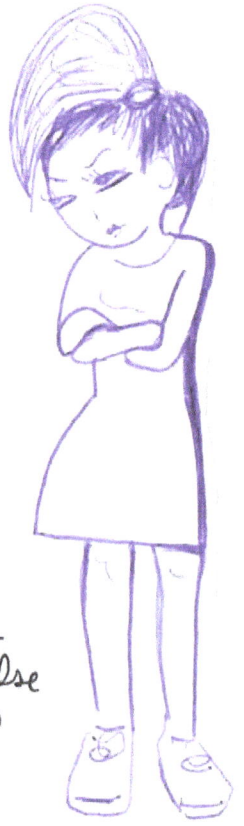

Flip OFF

but I don't have to be an asshole to everyone else till it goes away.

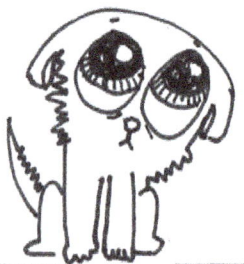

If your family doesn't love you, make your family of choice.

Oooh @ Precise

Suicide Ideology
= The idea of suicide as an answer and choice.

2.7.09 v.v.

I grew up alone and isolated in my own brain, Laha ValerieLand. I had to protect myself and stand up for myself. I was invalidated as a child, that made me quiet, in addition to being shy. My opinion did not mean anything. Moms friends always made sure to point out and make fun of me for being shy, because for some reason that was wrong. Later on, as a young adult, they made sure to tell me how beautiful I was, just like my mother and to her, they would comment on what a bitch I was. I grew up with death and suicide in a place that has an alcohol problem. When you grow up with too much of anything, you become desensitized to it. Nobody talks about how wrong suicide is or that it was because of alcohol and bad feelings. They just get drunk, and MORE SAD. Funeral = Loved for the 1st time.

If only there was a personality injection. Adam @ base of brain.

Suicide is never a good solution. The world needs you.

It will be painless. You will enjoy your life. You will be sparkley, people will like you and you will make friends easily.

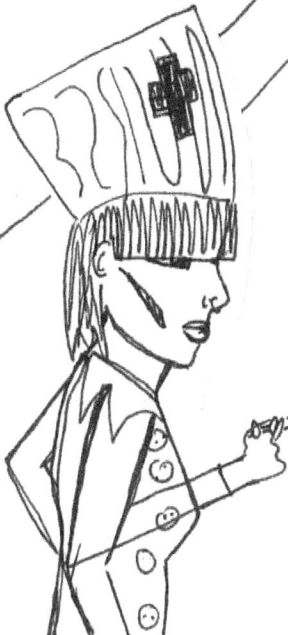

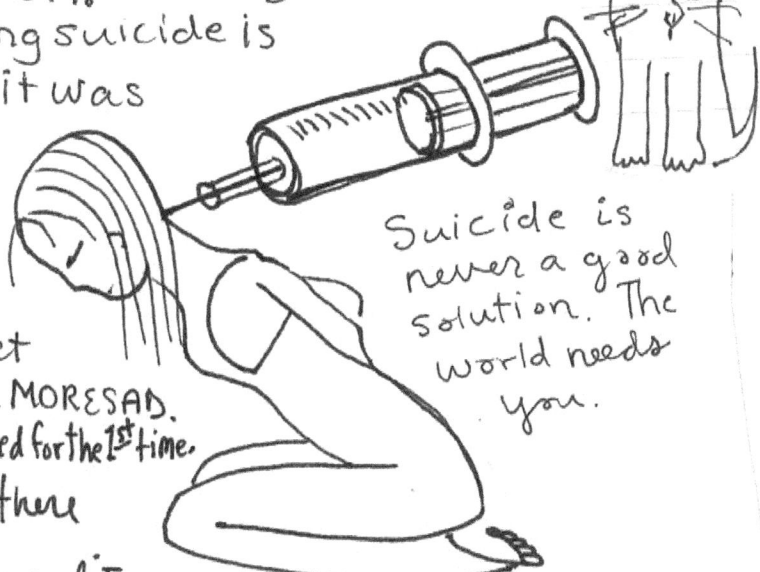

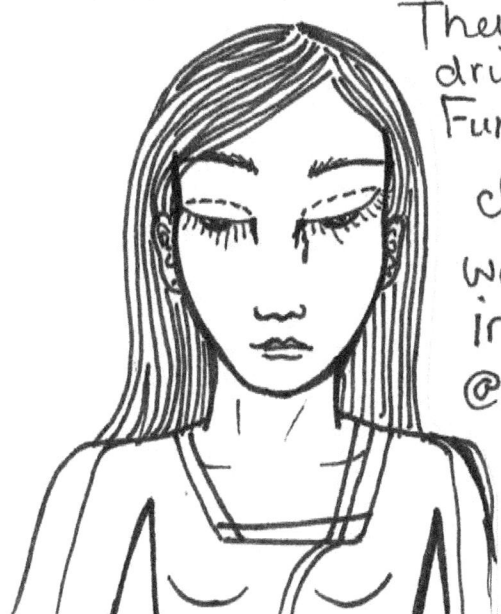

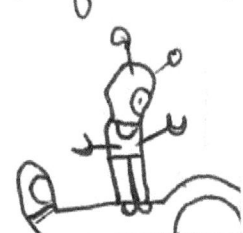

I have been suicidal since the age of 13, the age when mom abandoned us for Freedom in a Bottle. I had no social skills and felt like a freak more than usual. I started cutting (self injury) as a distraction from how I felt. I started with safety pins and went all the way to the straight razor. I ended up in the hospital for 3 days. I was put on antidepressants and told to do follow-up counseling. I was 30, before anyone got where I was coming from. It was a pain-in-the-ass for my parents, just like it was a pain in the ass when I would cry hysterically for no reason, and a pain in the ass for being angry and mean (which was my only emotional control when I was feeling crappy). I was left behind, my siblings knew love and I did not. No more counseling + no more antidepressants = Suicidal for 17 years. They didn't even care to notice till they HAD to when I almost killed myself at 30. They pretended to care for a minute, but went back to living in their glamours without me, like usual.

I learned the hard way that a person can love you and treat you like shit. Those people do not take care of THEIR OWN PROBLEMS.

give up give up give up give up give up give up give up give up give up
19 should I?

At 13, I turned into a promiscuous sad bitch. I was never going to be rich, powerful, and beautiful by societal standards. It made me angry because I didn't know what was wanted of me.

1/14/09 VL   O

53013

I learned to act "normal" and was good at it for awhile. I felt awful, like everyone hated me, I was a freak, yet somehow, other people thought I was the nicest person. They did not know I was suicidal, depressed, and freaking-out-anxiety inside. I never knew when my sadness would show up or how long it would last, this time. I still get the Sadness. My own brain turns against me and I feel like shit, and it still pisses me off every time. It reminds me that I have a Disorder (consistent anxiety) and my brain is not like everyone elses. I can't want to be happy, and just be happy. I have to distract my concentration from the yuck. I try to do it until it goes away. This is called meditation.

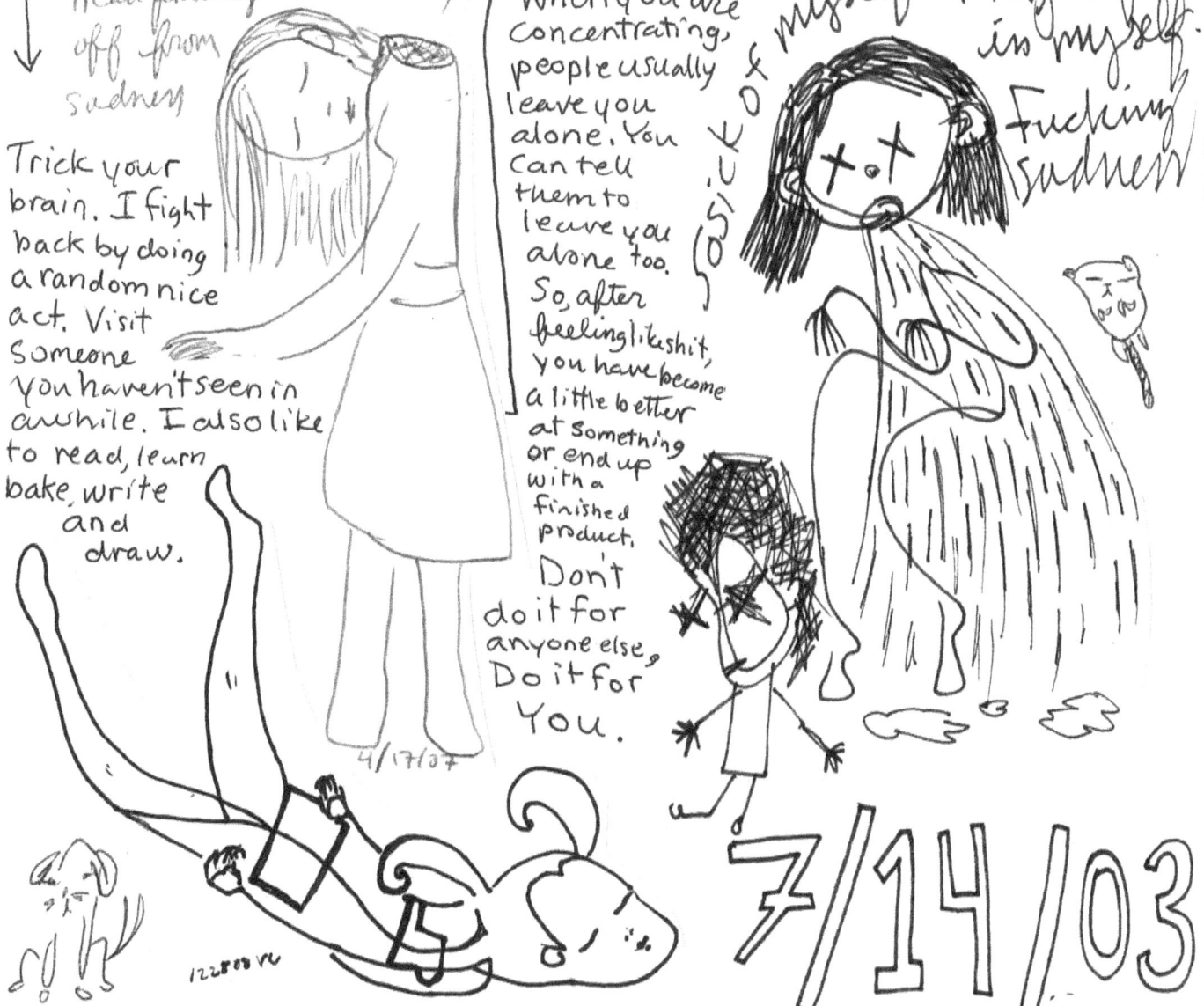

↓ Head falling off from sadness

Trick your brain. I fight back by doing a random nice act. Visit someone you haven't seen in awhile. I also like to read, learn bake, write and draw.

when you are concentrating, people usually leave you alone. You can tell them to leave you alone too. So, after feeling like shit, you have become a little better at something or end up with a finished product. Don't do it for anyone else, Do it for You.

so sick of myself on myself in myself.

Fucking sadness

4/17/07

7/14/03

The scientific explanation for distraction and why it usually works is this: The back part of your brain is the emotional side. The front of your brain is the thinking/concentrating side. When you are overwhelmed -emotional-with-no-control-over-it, the blood in your brain is concentrated on the emotional side. I call it my electric out. Can't turn it on till whatever it is decides to let off. There is nothing else I can do but be an asshole, which makes people leave me alone. I do stuff. When you use your thinking/concentrating part of your brain, more blood flow goes to that part than to the emotional part.

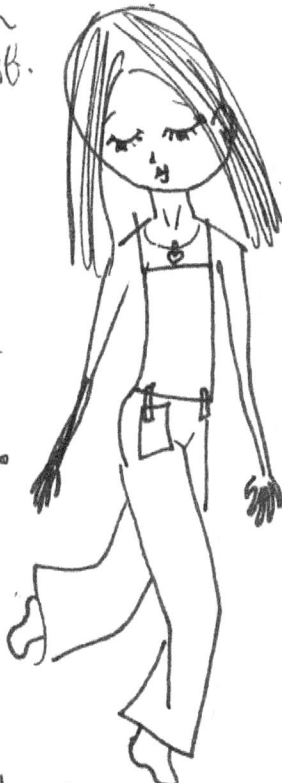

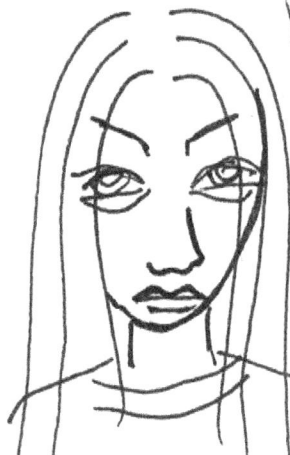

I wanted to die for so long, but not for any reason I knew about. I just felt like shit all the time and I didn't know why. I was tired of it; I just fucking sucked.

I was sad and mean/angry a lot. I knew what "it" was, but not really. I was a victim of my emotions.

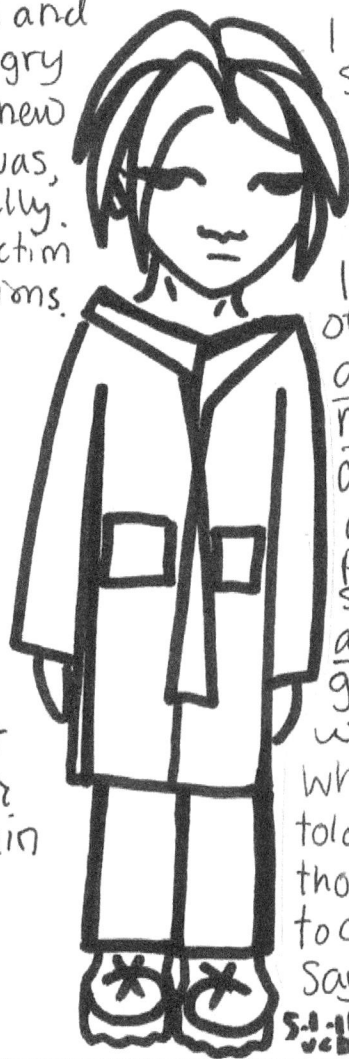

I believed that since I felt bad, I was bad. Not True. When you feel like a piece of shit, you are not actually a piece of shit. You are a good person who feels like shit. When I was 24, someone told me I was not who I thought I was. I learned to confront people and say what I really want and what I mean

I'm gonna die
I'm gonna die
I'm gonna die
I'm gonna die
I'm gonna die
die

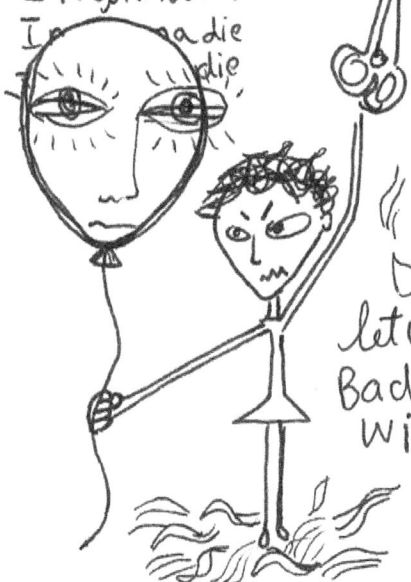

Don't let your Bad Brain win.

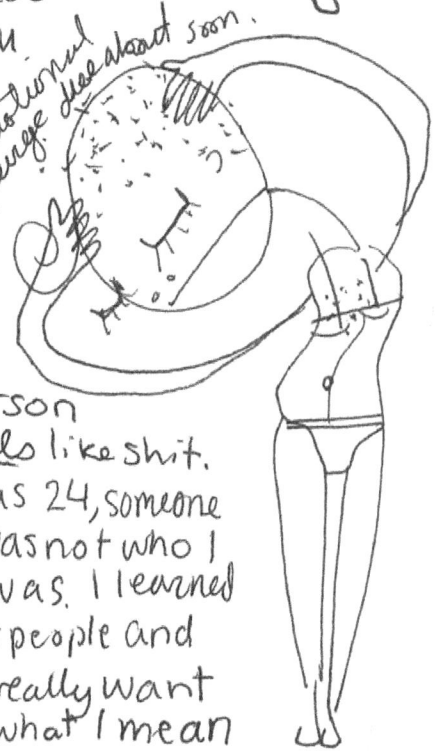

Emotional purge about soon.

I lived this way for more than a decade. An angel in disguise saw I had what she had, but I didn't know it until she told me flat-out, You have PTSD. I am going on two years of treatment for my disorder, depression and anxiety, and I feel and know I exist in reality as a good person. (I am not my feelings) My perception of what is actually going on in reality was twisted around in my brain to make everything and everyone seems against and out to get me. If your tricks of distraction are not working and you are being an intolerable butthole, put yourself to bed. Go to sleep. Don't get drunk or you may not wake up the next day.

There are living people who need your existence, to love them. Family, friends, teachers & people you have ever shared a smile with. When you kill yourself, all of these people feel like FAILURES.

ANGER.
Unsubstantiated Anger. Why? I feel crappy. That's why. Now I'm ok.

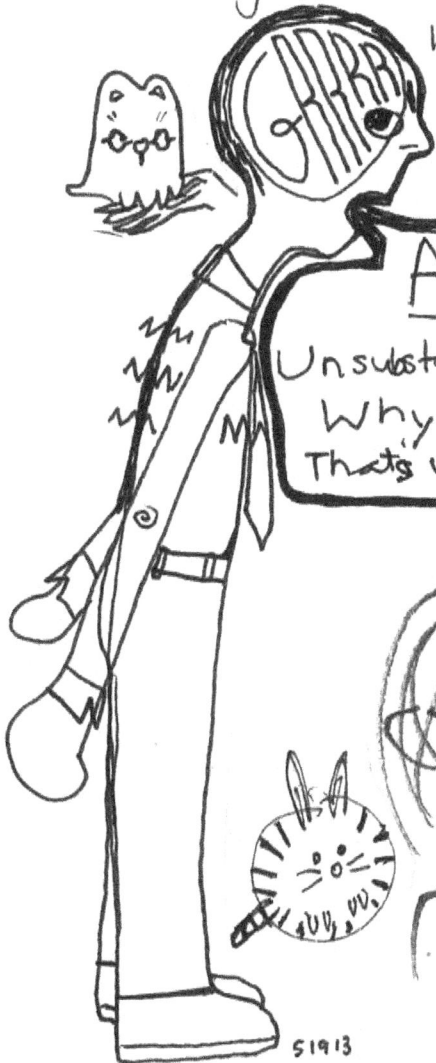

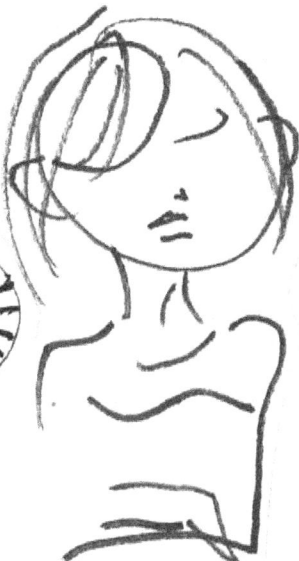

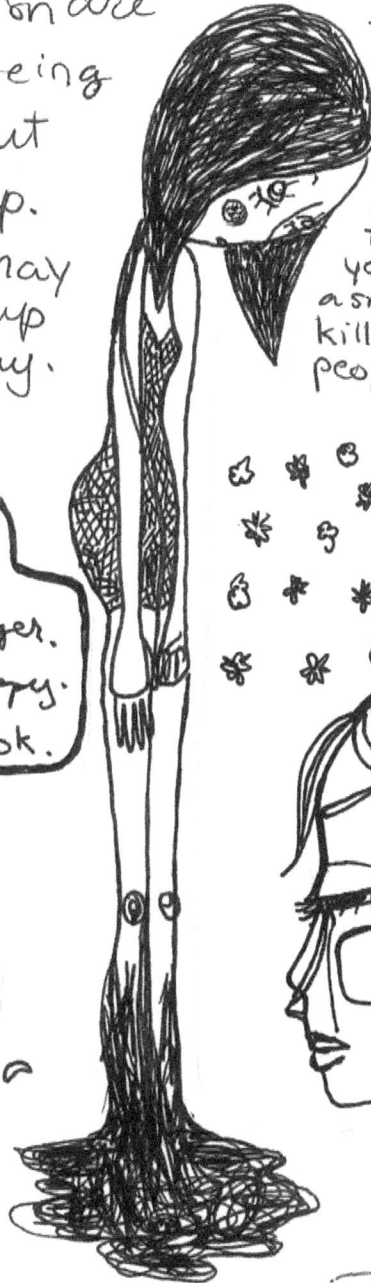

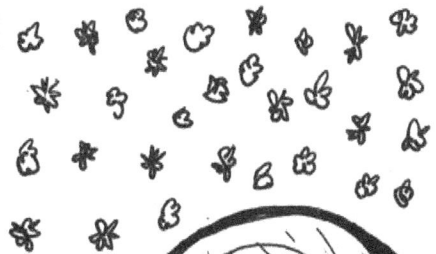

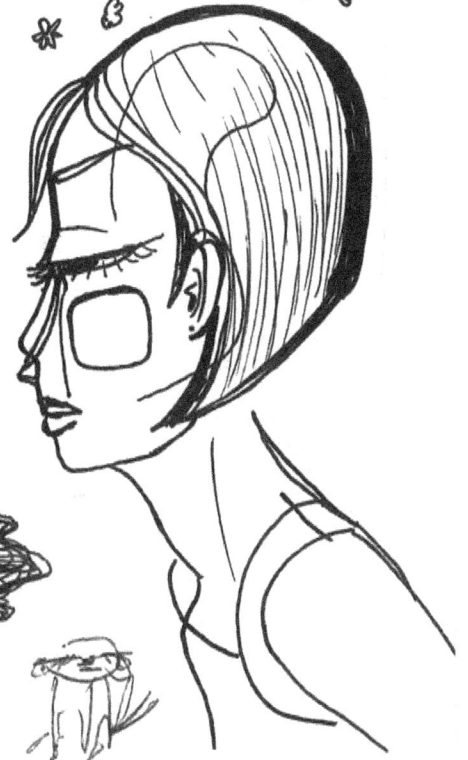

51913

PTSD is consistent anxiety. Anxiety is the gogogo feeling. You need to do something, anything. You are worried about nothing specific, your adrenaline is on the attack.

It is an all-is-not-right-in-the-world feeling. For me, I imagine it as the sound of a beehive or the black and white fuzz on an old TV.

As a child, very bad things happened to me and around me! Neglect, abuse, and addiction. My anxiety dial got stuck on High. My brain system adapted to the point where I have a disorder.

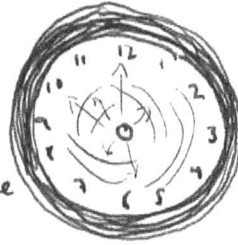

LaLa
Dun Dun Dun
LaLa
Dun Dun Dun

GOGOGOGO
GOGOGOGO
GOGOGO
GOGO

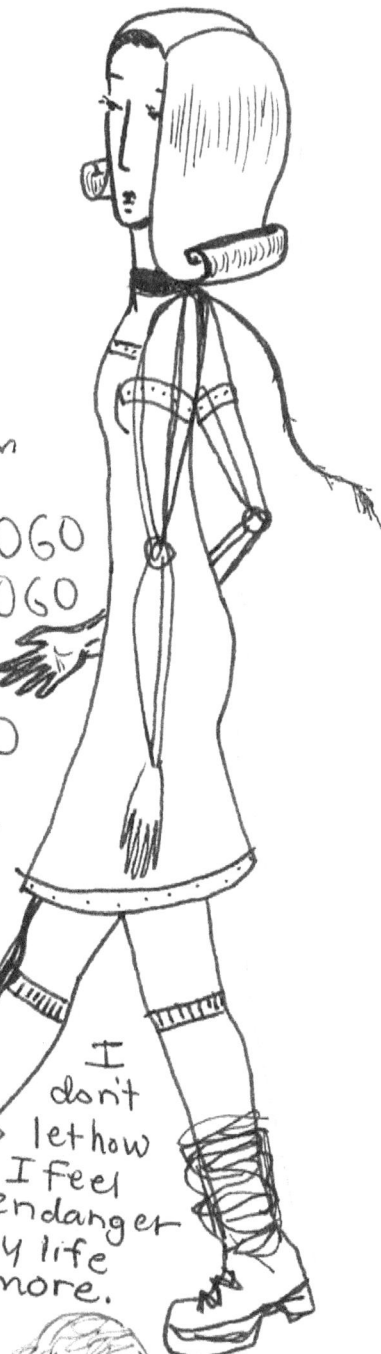

Hurry... dam always in a hurry and always doing something. I am a perfectionist, I like baking because of the required precision. Various medicines help me be calm. I'm on a high dose of a lot of things and I still get sad, angry, and suicidal once in a while.

up...

MUST RUN!!
Zoom Zoom

I don't let how I feel endanger my life anymore.

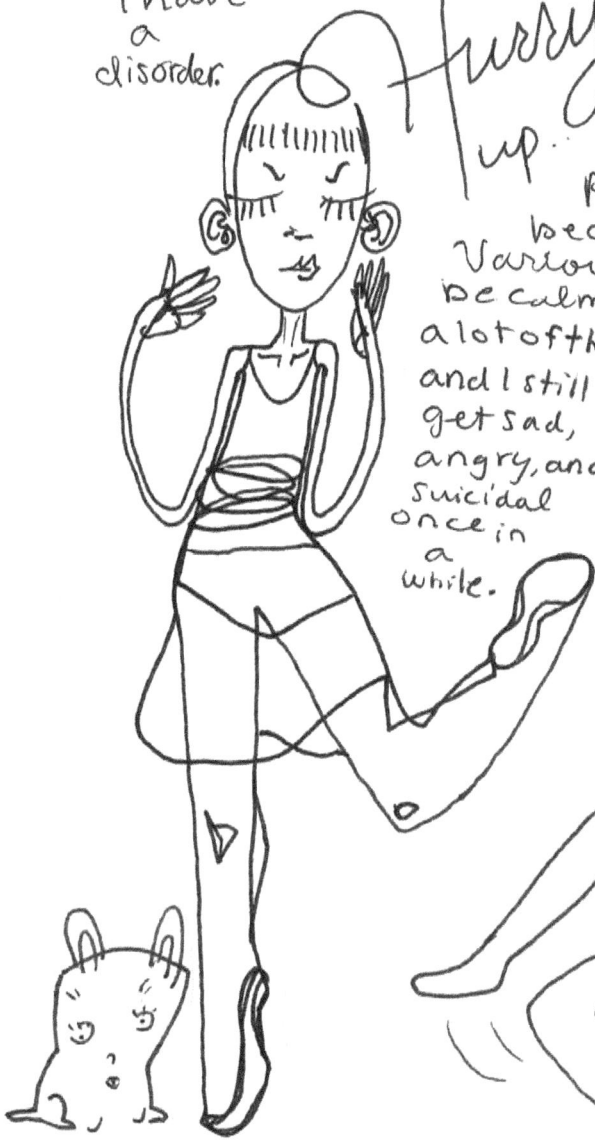

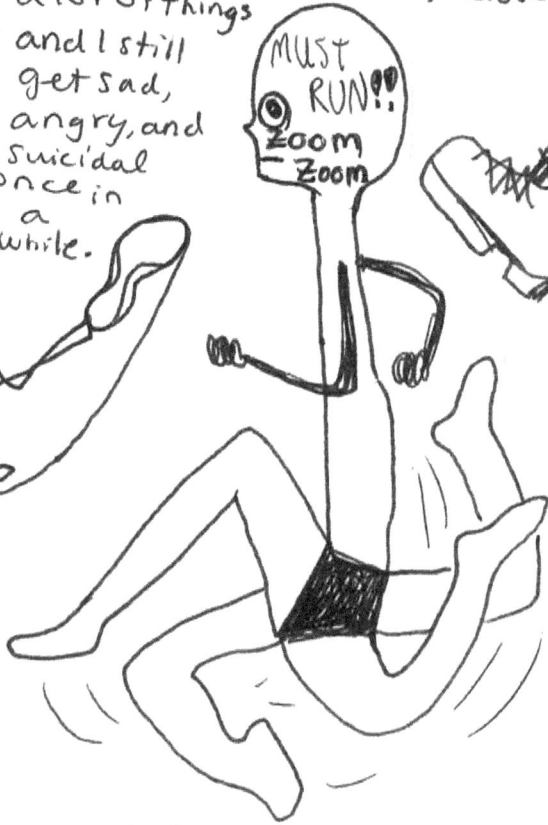

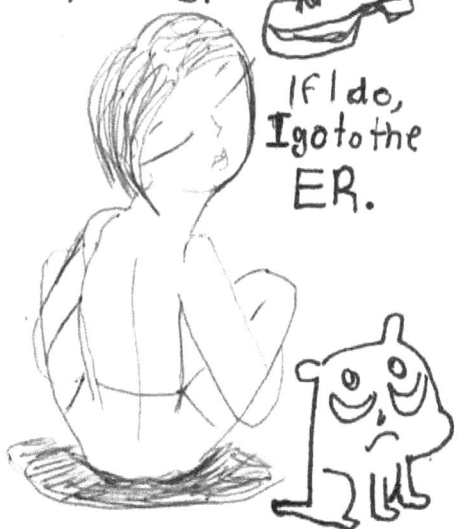

If I do, I go to the ER.

Depression. Everyone gets depressed at least once in their lifetimes. Time heals depression for a lot of people, the fortunate ones. Depression is like being on another plane. Days seem endless, you feel worthless and inadequate. Hope goes away and you want to go away. Nothing is enjoyable, efforts to make yourself feel better are useless. It is a sad that consumes your life. It doesn't feel good and it sucks having it. Thankfully, science and medicines have led to a better understanding of what causes it and treatments that work. It is true that there is _still_ stigma that surrounds mental health unbalance. Your brain chemistry is unbalanced, medicines can balance them to a point where you can live your life without staying in bed all day. Medicine takes time to work effectively and it is hard work processing unacknowledged emotions with a counselor, therapist or psychiatrist. Forward is Forward. It is worth the work becoming who you are and understanding why you are the way you are. You are [not] crazy. Don't let others make you believe it.

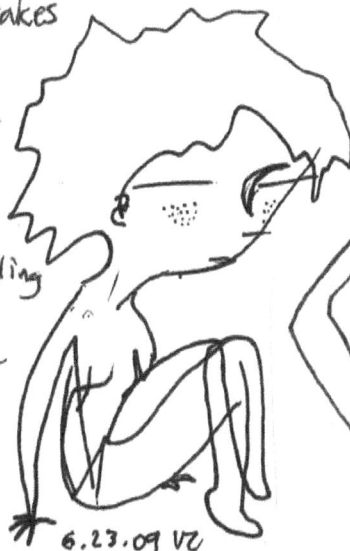

6.23.09 VC

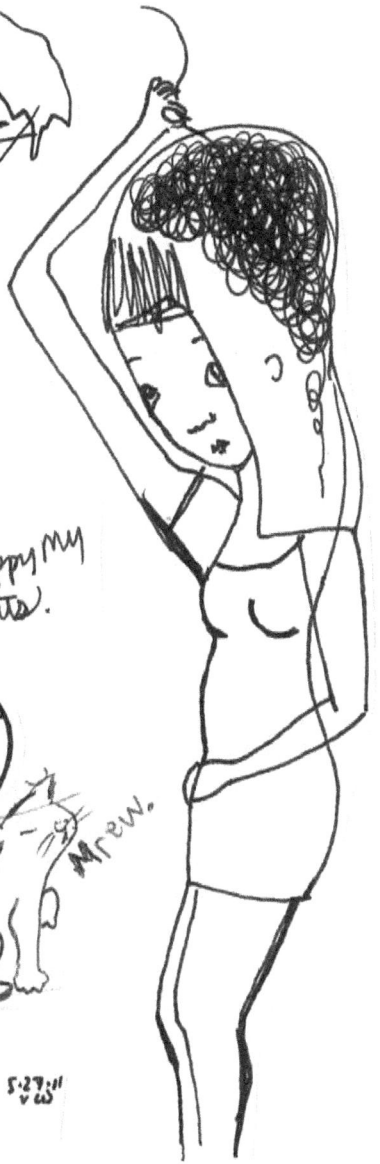

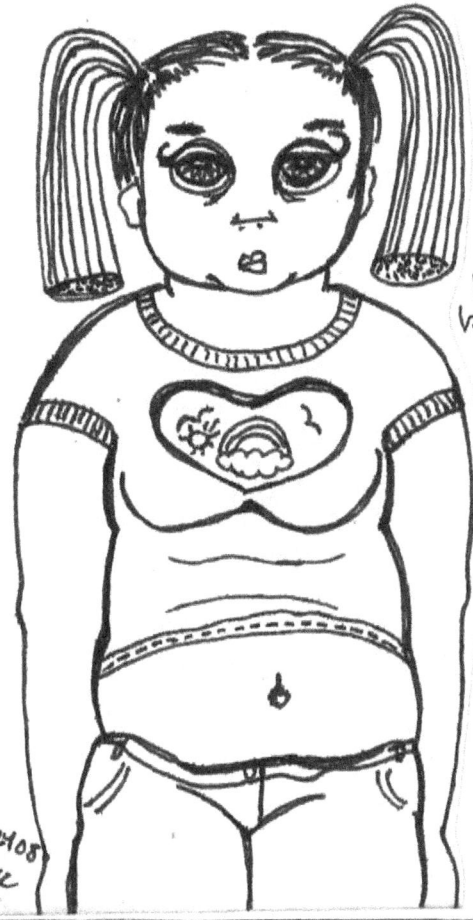

3.24.08
VC

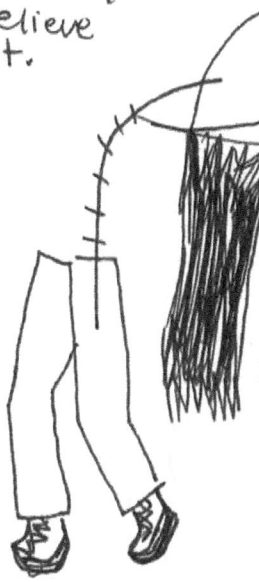

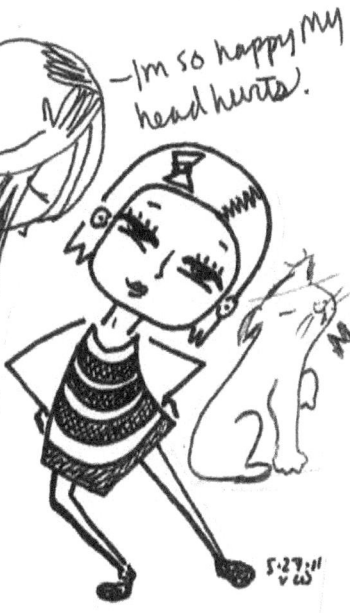

—I'm so happy my head hurts.

Mrew.

5.27.11
VC

Alcohol is suicide juice.

People drink alcohol when they are sad because people don't want to feel. Your darkest feelings come to the surface where you can think about them. It makes your feelings more real. Alcohol makes a person carefree and they forget about their problems and badness. It also makes your memory and judgement Flatline. When you don't know what you're doing, you might miss the fact that DEAD IS FOREVER.

When you think that things would be better without you, you are wrong. People will be sad but they cannot do anything about you when you die. You stop all of your future potential, all of your stories, and your memory of your real self is forgotten with time.

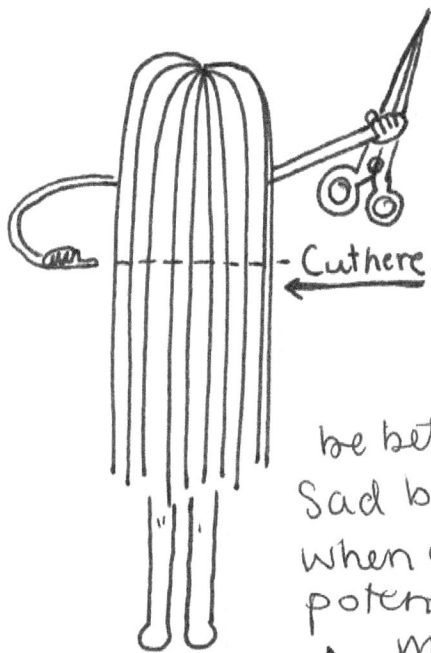

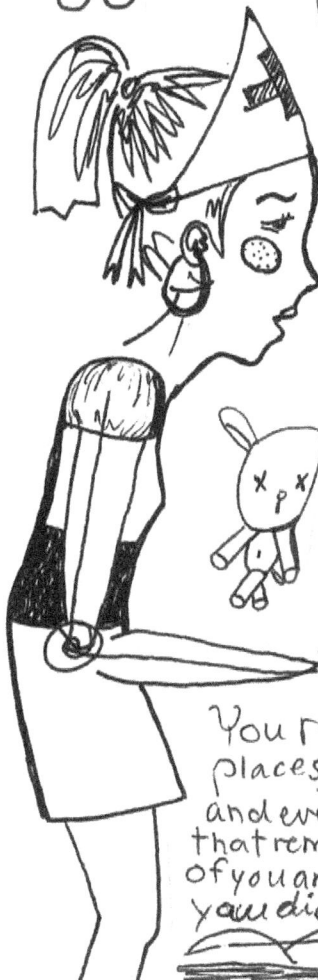

← Cut here

uuuh, it looks like you have a broken,... heart?

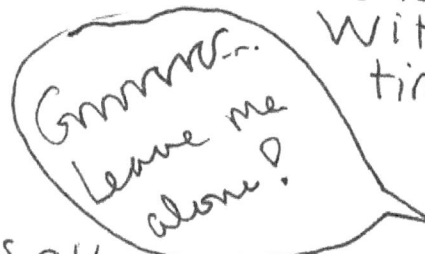

Time fades all things. Memories in a persons' head only last till they die, if they are lucky. Friends and family might resent you for doing something so selfish. Some of them may commit suicide themselves.

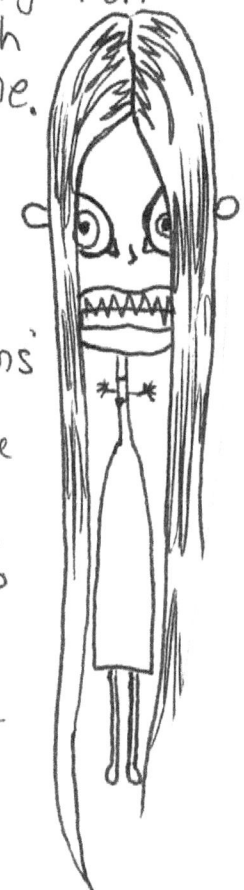

Grnnnnn.. leave me alone!

MY Life

You ruin people, places, anniversaries and everything that reminds them of you and what you did.

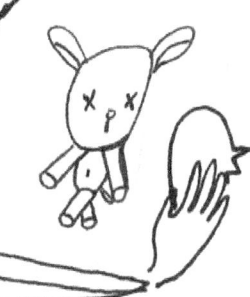

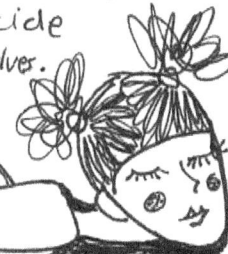

filet

There are many reasons people may want to kill themselves.

— Untreated chemical brain imbalance or mood disorder. Medicines prescribed by a psychiatrist help a lot.

— Physical pain. They may have a terminal illness or they may be an addict. Addicts in pain from withdrawel pray for death.

— Lonliness. Older men have a high rate of suicide. Sometimes people feel like there is nobody out there for them. The secret is to get well, get out and do things you love or used to love. When YOU are happy, love will come. Love attracts love.

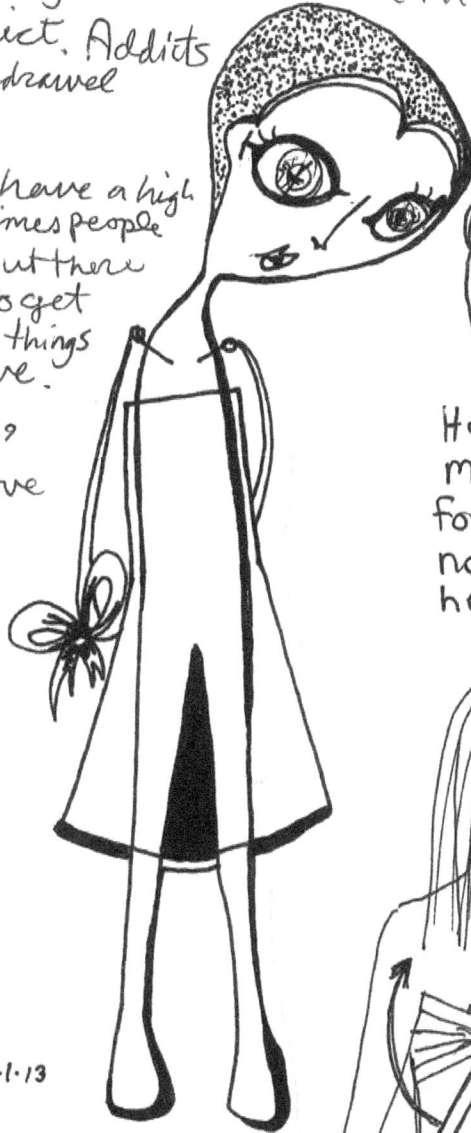

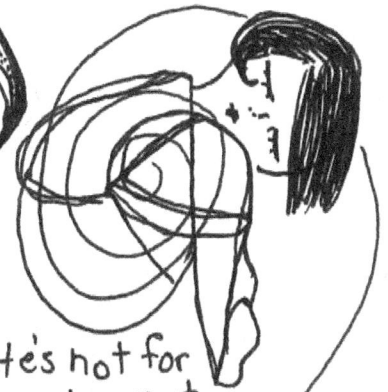

5·1·13

He's not for me hes not for me hes not for me hes not for me.

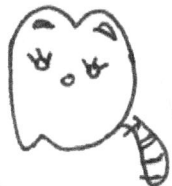

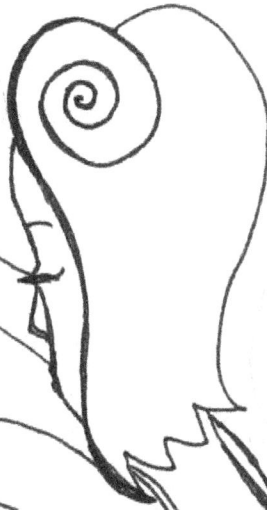

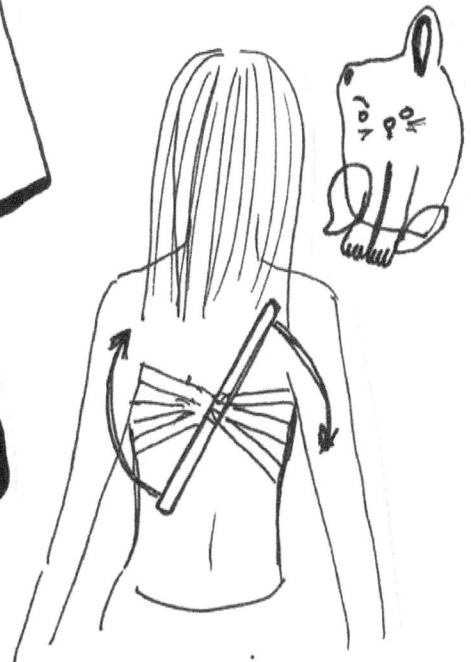

Clockwise to Tighten.

—They will never be what society wants them to be: Successful, powerful, popular, and beautiful.
★★ None of THAT is
happiness

2·7·09 VC

5-12·06

— The feeling of no future, because you can never be "good enough" and you feel like you don't exist. You are not letting yourself exist if you suffer alone. People love you, pets love you, so learn to let them. The closest future that matters is when you wake up alive day by day. The future is always coming and change is always happening. Sometimes for better, sometimes for worse. That is life.

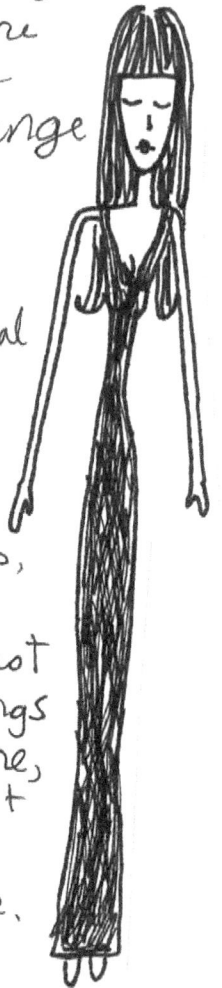

— Being a victim of verbal, emotional and physical abuse.
— Being a victim of abusers who threaten or intimidate.
— Being a victim of rumors, gossip, and blackmail (which is a felony).
— Guilt. Guilt over things that cannot be changed, guilt over things they have done, and guilt over a close suicide.

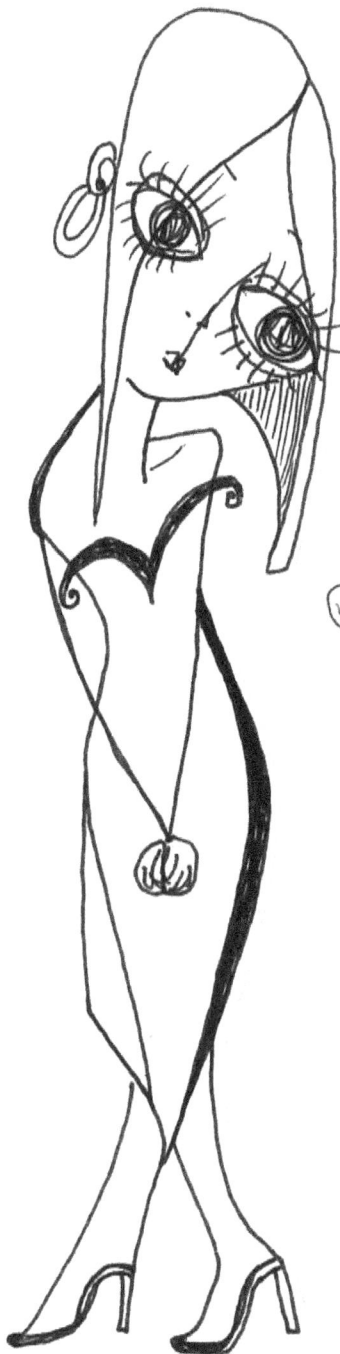

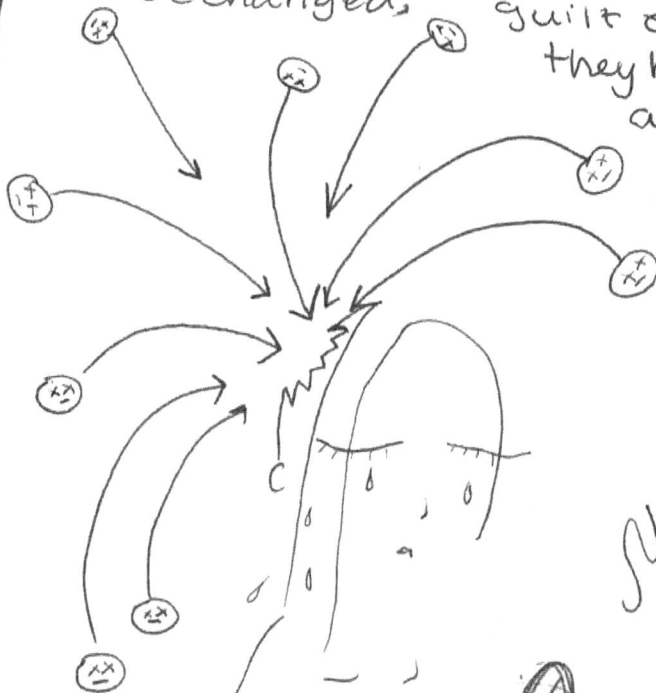

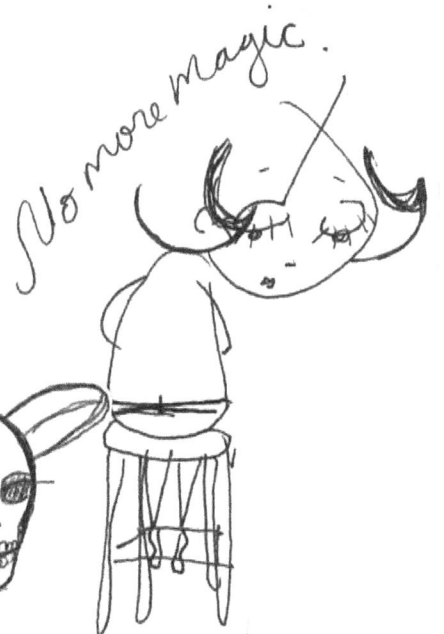

No more magic.

— Emotional pain. Cheating, fighting, and relationship Break-ups happen. It sucks but it happens all the time. Death happens too. Many commit suicide over the death of someone close.

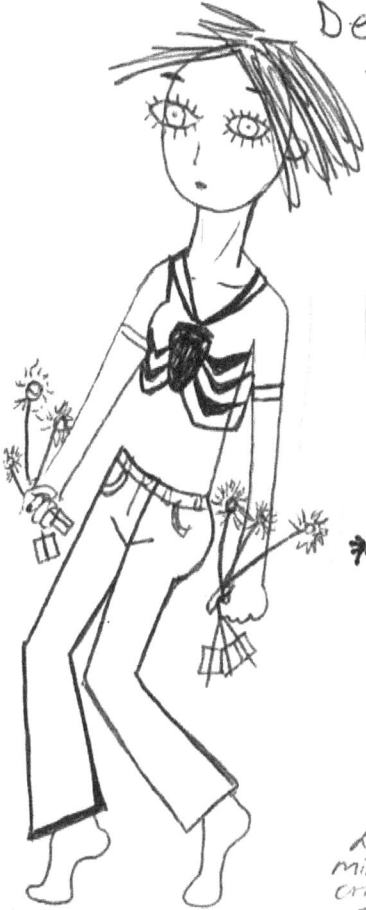

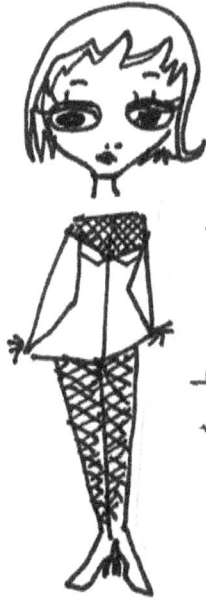

You can't bring anyone back to life or make someone love you. If they don't want to be with you, it is not the end of the world. Heartbreak hurts and sometimes you really feel like killing yourself. The person you kill yourself over goes on, just like they have been for some time now. It is ok to be sad.

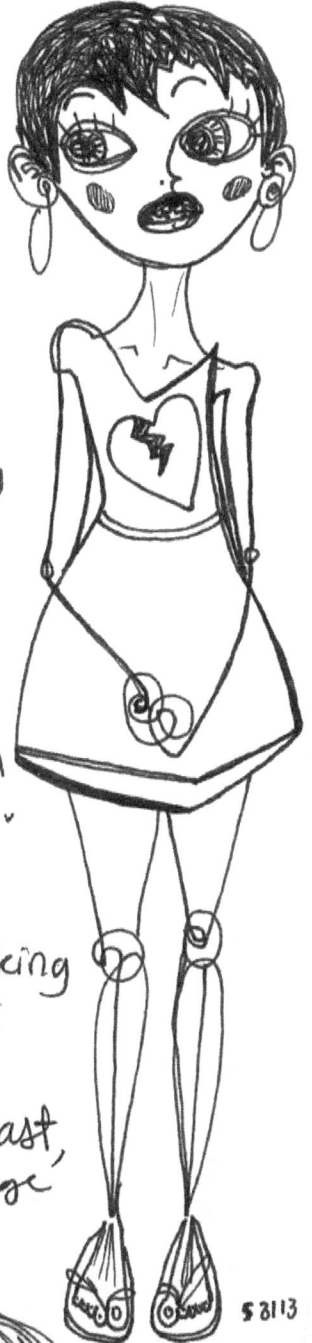

Losing my mind like a fire cracker 2/17/06 ©

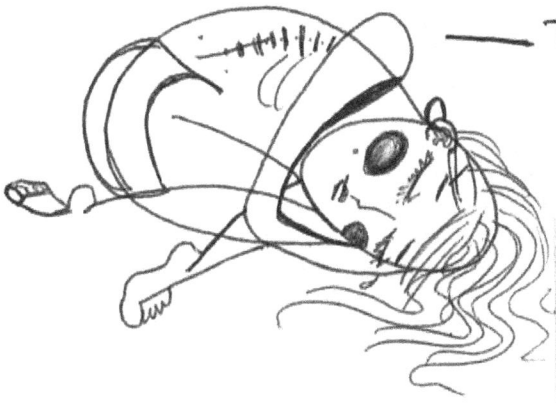

— They are depressed, drinking alone, blacked-out, and suicidal.

You cannot undo the past, but you can acknowledge and process it. If you don't process feelings Change is ↓ Difficult, but not impossible.

Today he wrote to me I'm still beautiful. I'm contemplating DEATH!

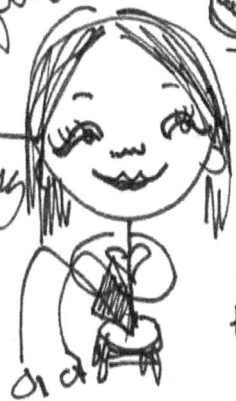

I'm not sure if I want to do this any more...

2/20/06

The present is lost to them. They are stuck in the past and worried about the future.

5/31/13

I am a Suicidal Survivor. I have emotional damage, an old battle-scarred soul. I was suicidal off and on for 17 years. it sucked and nobody knew-knew. I survived through all of the factors against me. I didn't die and I did not become an alcoholic like my mother.

[Factors]:
- I am left handed. Left-handedness is the result of the mothers stress throughout her pregnancy. I love being a Leftie. I have had anxiety since birth, though.
- My family genetics. Addiction and mood disorders are inherited.
- I never felt normal, cared about, or loved. I didn't even know God loved me as his own child, 'till I was 30.
- I felt alone, so I thought I was alone. Not true. Although experience and perception differ from person to person, so many people know what it is like to feel like I did. Any person is not alone and never will be. The way you feel about yourself is not real.

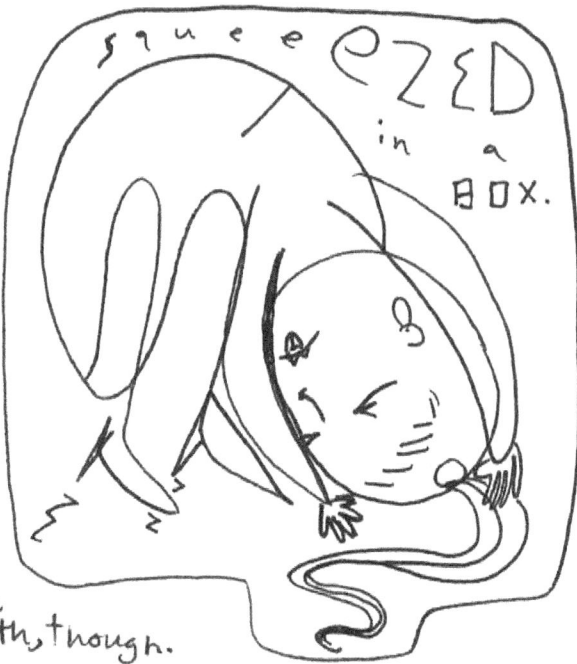
squeeeZED in a BOX.

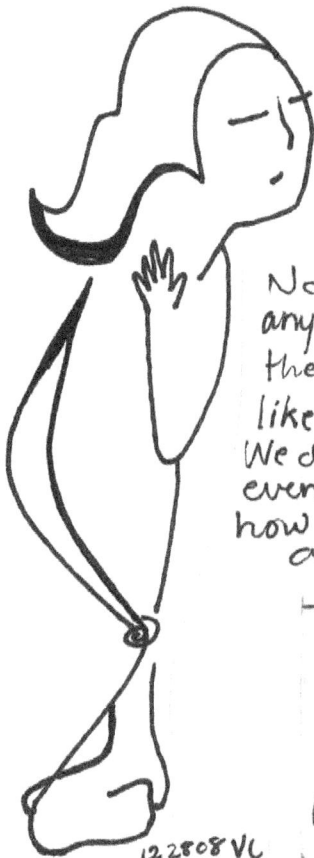

No person has any idea what they look like to others, We don't even realize how we are.

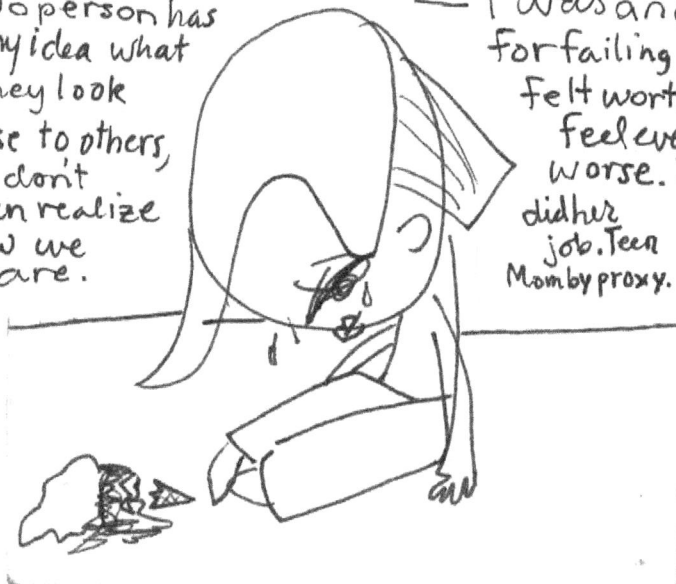

122808 VC

- I was angry at my mother for failing to rescue me. I felt worthless, she made me feel even worse. I did her job. Teen Mom by proxy.

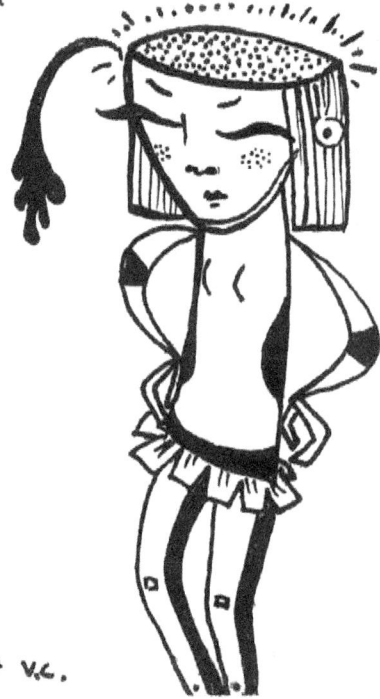

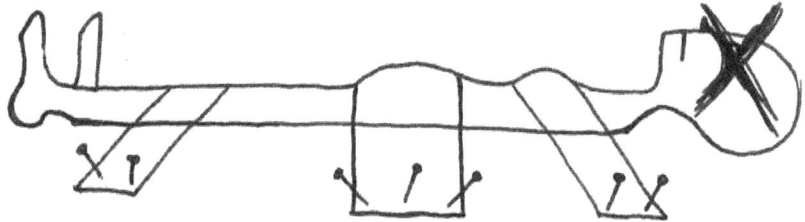

6-8-07 VC.

Factors continued

— I was not raised with religion or spirituality. I went to church but that was that. I did learn prayers, but they had no meaning to me.

— I didn't learn of The Gospels till I was 30. (Story of Jesus.) I also acknowledged Him in my heart, he was there the whole time, I just didn't know.

— An alcoholic parent. Alcoholic parents are emotionally unavailable. They don't care about their children, they don't encourage them, and they don't let them know they exist and are loved. Alcoholic parents fuck their kids up and they don't even know until their kid commits suicide, becomes a criminal, or runs away from home.

* Kids run away from home all the time. They are usually being smart and removing themselves from whatever abusive situation they are in. Running away is better than killing yourself. If you run away from home for a good reason, KNOW that people want to protect you from having to use your body to get what you need to survive.

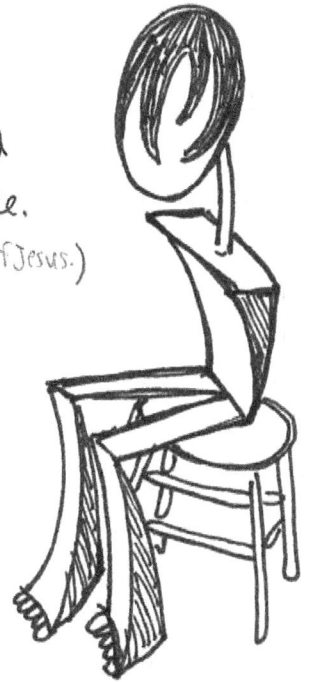

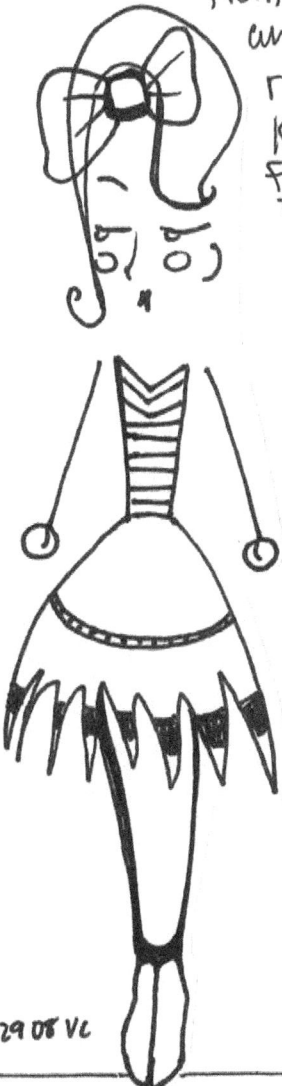

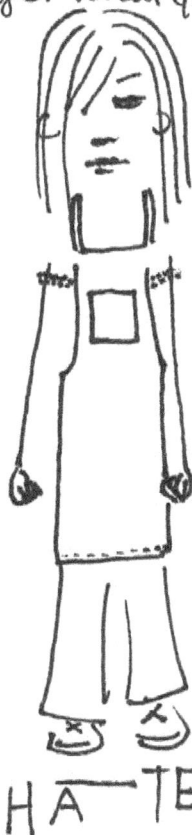

There are people who WANT to help you. They will give you a risk-rape-free place to sleep. They will give you food, whatever you need.

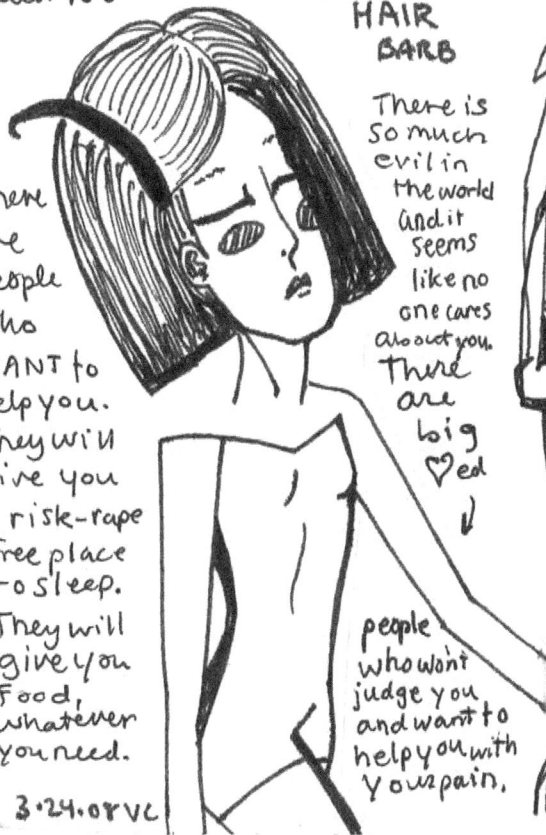

BIG HAIR BARB

There is so much evil in the world and it seems like no one cares about you. There are big ♡ed

people who won't judge you and want to help you with your pain.

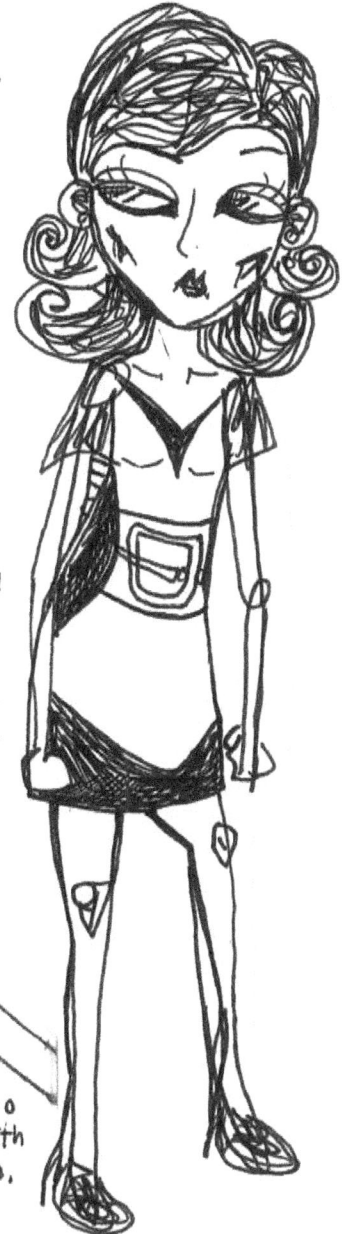

HA TE

— I never felt ok to be me. I was shy, people made fun of me for it. Mom was embarrassed by it. My teeth were crooked and that was wrong. I went through 4 permanent tooth extractions and 2.5 years of braces and headgear. When I was a young adult, mom told me they were considering a cosemetic nose surgerys for me. I was never beautiful enough. I didn't feel beautiful until I was 21, when someone actually told me.

— I was invalidated a lot. I would tell mom I was sick, she would tell me I'm fine.

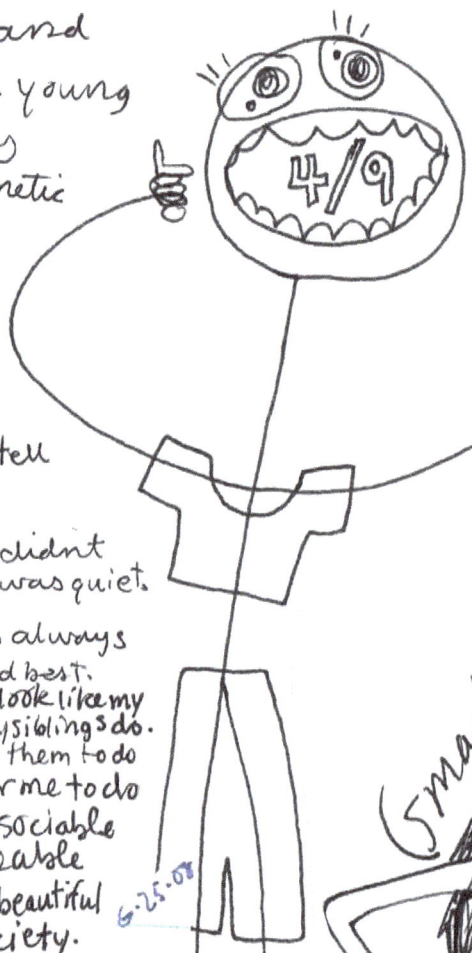

4/9

— I was a blacksheep and scapegoat. I always "took one for the team"

I was used to being scolded and yelled at. At 8, I learned to fight back. My threats to call the police protected me. My threats were always serious.

My opinion didn't matter so I was quiet.

— I was always second best. I do not look like my Father, my siblings do. What is ok for them to do was not ok for me to do. They were sociable likeable and beautiful in society. I was not. Now, I am ok with that.

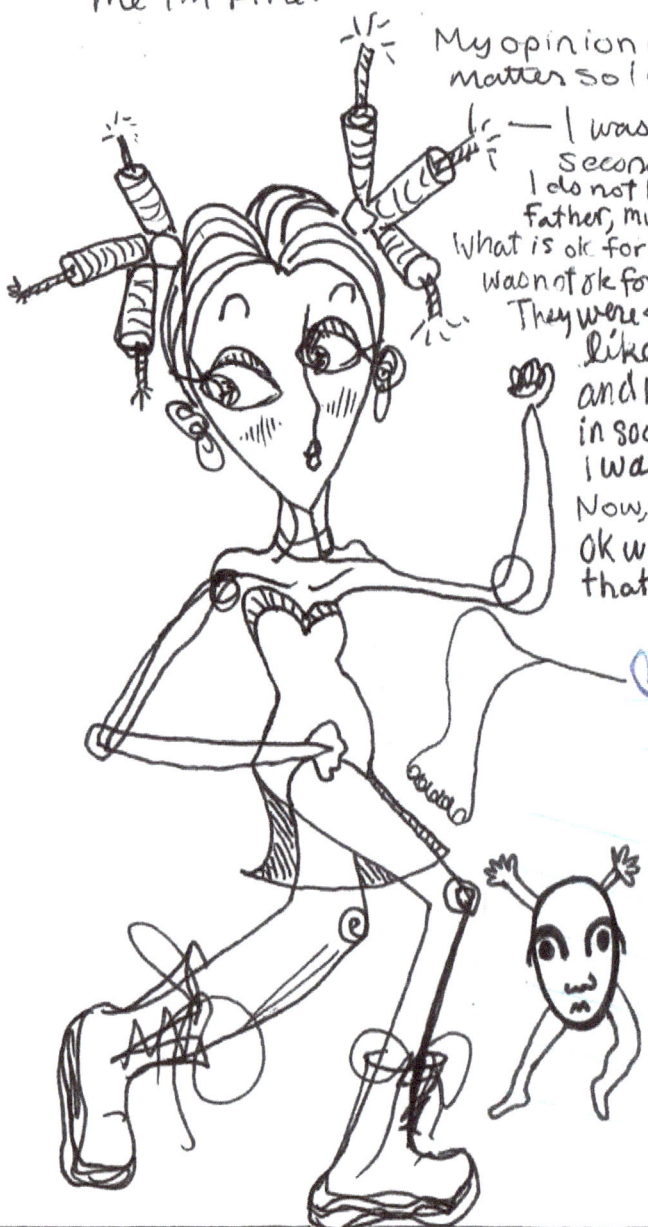

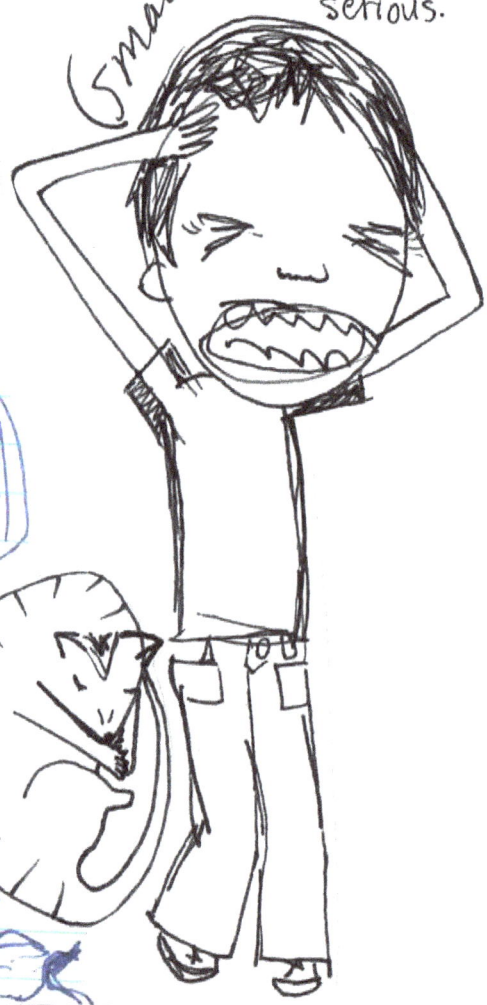

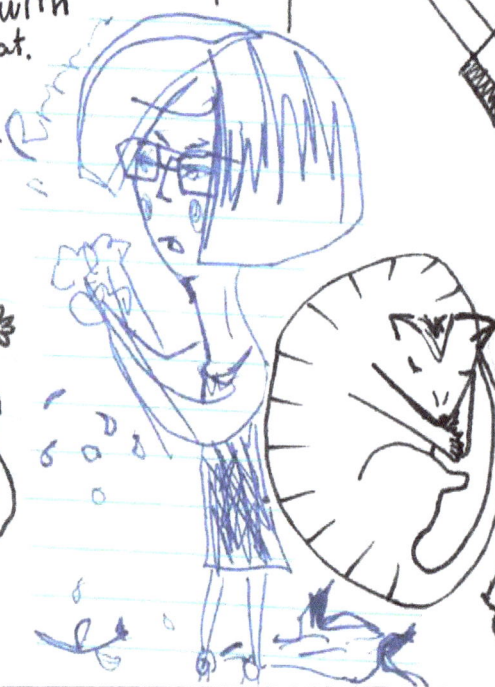

6-25-08

(smack.)

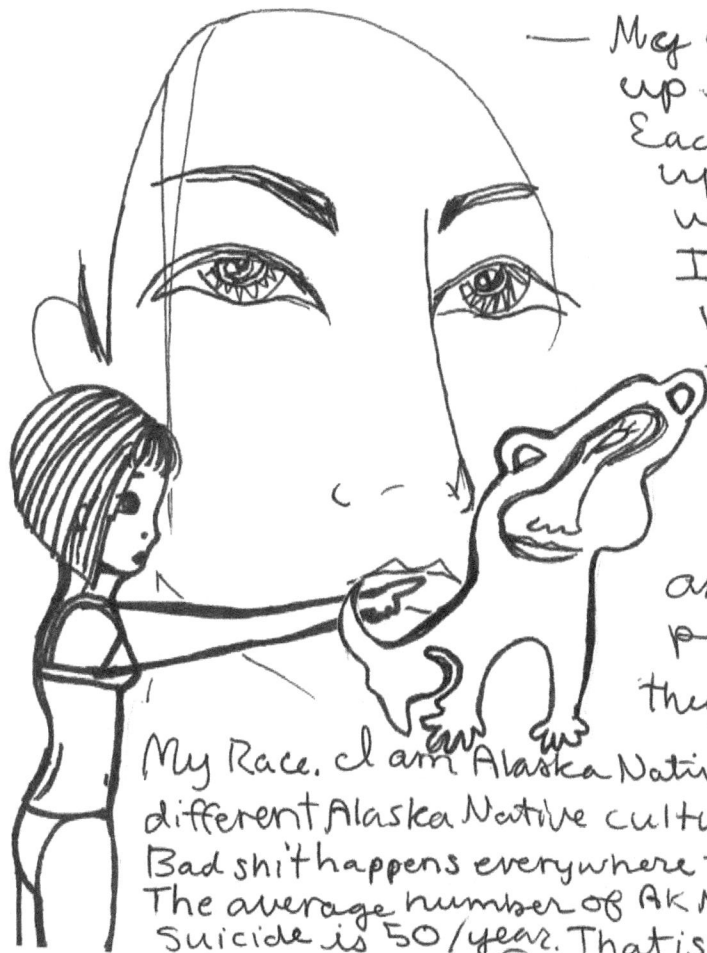

— My childhood environment. I grew up with every disaster, involving suicides. Each one was alcohol related. I grew up around alcoholics. When dad was gone, the party was at our house. I have seen so many dead bodies in my lifetime. I thought it was weird when my 30ish-year-old friend said that he had never seen a dead body. At every single event, celebration, and funeral there were drunk people. I learned it was ok because they never got kicked out.

My Race. I am Alaska Native. Alcohol abuse is prevalant in different Alaska Native cultures throughout Alaska. Bad shit happens everywhere there is alcohol present. The average number of AK Natives who commit suicide is 50/year. That is one every 8 days.

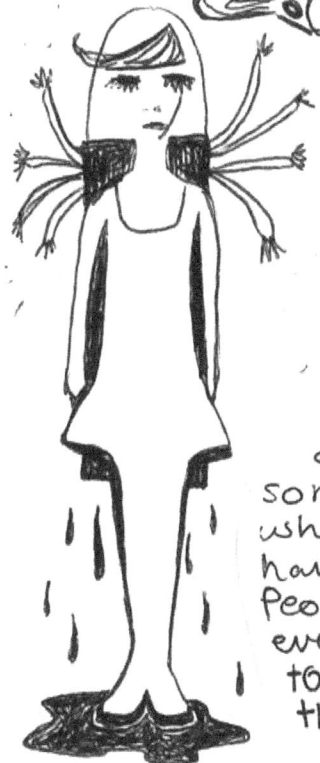

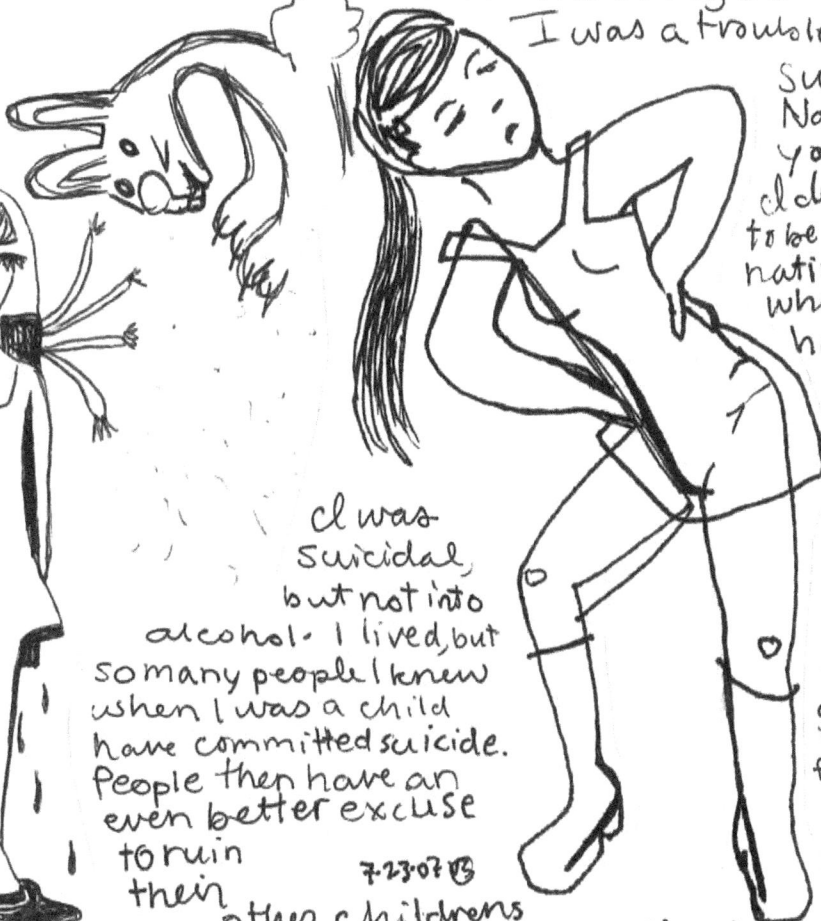

I was a troubled, suicidal native youth, but I didn't want to be another native youth who couldn't handle life

I was suicidal, but not into alcohol. I lived, but so many people I knew when I was a child have committed suicide. People then have an even better excuse to ruin their other childrens lives the SAME WAY.

7-23-07 B

2/24/06 B

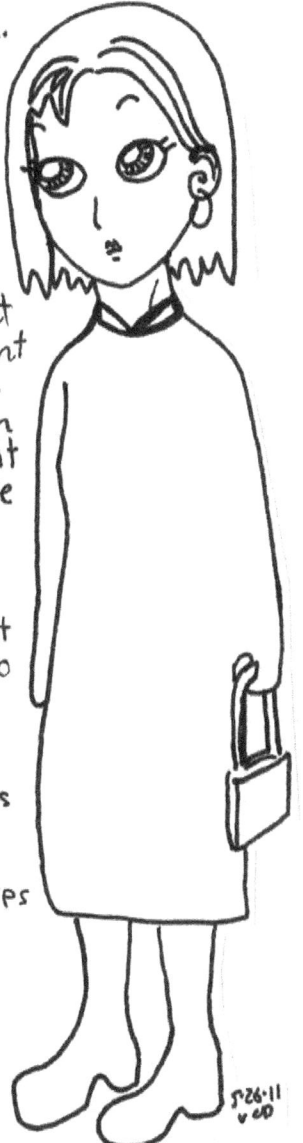

I didn't want to be a single mother who has "teen" grade relationships for the rest of their lives.

5-26-11
v.d.

Moving to the city was traumatic, Cultural Shock. Despite being Totally Native, I still had friends and I wanted to learn. When I had to do a placement test, I cried because I was embarrassed, I didn't know math. Sixth grade. That was also the first time I was confronted by an adult. I had given up on my parents and I was afraid to ask them for anything. I had to protect myself so I became defensive and mean. I effectively stopped anyone who tried to fuck with me. I grew up feeling like a freak, getting thrown into normal society compounded that. My alcoholic mom would call me weird and pitiful when I couldn't stop crying.

She abandoned us when I was 13 to live her life however she wanted.

No more pesky kids to babysit or get in the way of being with her friends. She was forced through treatment as a last ditch effort to keep her around. All of her friends assured her that they would have a beer waiting for her as soon as she got back.

Those friends are still alive and know their grandchildren. My mom died.

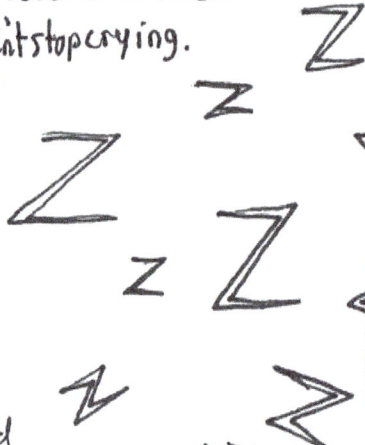

I was a Sister Mommy. I left when I was 19. I am out, I was never in. I stopped my fruitless search for validation when I was 30.

I only worship God. No one can love and worship money and God. Money and material things are not important to me.

yaya

They are dead weight, the absence of them make change easier.

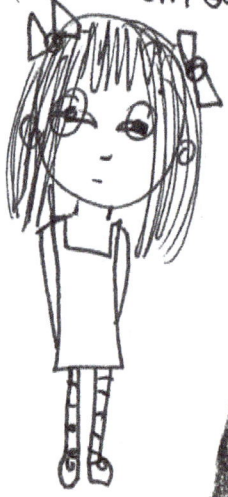

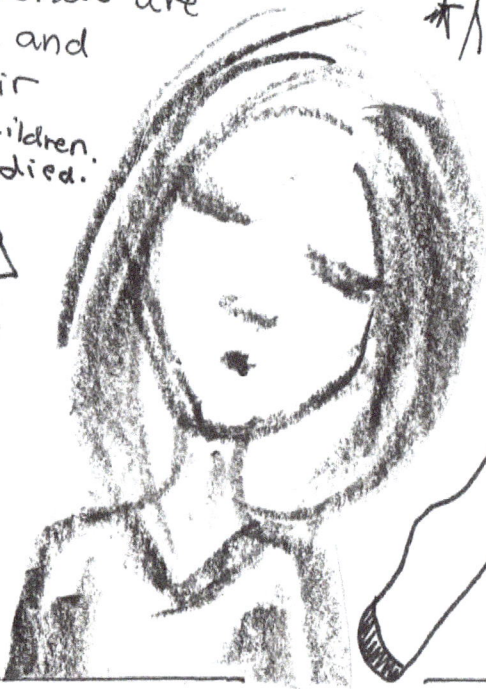

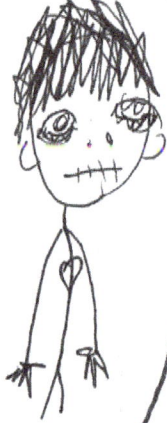

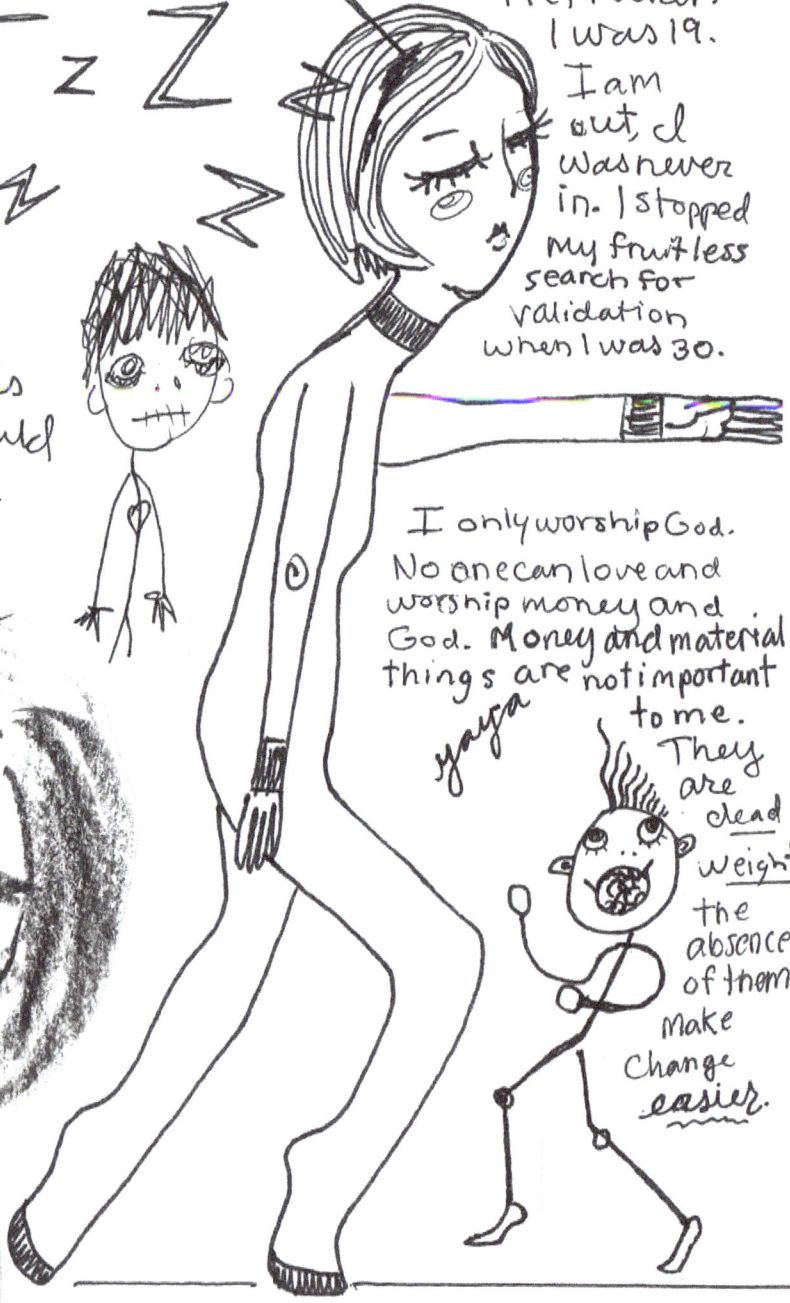

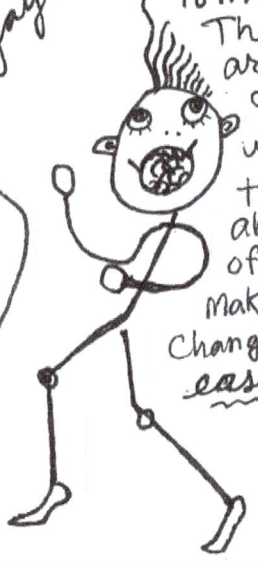

My theory of the Suicide Cycle

The root of suicidality starts in childhood. This is when you learn to feel unimportant and/or inadequate. Nothing you do is right and you will never be good enough for anyone or anything. When children are uncared about, they turn into a wild trouble-maker. It is easier for them to get addicted to drugs or alcohol. They are also at a higher risk for committing suicide or crime. In cases like that, isolation, uncharacteristic behavior, and suicidal clues go unnoticed when a parent doesn't care about their kids.

The result from that can cause suicide. Chances are, they were raised by older wild kids, grandparents, or siblings.

The basis of gangs is family and belonging, things many people grow up without. Humans are a social animal. We NEED to FEEL a sense of purpose and acceptance. If a persons' childhood sucked, they yearn for a family they can depend on, no matter what.

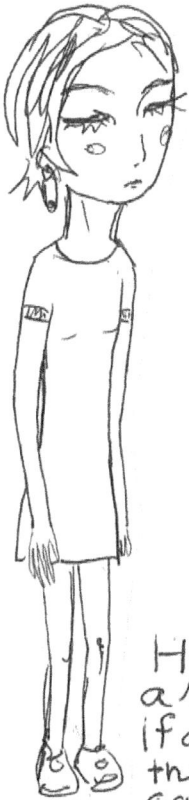

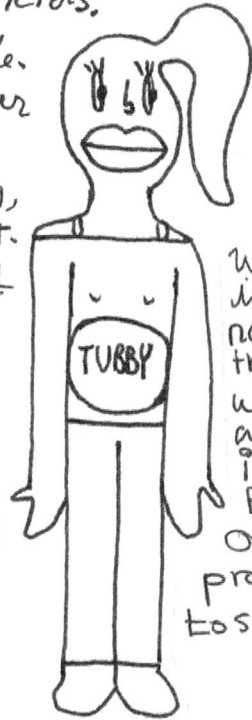

When one is lost with no direction, the first one who offers a path is Followed, or they progress to suicide.

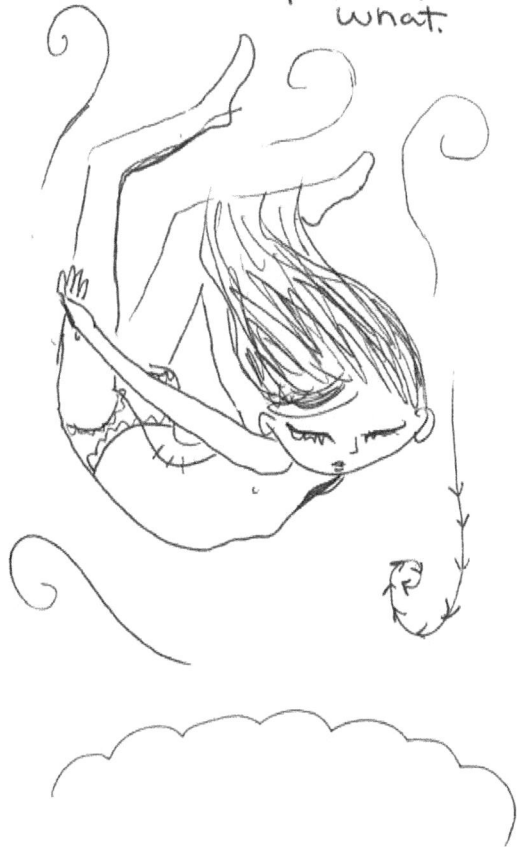

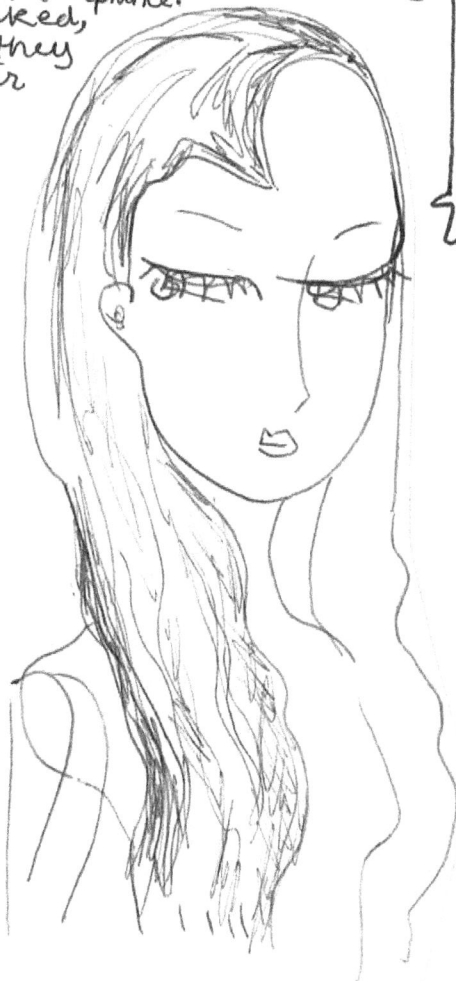

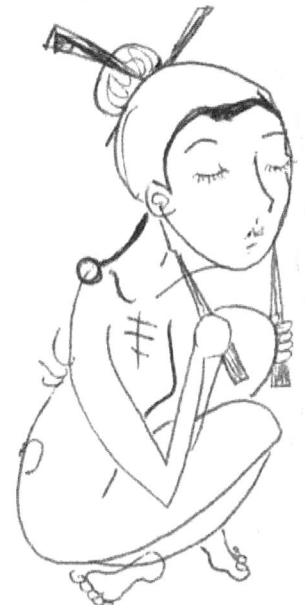

TUBBY

2/9/06
vc

When abuse and neglect continue, despite many people knowing about it, alcohol-related death is predictable. When a suicide victim dies where I grew up, people are there to get wasted with you. When the victim is alive, "It is nobodys business" and they talk behind backs. Suicide happens, people drink more, more suicide. They obsess over "Why oh whyyy is this happening to them?" They never wonder "Why did I ruin my childs' life?" which would be more appropriate. Then they drink the same thing that killed their child and continue to be emotionally unavailable to their other kids, who's lives are also at stake. Horrible, unspeakable, and depraved things go on (present tense), and keep going on.

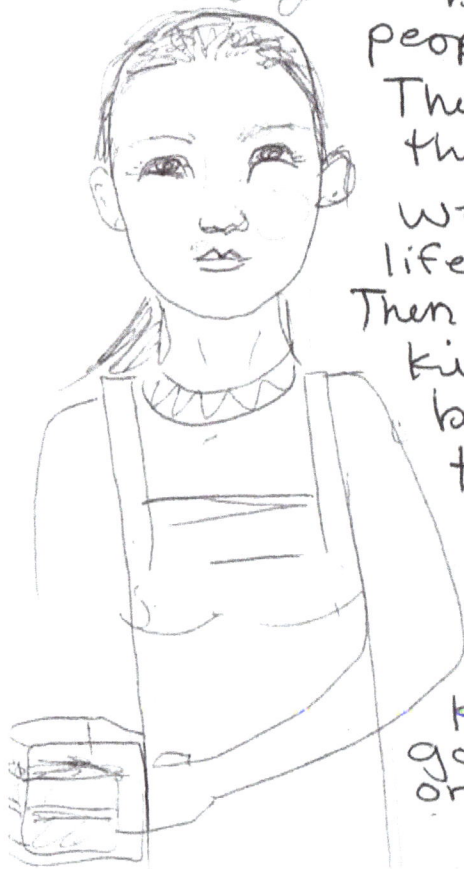

mmm chocolate cakes

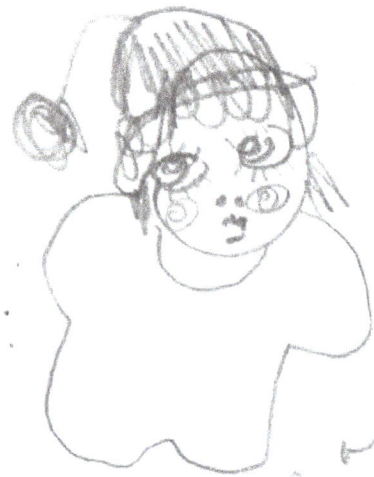

I am a Blob

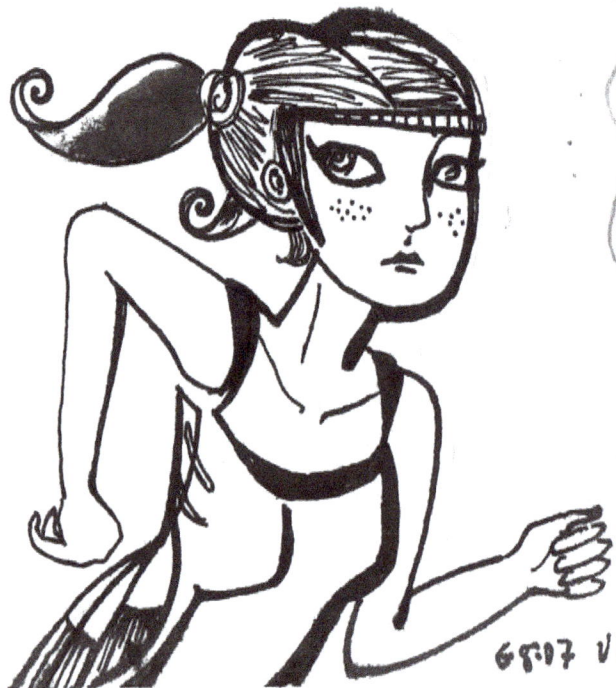

Classic.

GF07 VC

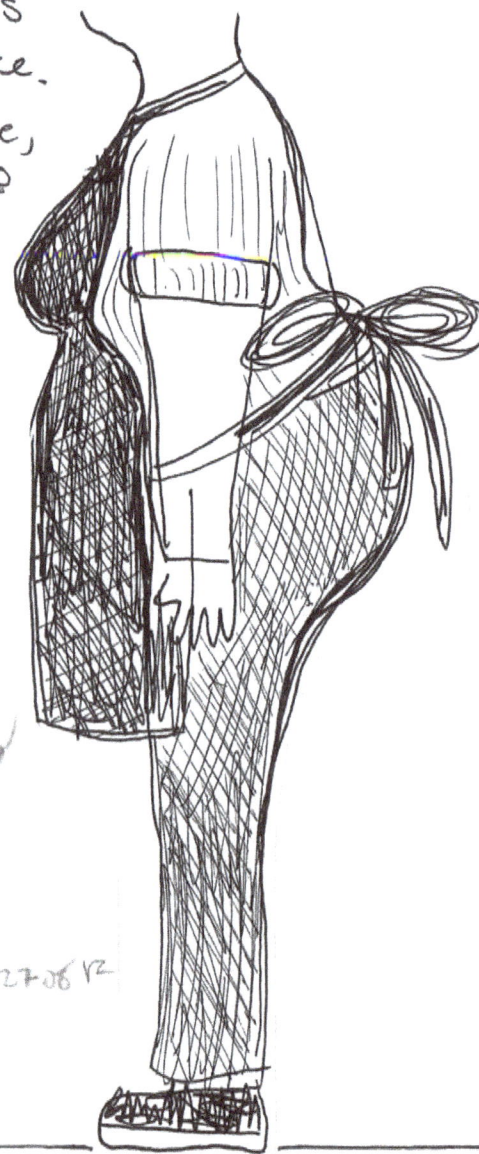

12/27/06 V2

How to fight back. The best way to fight back is to confuse your abuser with compassion. Tell them that if they feel like they need to treat you like shit to relieve _their_ suffering, then as a good and compassionate person, you will endure it, for them. Also, if they are going to use violence, tell them you will call law enforcement. If you're just tired of their harpy shit tell them and yourself:

10/8/06

I am going to live my life. You do not care about me now, you _never_ have, and maybe never will. The least you could have done was tell me that things are ok or going to be ok. I became ok without you. I know the way you treat me is NOT ok. You do not own me and I do not owe you anything.

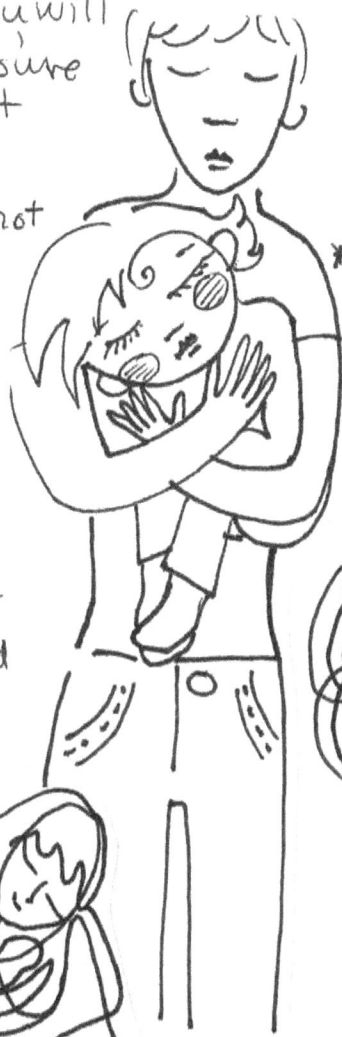

Use your tricks to fight yourself and your butthead brain to expel Massive Suicidal from your feelings.

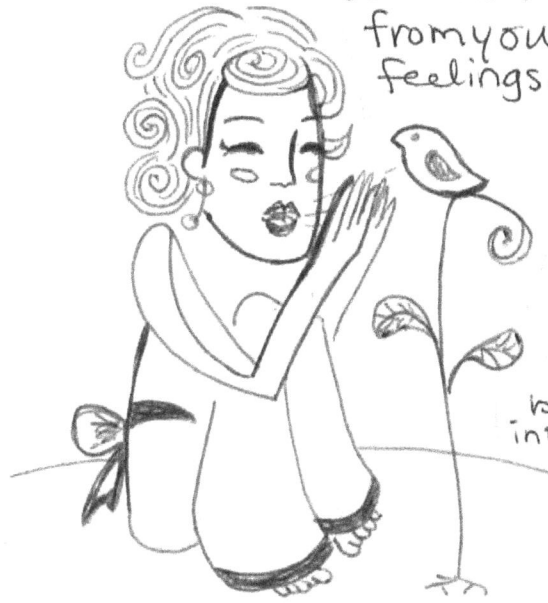

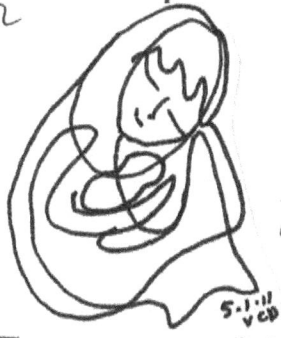

PAT *PAT*
Everything will be fine.

5-1-11 VCD

Turn bad energy into good or productive energy. It takes practice.
Learn,
Change,
Adapt.
Be a survivor.

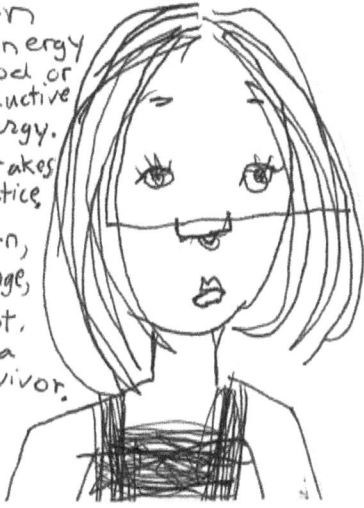

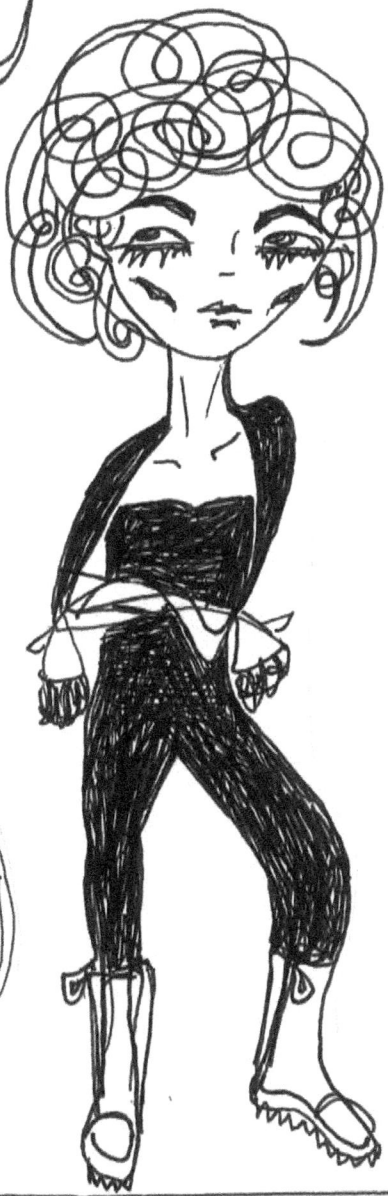

My psychiatrist and mentor taught me this:

Imagine a room that is yours. You can make this room your dream come true. You can let in or not let in whoever you want, that gives you control. Abusers want to destroy your room, do not let them. Even though your room is your dream come true, it is imperfect, because you are imperfect. In my case, the electricians did a bad job and the electric goes out and I am in the dark. There is nothing I can do but wait for it to come back. When my electric comes back on, my room is still the same, somewhere I can be happy.

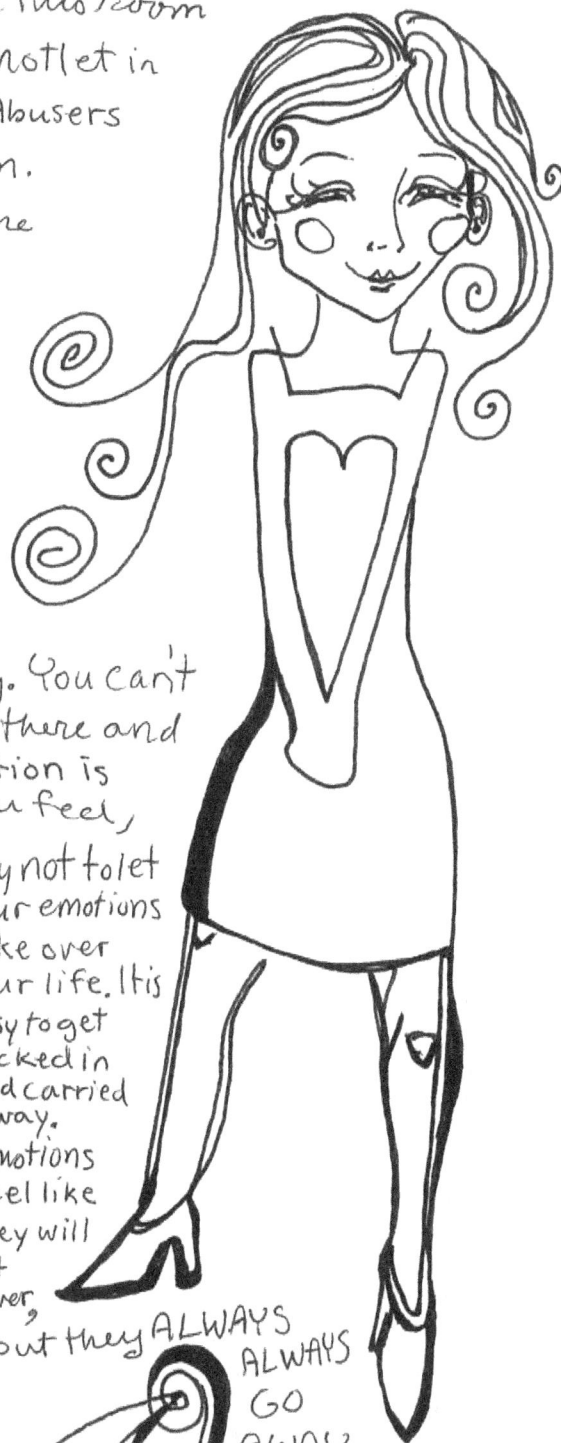

Maybe you have a structural imperfection or the inside work was not done correctly. You can't keep these from happening, they are already there and exist until you repair them. The imperfection is your emotions. You can't control the way you feel, but you can adapt, learn skills, and accept that you will never be perfect, like everyone else.

Well, I'm working on a book about Suicide.

Use your tricks. Trick your feelings. Don't forget that when you are alone in your head, you exist and are loved by more people than you realize. Know That ♡

9.24.12 5.8.11

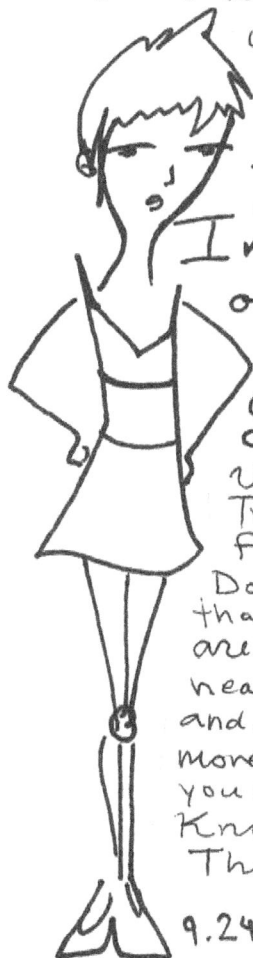

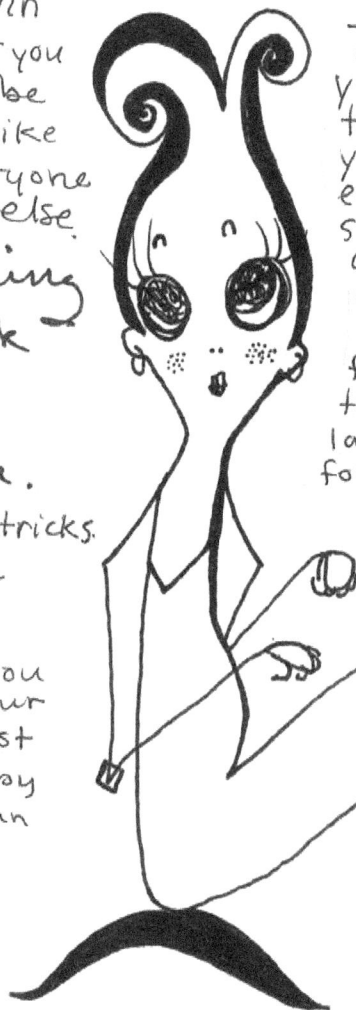

Try not to let your emotions take over your life. It is easy to get sucked in and carried away. Emotions feel like they will last forever, but they ALWAYS ALWAYS GO AWAY. Killing yourself is never a good answer. Dead is Forever. Nothing can be fixed after you are gone.

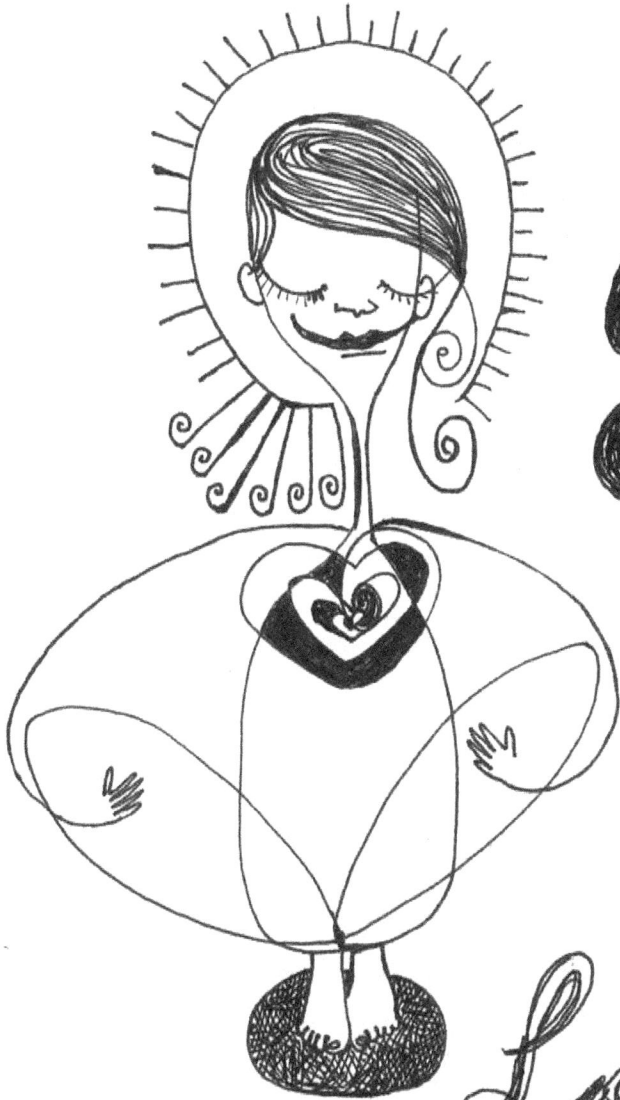

Self

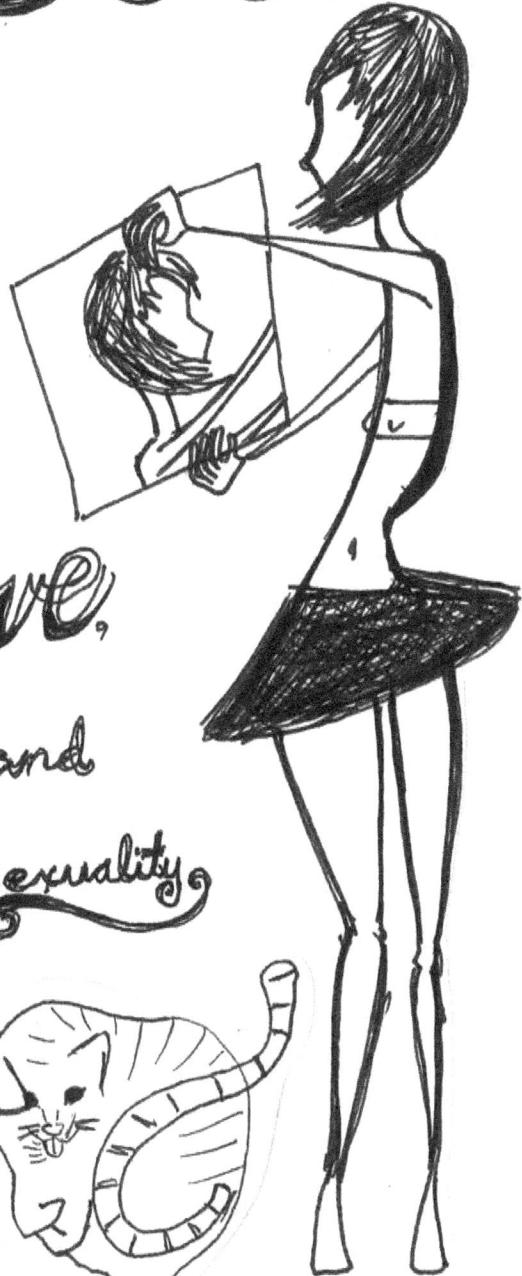

Love,

and

Sexuality

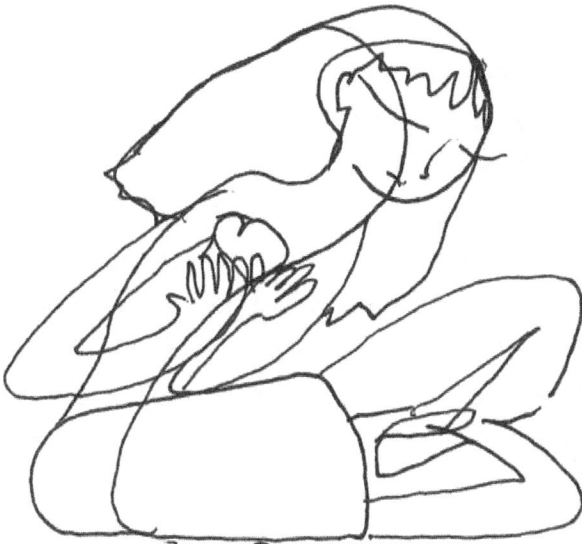

G2309 V2

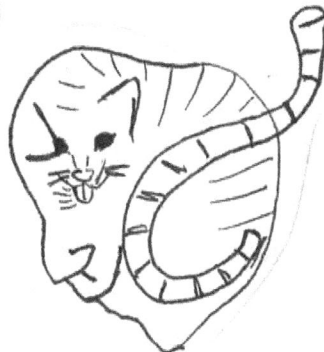

You are a living person who is powered by a functioning BRAIN. Humans are a mammal. Our bodies are made of so many systems that work together to house our life force, or soul. A soul in a body = life. Every human body is the same, but each one is different and has a unique perspective. No one in the world is exactly like you, says Mr. Rogers. It is not for anyone to decide what is beautiful or unattractive. Our concept of Beauty is mirrored in media and the Western world. We all want to be beautiful, successful, powerful, desirable, and Perfect. This concept is ingrained in us since birth, The American Dream. They define beauty and sensuality. What looks good and how you need to be is always changing. They do not define You.

All this is only the surface of YOU, which diminishes with time.

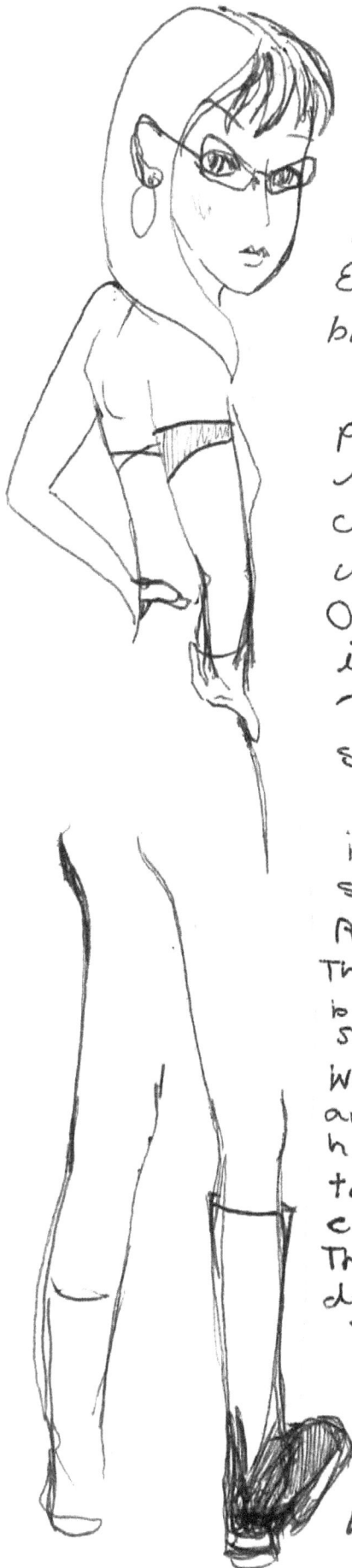

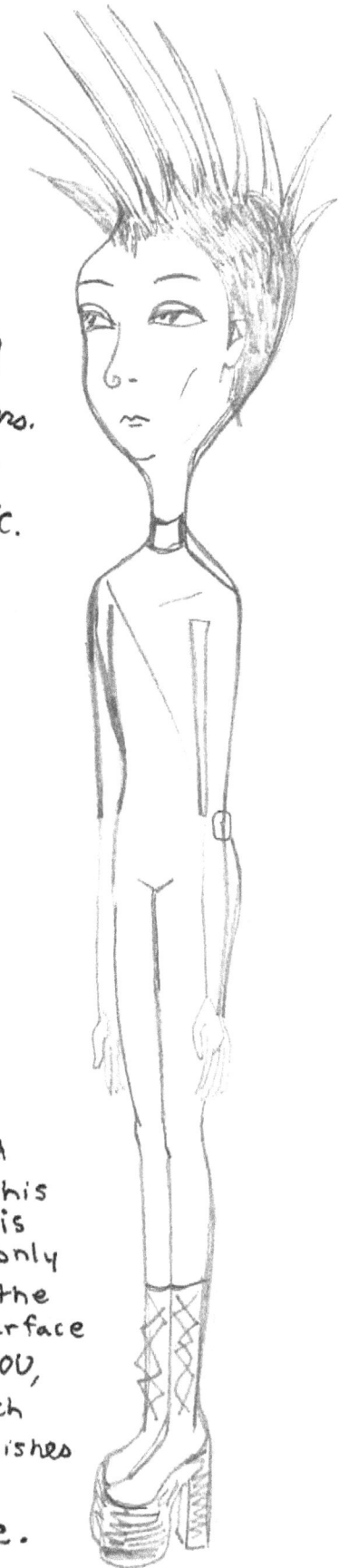

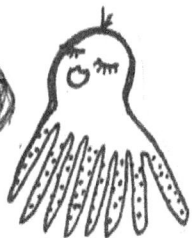

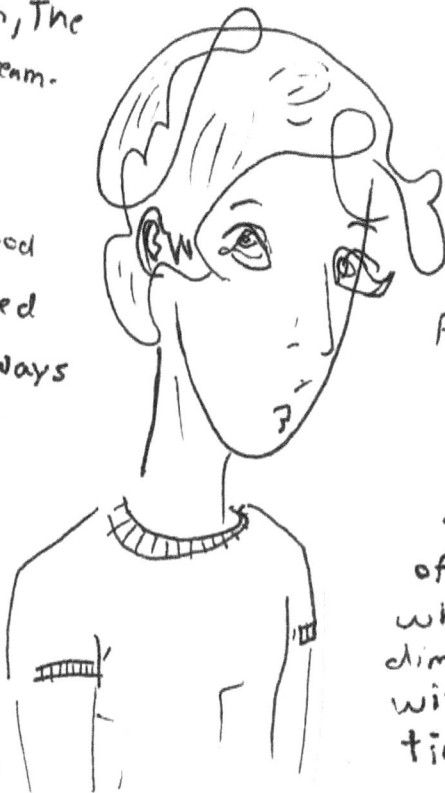

We want to look young and live longer. We believe makeup and creams can preserve our appearance, that expensive vitamins can prolong life, and that our futures need to be planned out. Tomorrow is never promised. All humans age and die. We live in a body that is subject to toxins, weather, and pollution. Our body systems and mind slow and eventually break down. No product can make you more beautiful. Beauty comes from the inside out.

The Secrets to Beauty:
- Eating and sleeping well
- Drinking water
- Wearing lotion
- Wearing sunscreen
- exercizing body and mind.
- Avoiding excess alcohol or drug consumption.
★ - Being happy with who you are and not stressing for the unattainable like everyone **else**.

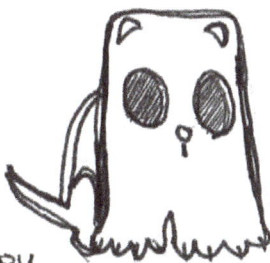

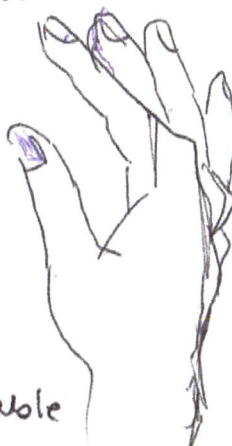

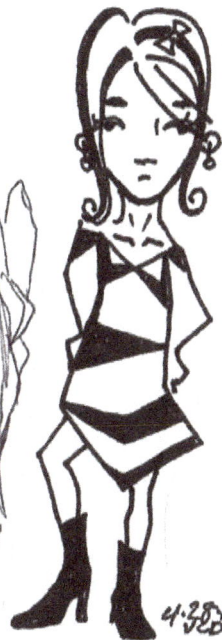

Until you realize these things, corporations and media will continue to prey on your insecurities.

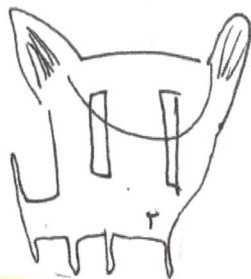

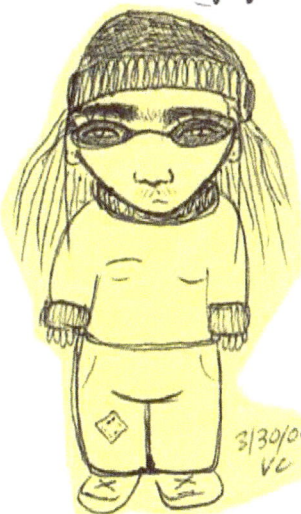

I am no Beauty . . . .

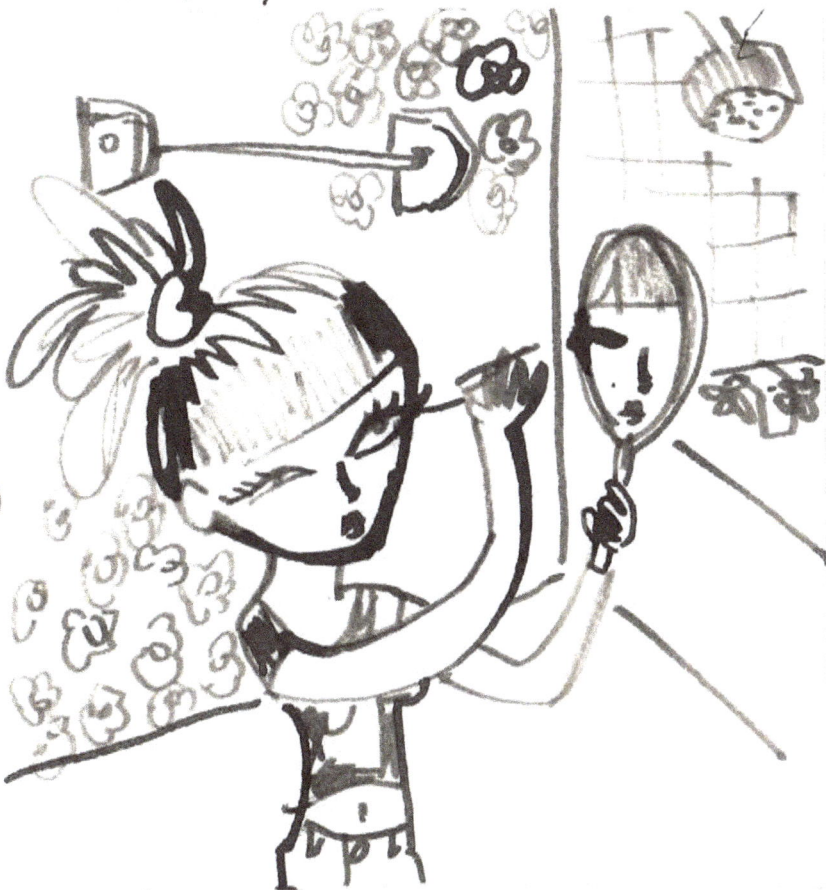

3/30/09
VC

4.28.11
JCO

I wanted for so long to be like other people who seem to have things figured out. I had braces and wore make up. Nobody tells you when you kind of look like a trashy whore. Some get trapped it this world of glamours. They define their lives with material posessions and spend their entire lives trying to aquire more. A shiny red apple is sometimes rotten in sad inside.

The most interesting people I know don't have it all figured out. They are people with disorders and diseases, recovering addicts, recovering victims of violence, and people who had a less than perfect life and knows how hopeless things can seem. The surface doesn't matter to them. People who suffer fast-forward to the end, to the secrets of life and purpose. Regular people spend their entire lives trying to find these things out. The secrets to a happy everything:

— Love
— Compassion
— Hope
♡

DOING GOOD

PRODUCES MORE GOOD. Doing good is a good reason to do anything. →

You've got to be kidding me.

Love your brother and sister humans. Share a smile or a laugh, it can go further than you can imagine is even possible.

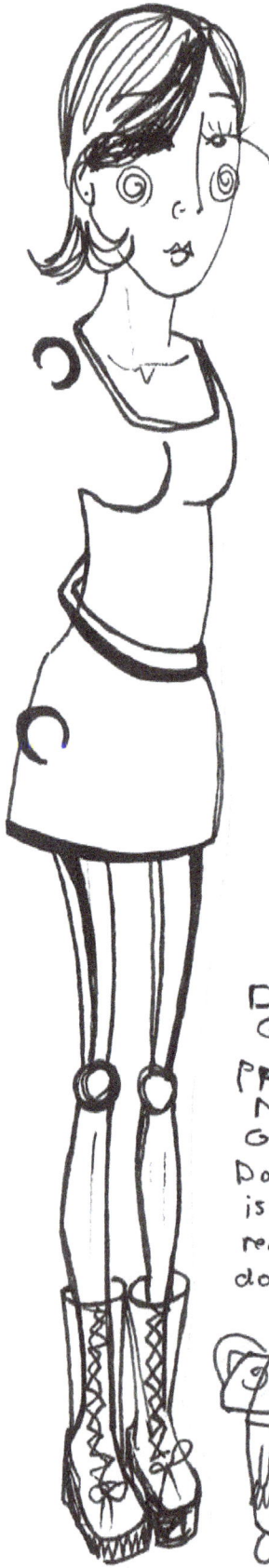

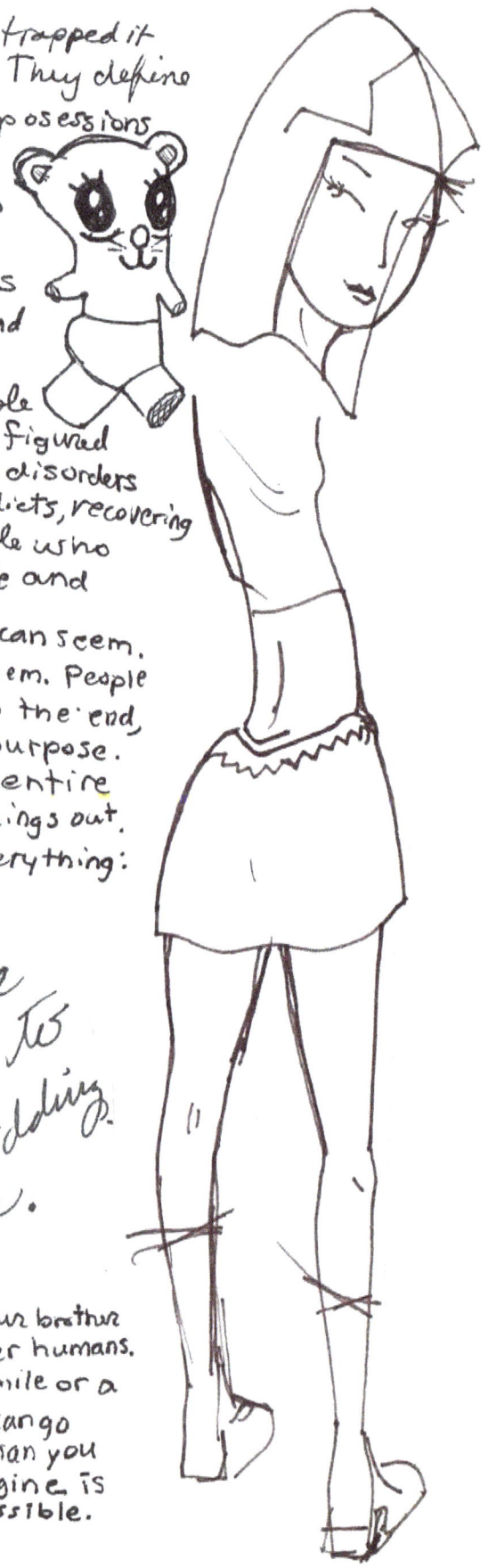

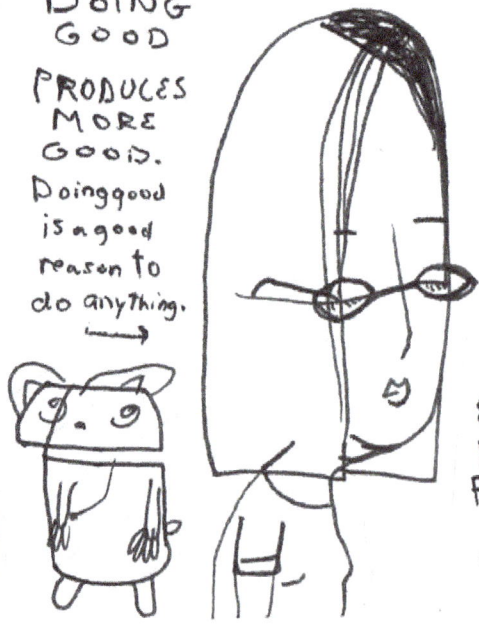

You should not have to look or be anything but yourself for people to like you. You are who you are and look like you look, people can take it or leave it. It has taken me 30 years to be ok with who I am. I am half Alaska Native. I am city, I moved when I was 10.

My being native carries many stereotypes that have affected me, just because I am unmistakenly Native-looking. I am alcohol abstinant, I don't "Party," I am not an alcoholic bum, I don't neglect my child, and I do not have a pack of kids from different baby daddies. Despite all that, I get yelled racial slurs from random vehicles, I get followed in retail shops, turned down for loans, and told to go home to my kids by complete strangers.

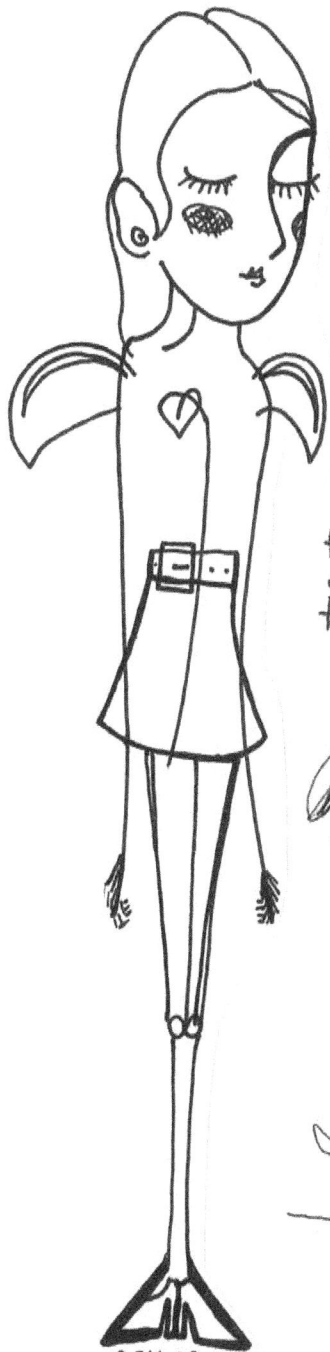

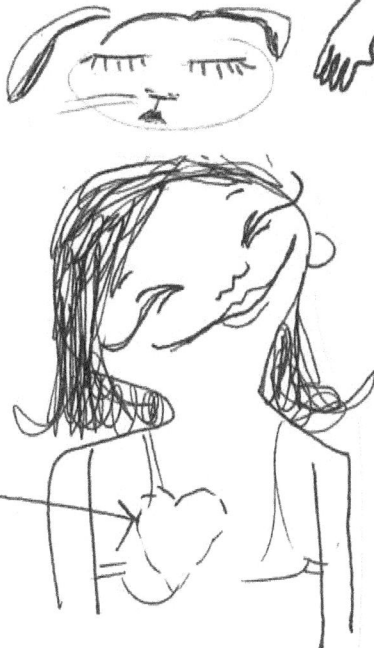

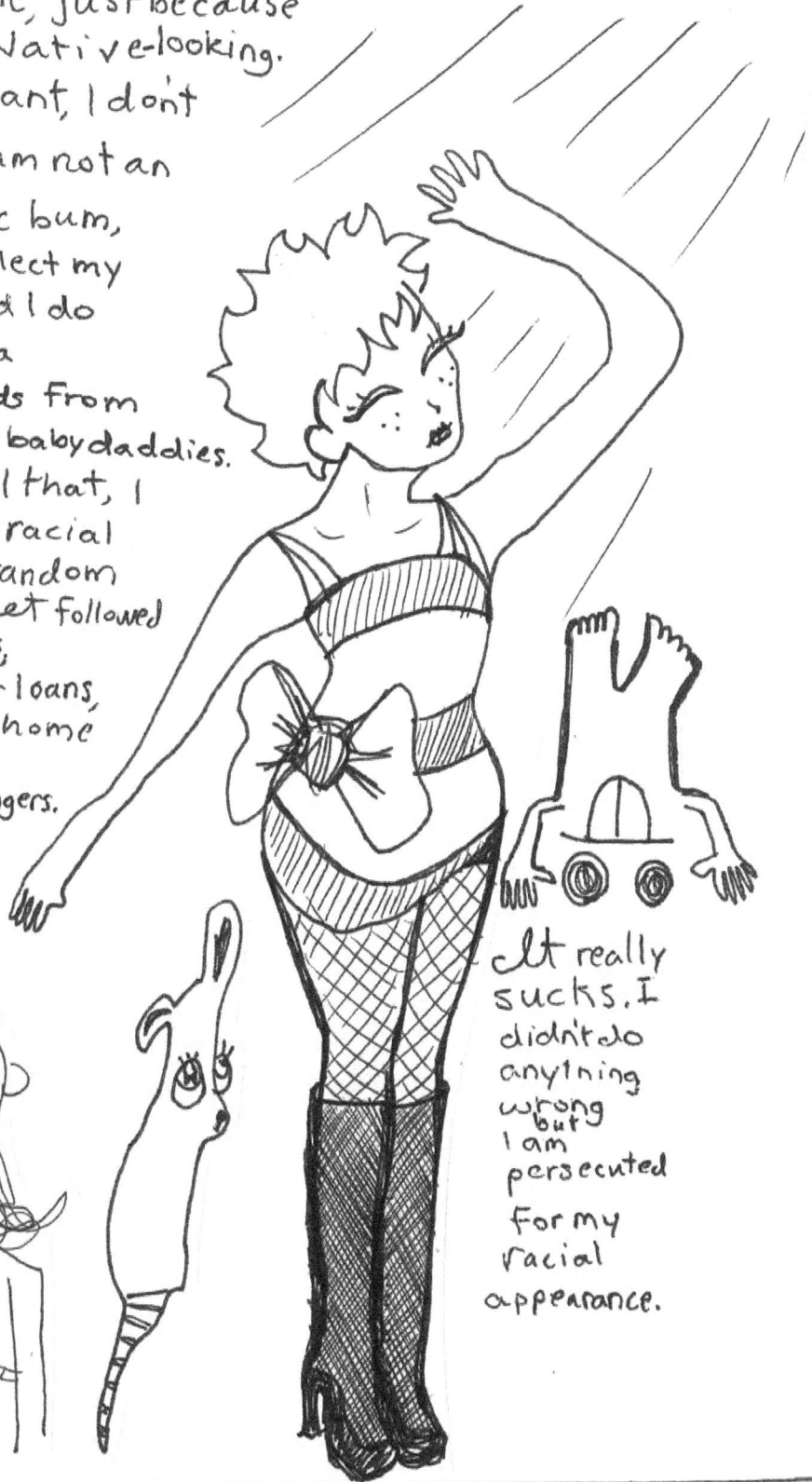

It really sucks. I didn't do anything wrong but I am persecuted for my racial appearance.

6 24 09 rz

I don't "feel" Native and I don't have a cultural identity. I AM an imperfect, individual, human being. A person is a person is a person. We are all born innocent and judgement free. We learn to judge people by society and our parents. When you learn to see people as living creatures, it becomes easier to not pass judgement on them. Instead, have compassion for them. Listen to whatever suffering they may be in or have been. When you are suffering yourself, think of how you would like to be listened to.

Everyone has Love and Light in their hearts, we are born with it. You can see them in smiles and good deeds. When your light is dim and far-seeming away, REMEMBER IT IS NOT OUT.

It is the tiniest blinking star among the other big shiny stars that demand to be looked at.

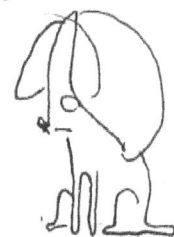

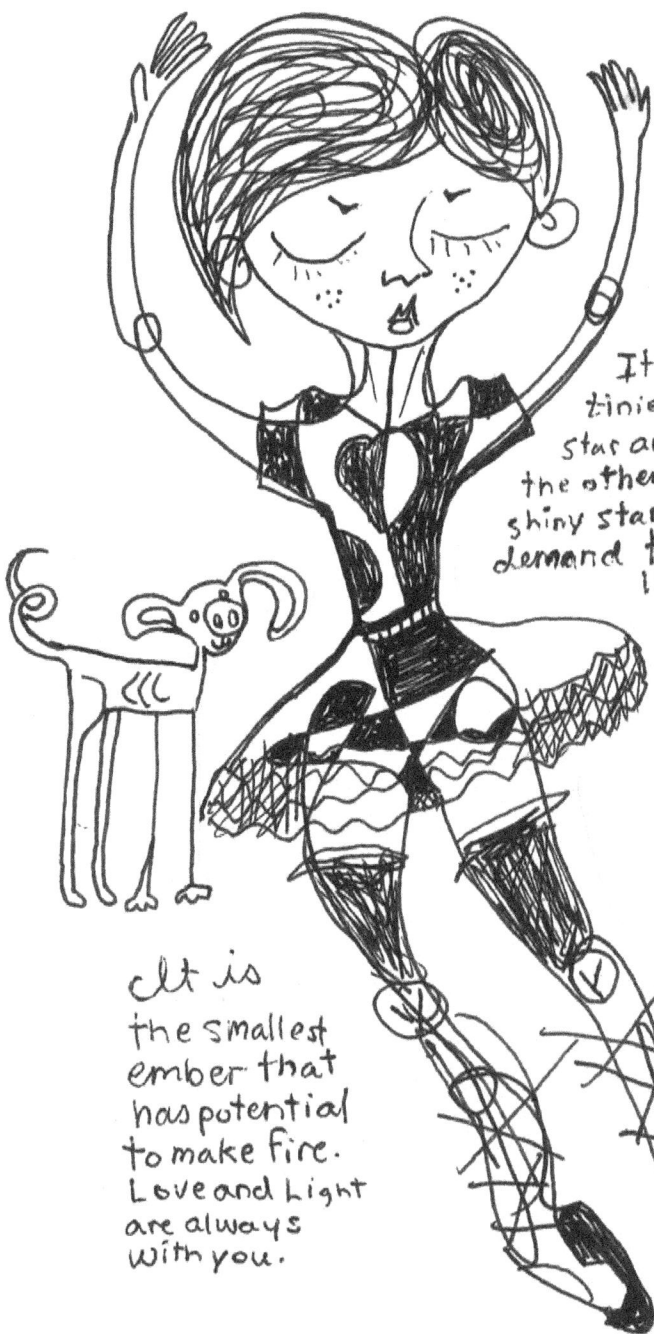

It is the smallest ember that has potential to make fire. Love and Light are always with you.

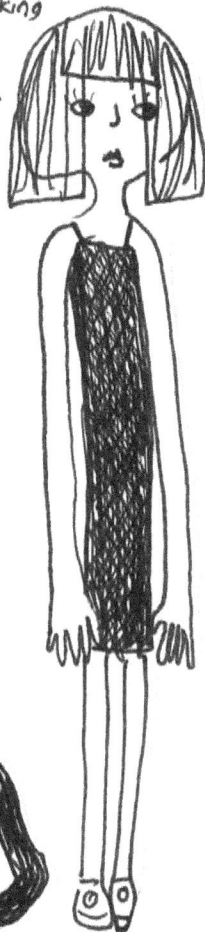

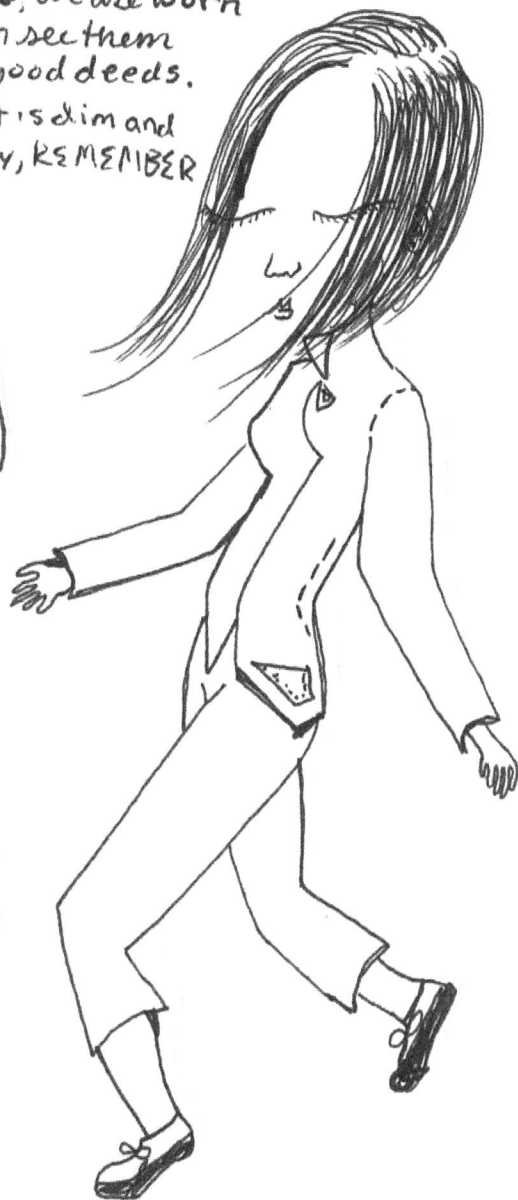

The world we live in is filled with SEX. Alcohol and hookups are portrayed as normal by media. We have been desensitized and over-stimulated, Sexual ADD. Sex is so romanticized that people feel like they need sex in a temporary relationship, or whenever the opportunity presents itself. Sex does not mean love. If it did, families would fuck each more than they already do. Sex does not make a person more grown-up, it doesn't make a person ANYTHING. Sex causes pregnancy and transmits disease and infection. diseases can not be cured, bacterial infections can. Unless these are medically treated, they can spread to others and cause reproductive damage As they go down the line, they mutate and become treatment resistant.

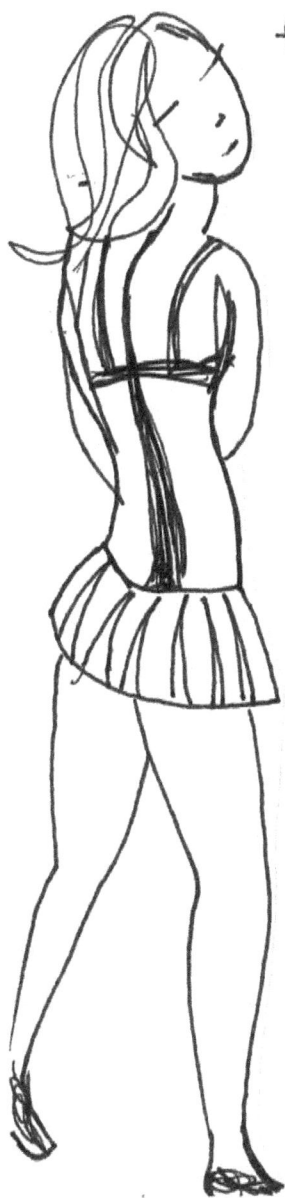

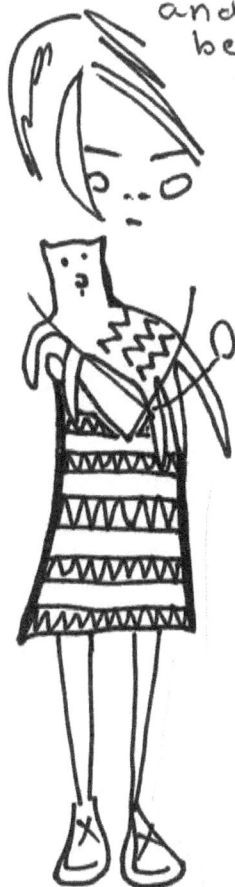

12 29 08 VC

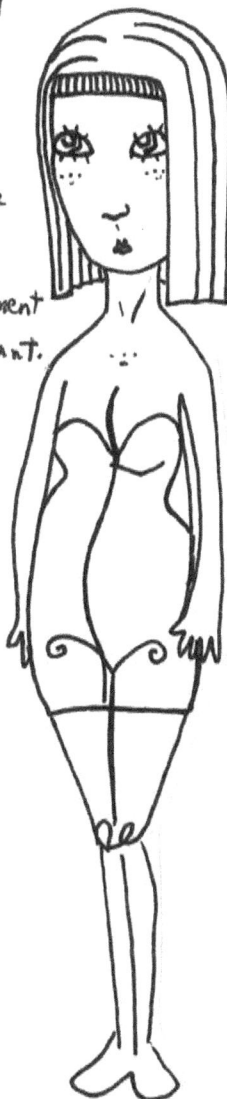

624 09 VC

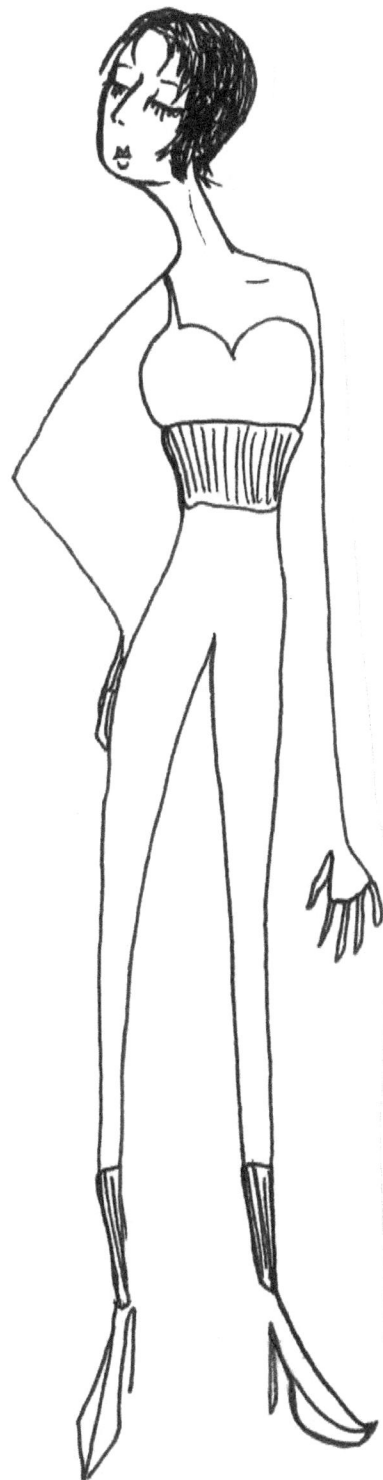

Abstinence is the only 100% effective way to avoid infection and pregnancy, True. Sterilization and birth control do not protect against infection.

All people are born virgins, some stay that way until they meet their Special One. I gave up my card when I was 13 to some ugly older guy. i was not told about gossip, STI's, or how sacred my body was. Your body is the one thing in this world that you own. Don't give some A-hole bragging rights about taking your virginity and how much you sucked at doing whatever.

The purpose of sex is procreation. It is a survivalist animal behavior and drive that is meant to create offspring.

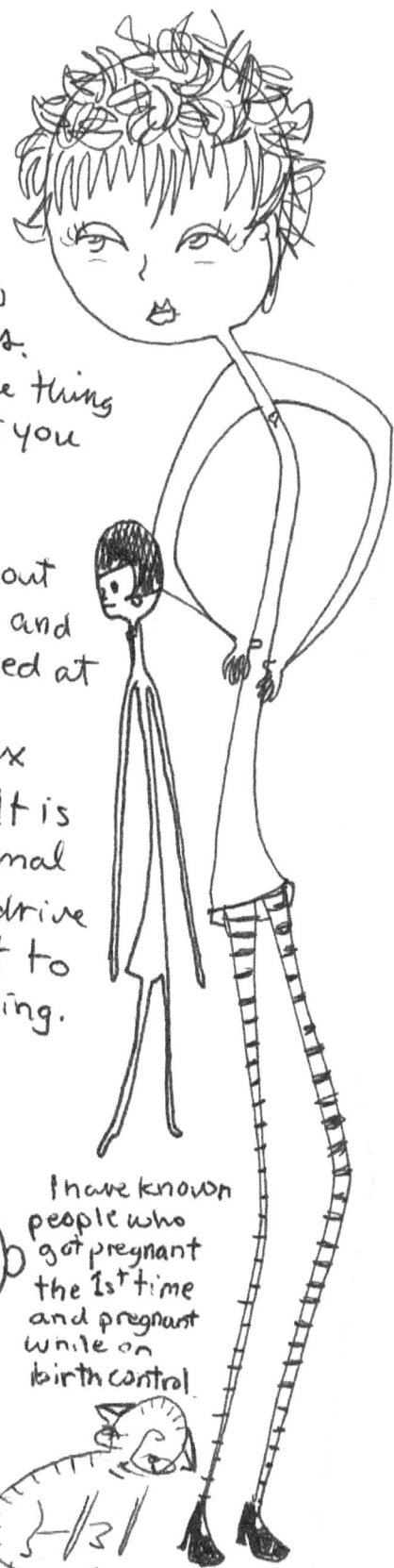

I have known people who got pregnant the 1st time and pregnant while on birth control.

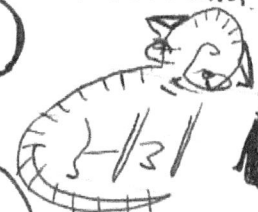

Do not underestimate natures powerful forces.

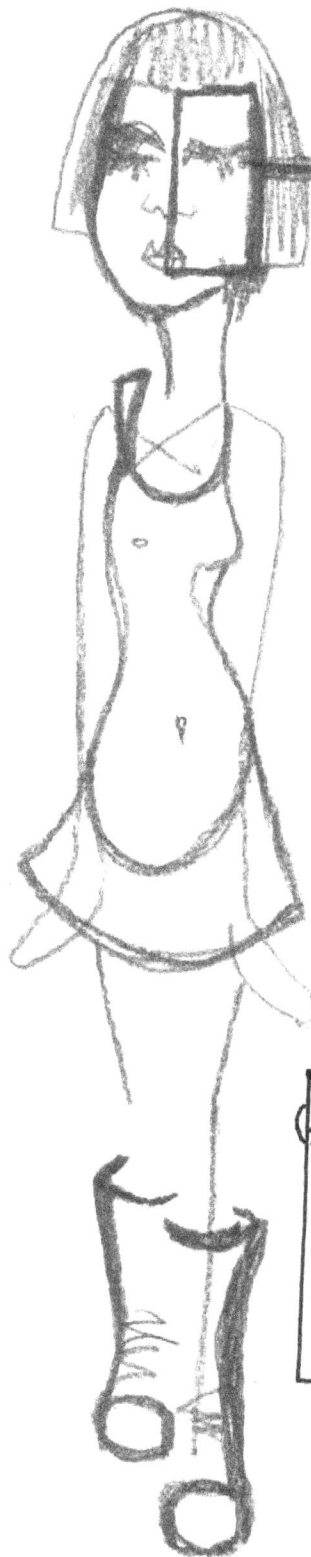

Fuckin 80s!

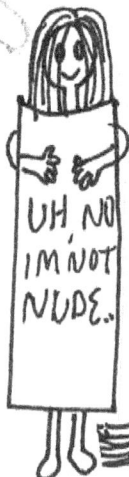

UH NO IM NOT NUDE.

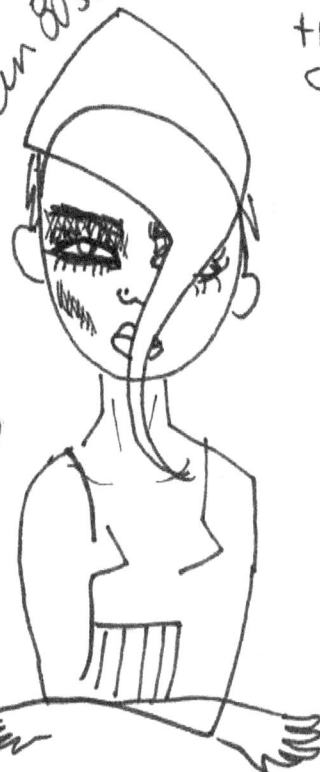

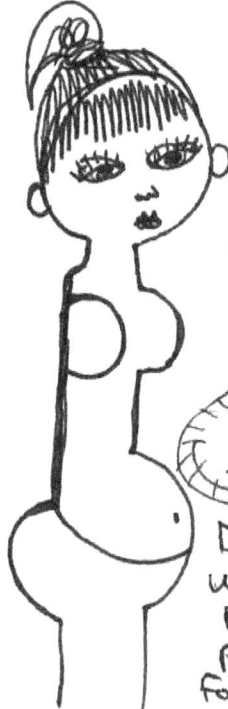

Young adult bodies go through dramatic changes and the reproductive systems mature. Hormones are at their peak. You turn into a fully developed human that can produce babies. Having a baby while you are young can result in premature birth. Most babies survive from as early as 25 weeks, others have life-long health problems. My own son was born at 27 weeks and had to spend 3 months in the Neonatal Intensive Care Unit (NICU). I have seen everything that can go wrong with babies and there were many young mothers and fathers there. Having a baby is never a wrong choice, you made another HUMAN. This particular human depends on you for their survival and growth, so your life is no longer about you. Girls have a reputation for trying to keep a guy, by having their baby.

GUYS DO IT TOO!

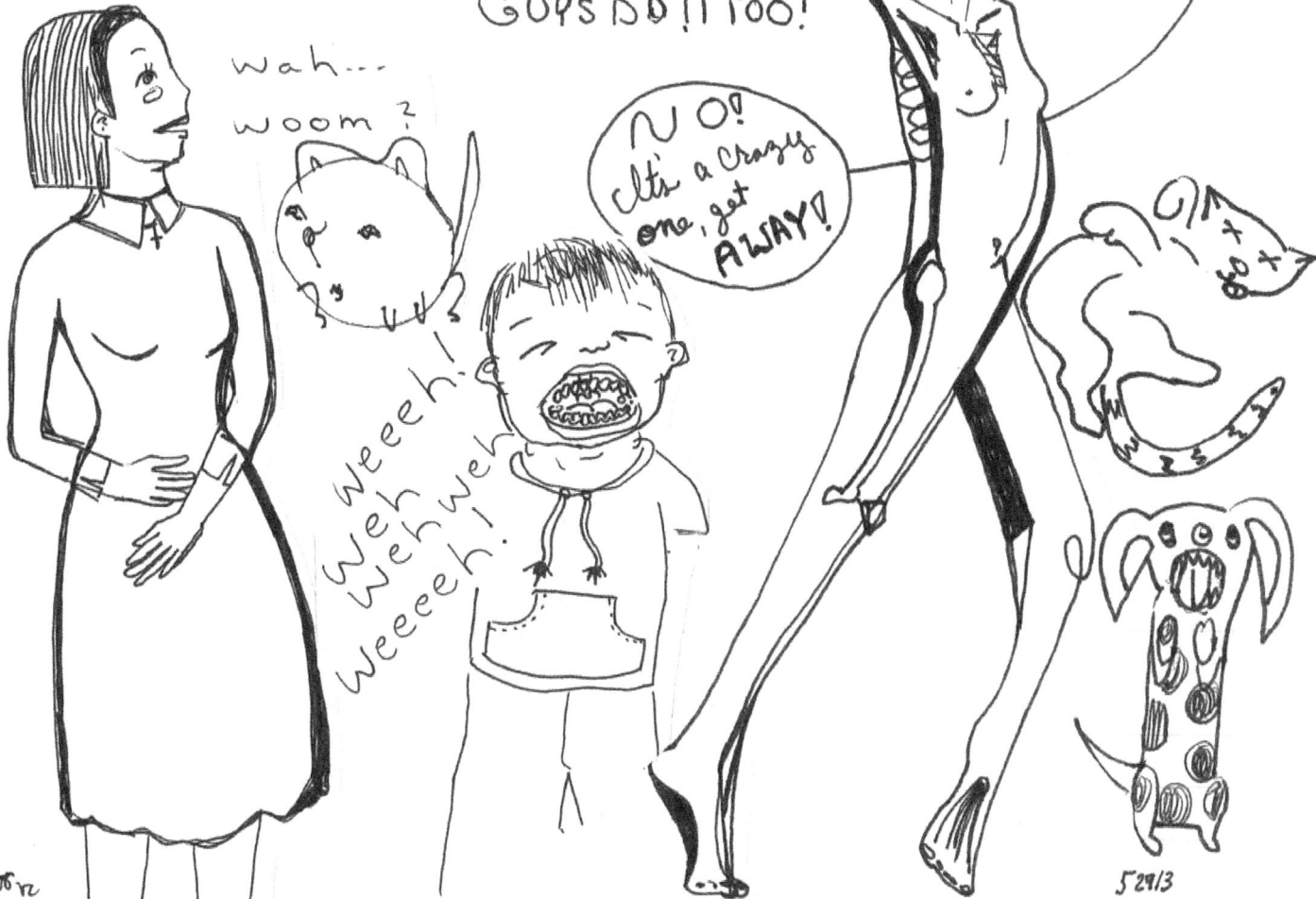

Wah... woom?

NO! It's a crazy one, get AWAY!

weeeeh! weh weh weh weeeeh!

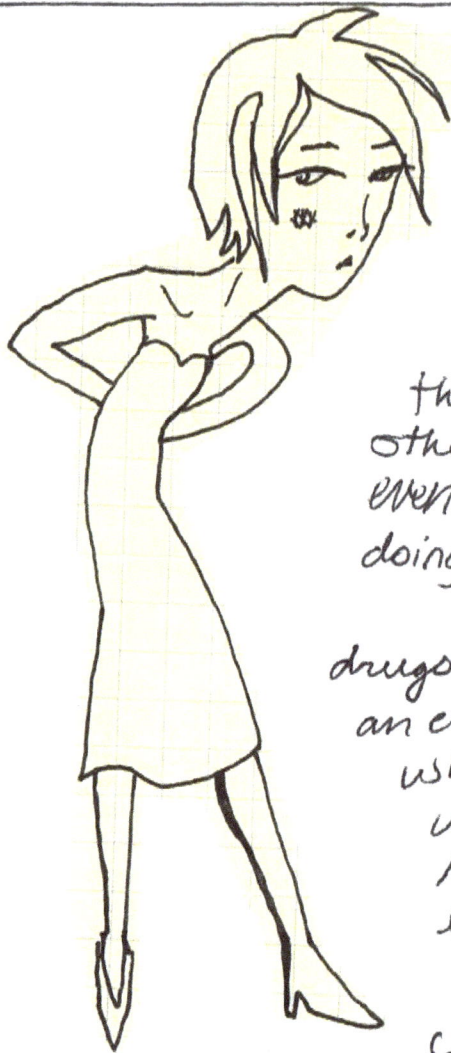

9 12 0 8   Sex is not everything it portrays. It is clumsy with elbows, knees, and limbs. Sex is slimy and you exchange body fluids.

You don't give a sample of sweat, saliva, semen or vaginal mucus to a stranger then expect them to drink half and put the other half in their vagina or penis. Who even cares about "technical" virginity when you're doing all the other nasty stuff anyway. Alcohol is involved in reckless sexual behavior, so are drugs. Being drunk is never sexy and NEVER an excuse to screw somebody. You don't know where they've been, or whose been in. Drunk sex is rape. Alcohol or drugs can cause dryness and erectile dysfunction too. Being slutty gives you a bad reputation.

It starts with house parties, then you graduate to being a barslut. Guys and girls will seek out the drunk vapid whores, the ones with no self-esteem and no self-respect. Do you really want the party to start when you arrive and start doing crazier things you wont remember?

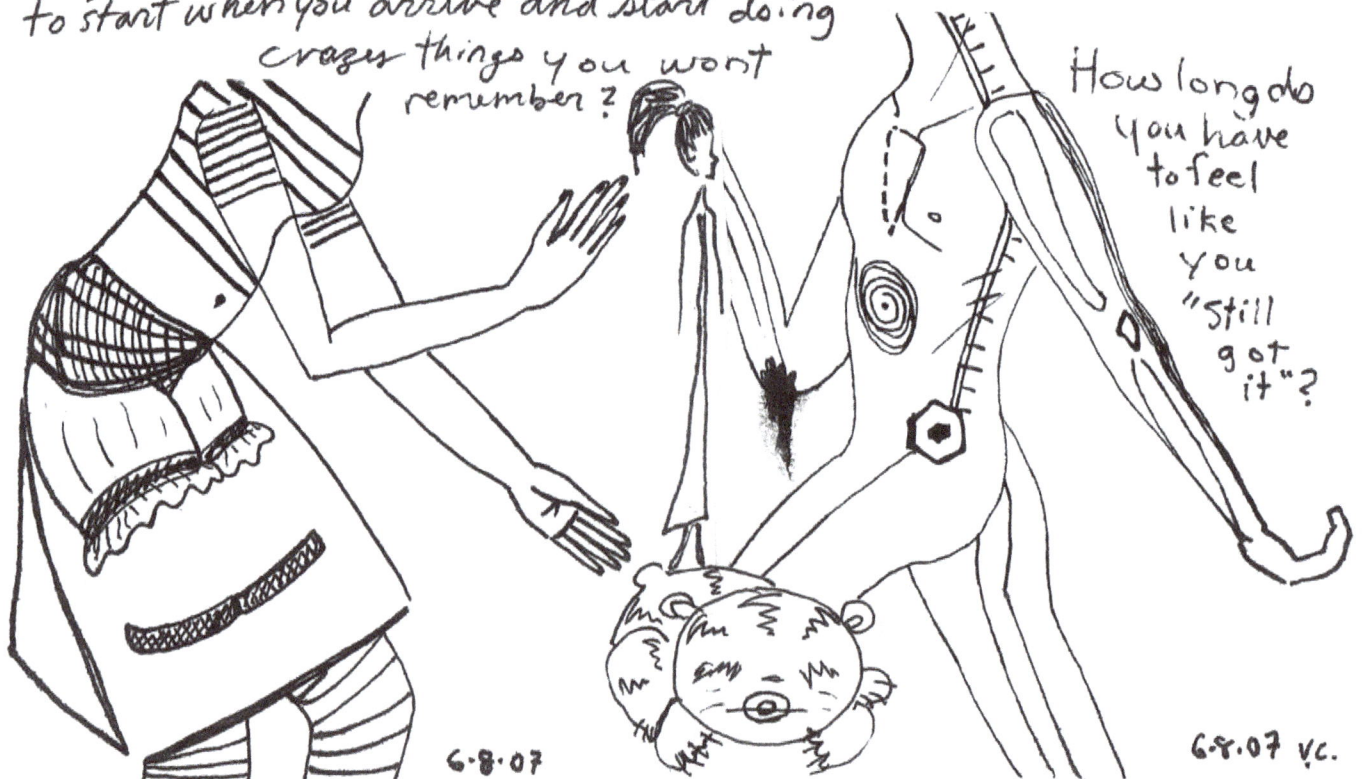

How long do you have to feel like you "still got it"?

6·8·07

6·8·07 v.c.

If your father or mother were either absent or inadequate, please don't fall for the older married person who "knows exactly what you are going through." They are not in it for love, just lust. They look for the empty sad girls and will tell you how amazing and beautiful you are. Guys too. Your adoration and need is easy for them to fulfull and they are more than willing to hold you and kiss you, and have sex with you. You end up with nothing but heartbreak if

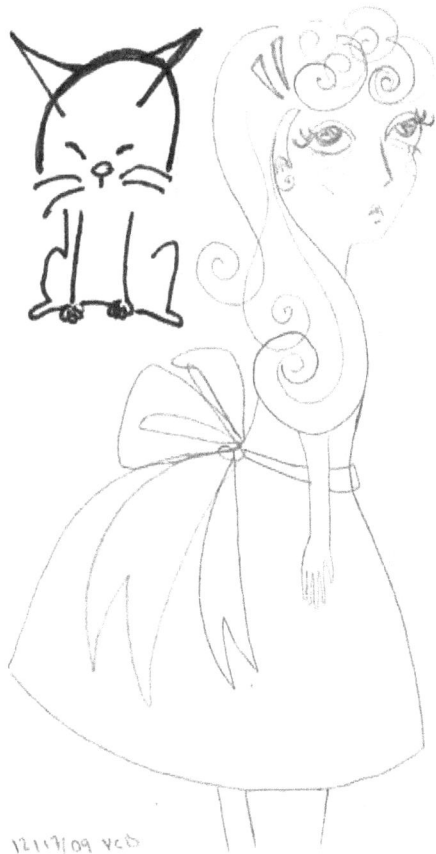

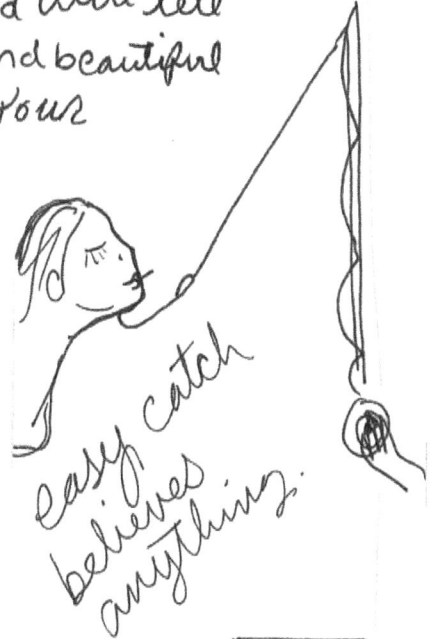

you fall for your daddy who loves you and treats you like a prize, A Trophy.

easy catch believes anything.

Bait Lies

NOT CAMERA SHY.

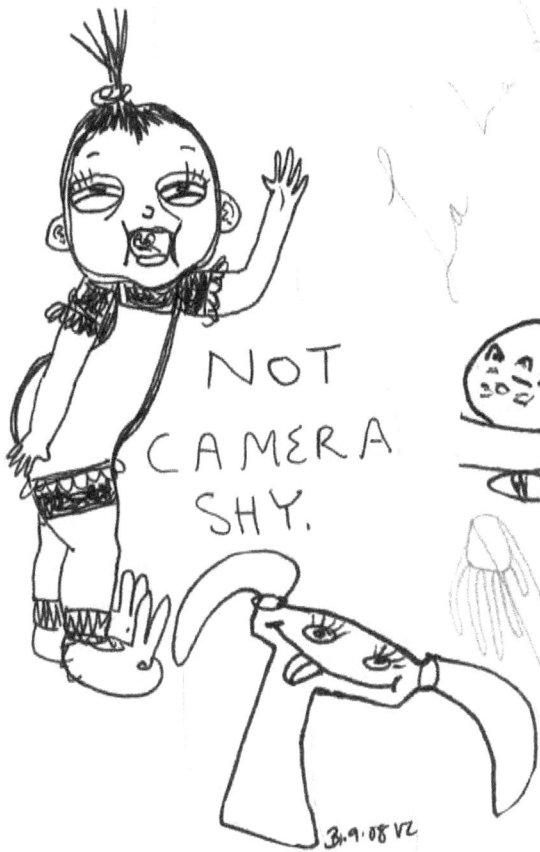

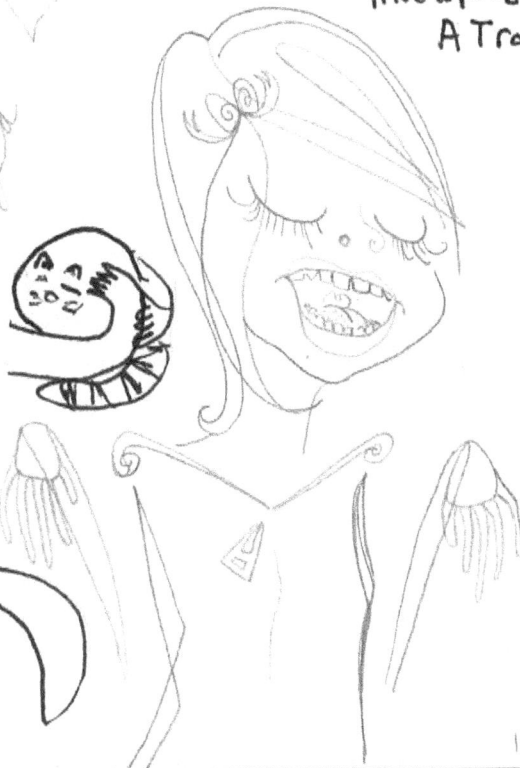

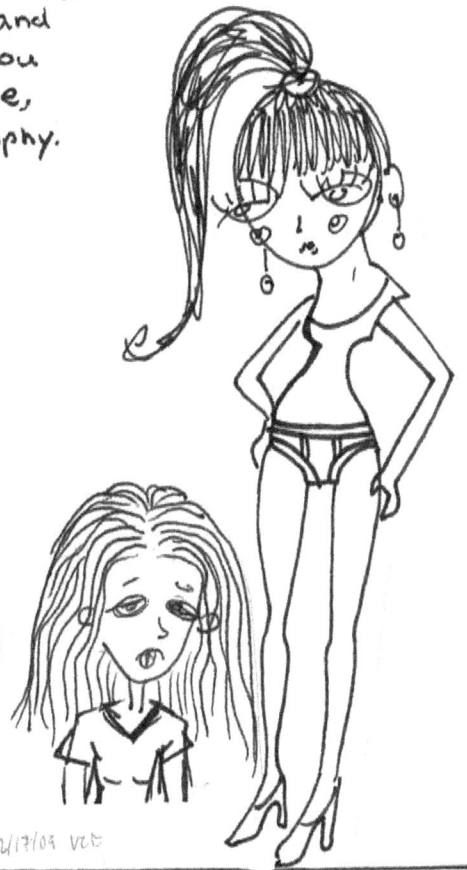

12/17/09 VCD

3·9·08 V2

12/17/09 VCD

Grown adult sexual behavior is reckless and usually involves alcohol. When you drink alcohol, expect the possible rape or unexpected pregnancy. Intoxicated people feel gorgeous, powerful and irresistable in their perception. They also let themselves be fucked by Losers and raped by tutors. It doesn't matter how perfect a person may look, they might not know Love. Some don't feel like they exist if anyone wants to fuck them all the time. When you have 50 partners under your belt, nothing sexual is new. Every area has been explored, this can ruin a relationship. People are insecure. They worry if they are big enough or tight enough, or if they can ever live up to the other persons' Porn Star Standard. They might not like to do some things that other people do to them. For a serial sexer or cheater one person may not be enough for them and they end up cheating. Relationship Over.

Tell me I Look hot or I'll Pound You.

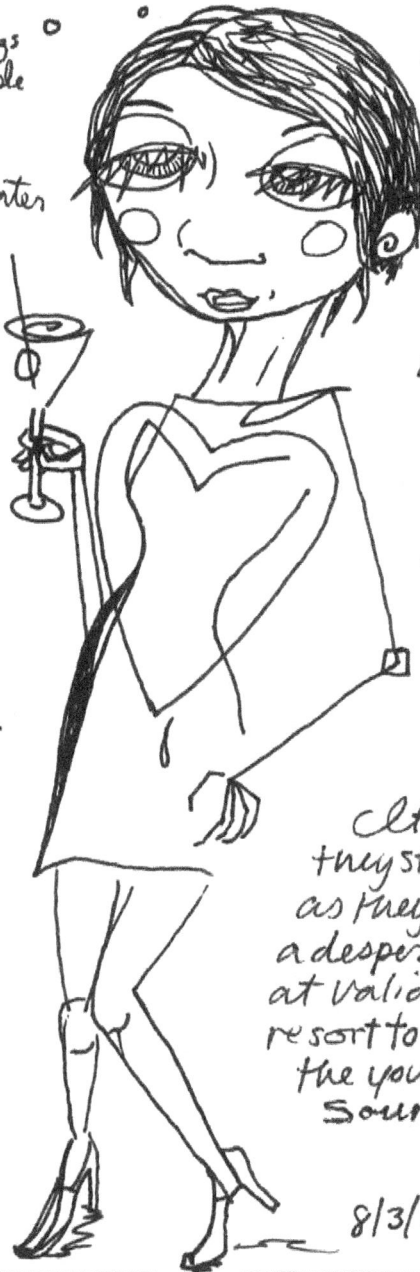

Modern Promiscuous Woman. She. Loves everything. Will fuck the living.

As long as SHE thinks she's Hot.

It is just sad, they stay the same as they age. Then, as a desperate attempt at validation, they resort to seeking out the younger crowd. Sound familiar?

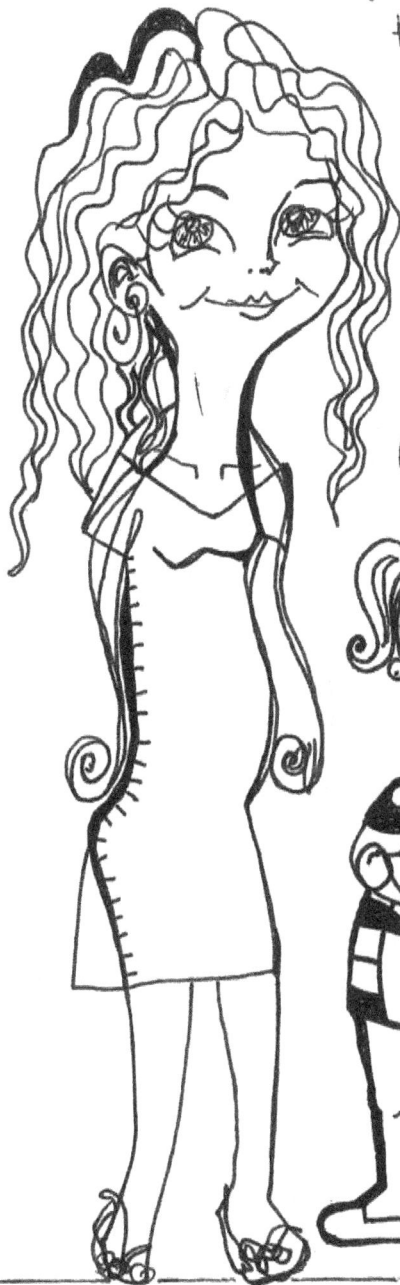

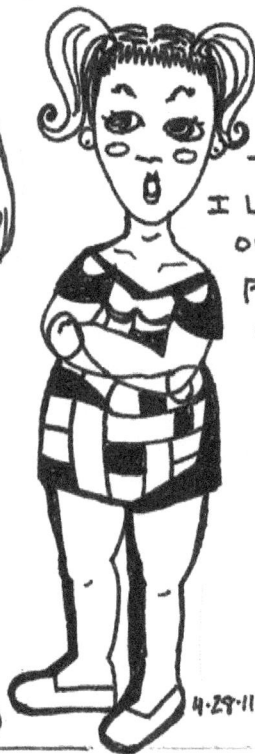

4-29-11 VCD

8/3/09

Your body is your business. Not one person needs to know that you are a virgin or abstinent, nobody needs to know what your naked body parts look like. Online it goes, and everyone knows.

Any digital media that gets to the online realm, stays there.

By putting whatever degrading sexual or intoxicated acts or you commit compromises your control. You can not control what people will say or do with those.

Everyone should have control over their body and be at least discerning over partners. Alcohol and drugs compromises that control. People can do anything to you when you are blacked-out or passed out. This can be anything from filming, taking photographs, or doing stuff to you: Rape to drawing cock and balls all over your face with permanent marker when you have to get up early and go to work. Promiscuity is an easy transition to prostitution. Prostitution is giving sex in return for a price. When you become somebodys bitch or ho, it is almost impossible to get out of their control over you if they have what you need, and they KNOW that. Drug dealing is a

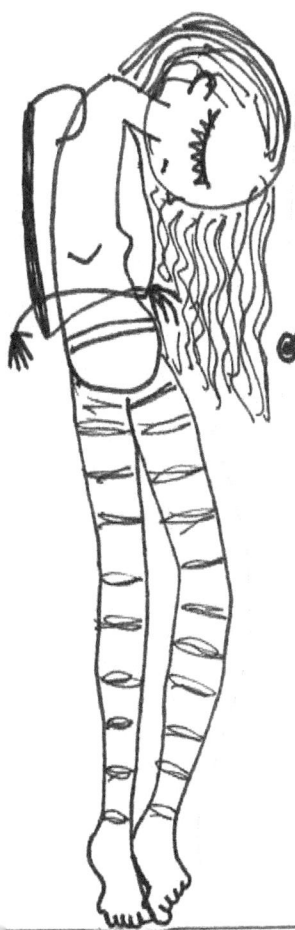

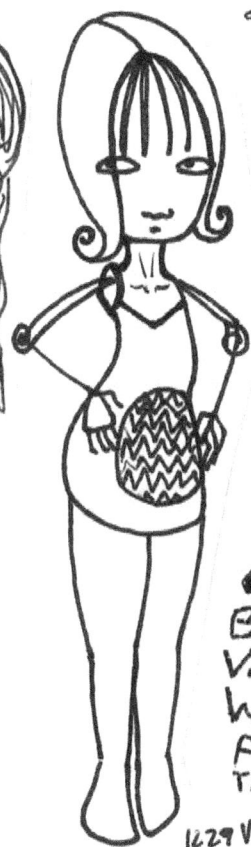

child molestors dream come true.

Grrr! Get out!

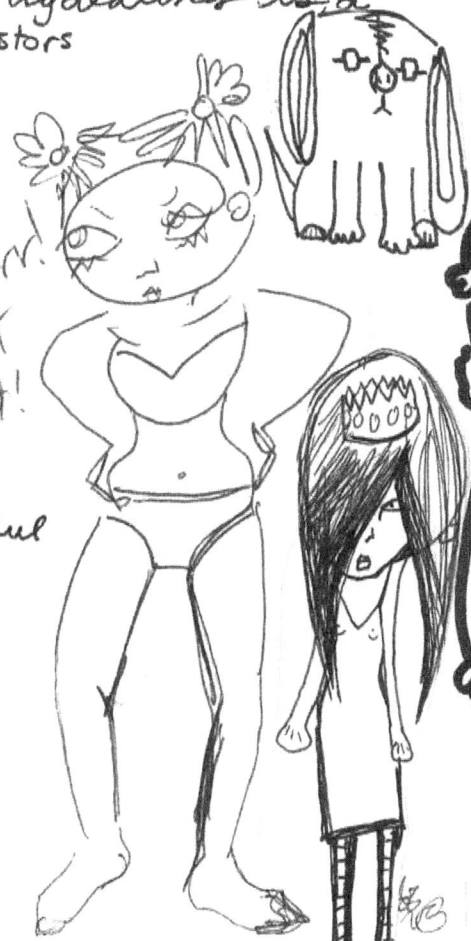

Beautiful
Mess
Crazy
Bitch
Vapid
Whore
Addict.
The end.

1229 VC

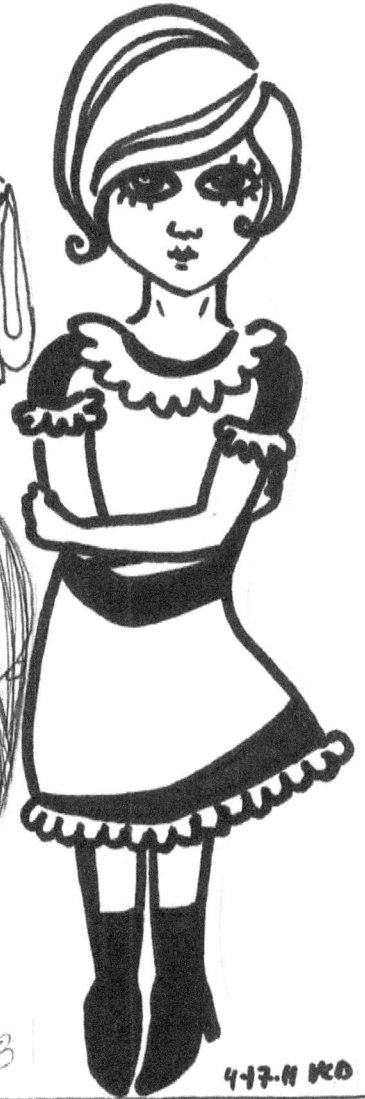

4-17-11 VCO

People have sex for many reasons. Sometimes it is by choice sometimes not. People have sex to make babies, make themselves feel important, something to brag about, to get drugs or money, to protect their siblings, vengence, being in an abusive relationship, sex slavery and human trafficing, mind or personality disorder, for attention, and to feel loved.

People also suffer through emotionally and physically abusive relationships. Both males and females are abusers and victims of domestic violence, name calling, bringing up the past, rape, stalking, harassing, threatening, making a person fearful and protective of their children, threatening you and using the children and pets to hurt you, threatening to commit suicide, and threaten your life, then wuss out and commit suicide. You do not have to be nice to them.

errr rr...

People do crazy things they will always regret when they are under emotional stress. They are usually under the influence of alcohol and try to say they are sorry. Yeah, know what? They are sorry.

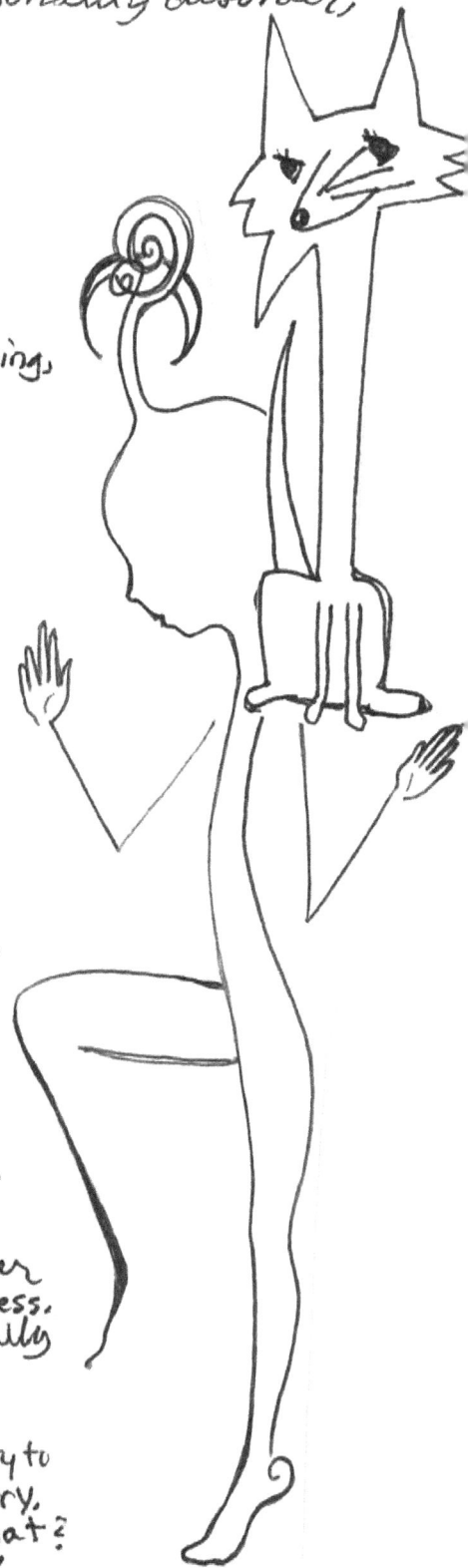

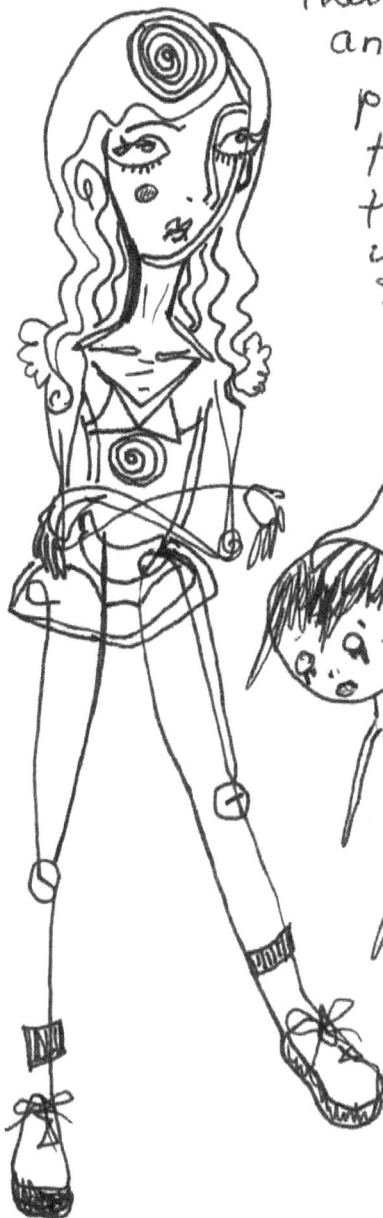

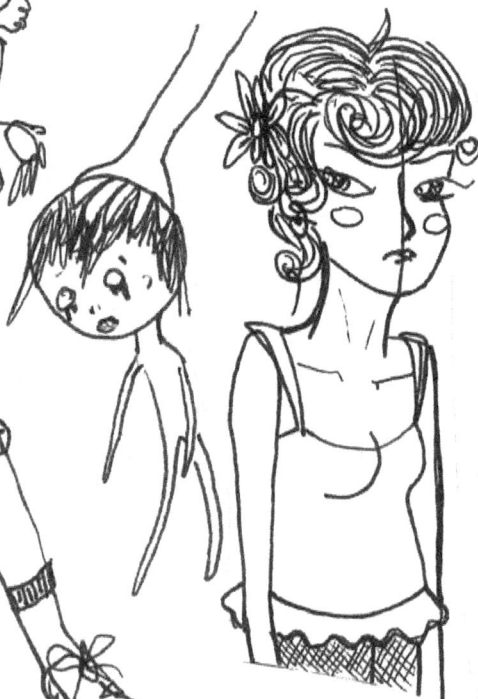

53113

6/1/09

No person has any right in the world to breach your personal boundaries by force, coercion, or threats. A person who rapes another person insults the victim by trying to apologize and come up with excuses. They cry, they get dramatic and suicidal. For example: "I'm fucked up because my cousin molested me." So fuckin what. That was then, this is NOW. HELLO, YOU JUST RAPED ME. Don't talk to me ever again, don't look at me, dont even think of me. One of my problems is that I am not confident and too nice. For example: me. My psycho ex nasty whatever was always always begging for me to have sex with him. Well, I woke up to him pathetically and unsuccesfully trying to have sex with me ... While I was fucking sleeping. He said he thought I was awake. BS. Then he turned into a crying blubbering drunk fool. Then he threatened suicide. Then he tried to kill us in the car.

He called me years later, drunk and suicidal. I talked his drunk-ass down, then he was feeling good enough to sing a shitty "rock" song he wrote. Dang social deviant rapists, yak. Don't be nice like me.

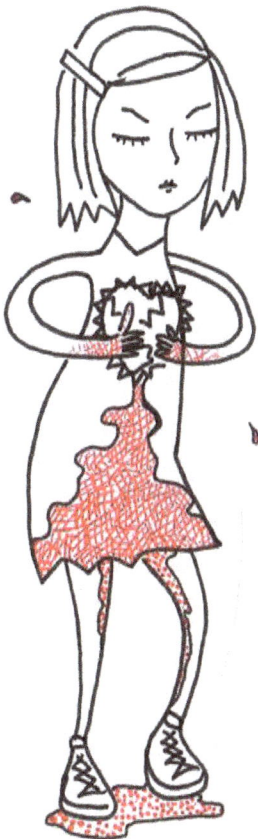

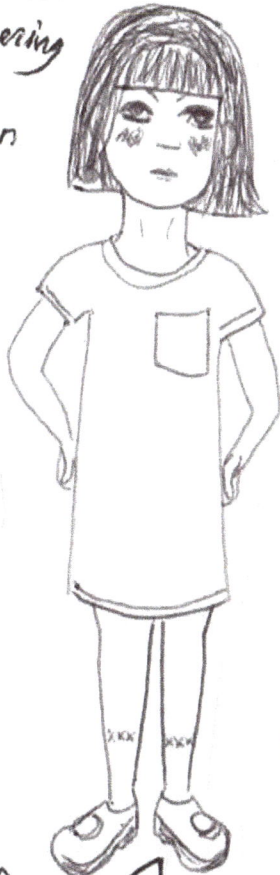

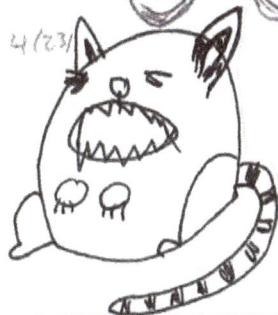

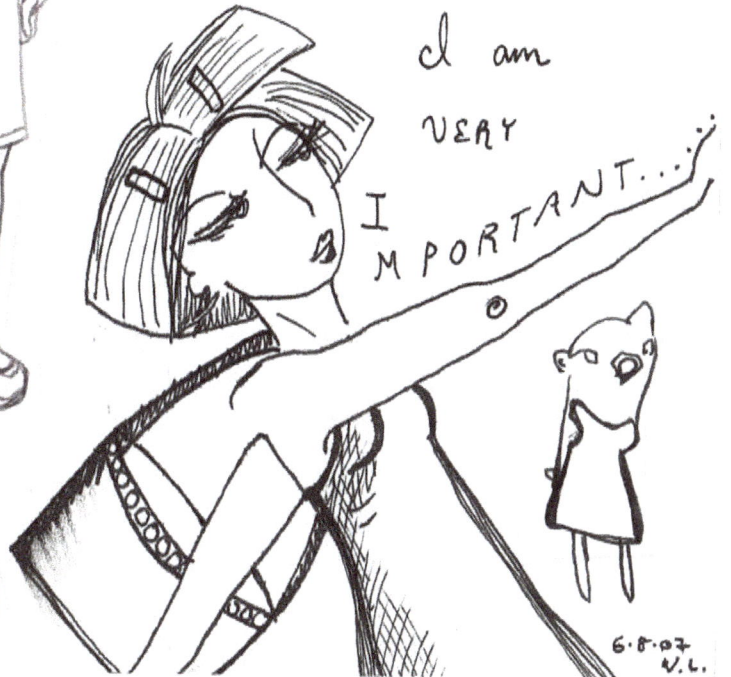

I am VERY IMPORTANT...

5·30·10 VCD

4/23/

6·8·07
V.L.

Sex does not get you anywhere and gets you nothing but trouble, Drama. A couple of sometimes-good-feeling-minutes can dramatically affect your life and potentially put a _dent_ in your life. Single mothers live in poverty and if they are not legally married, the dude can just take off anytime. HIV/AIDS and Hepatitus C kill people. Hep C destroys your liver and HIV/AIDS destroys your immune system. Sex is a choice that is in your face all the time in media. If you are gonna do what you're gonna do, at least use protection and don't drink alcohol and let someone rape you. You would not go outside in Disease Rain without a raincoat would you? Not me.

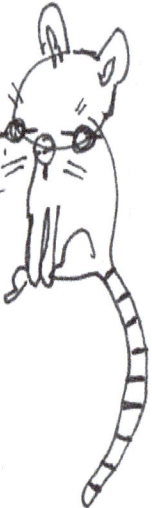

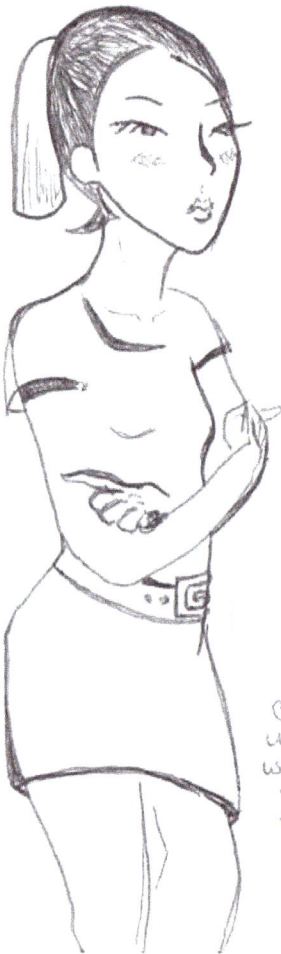

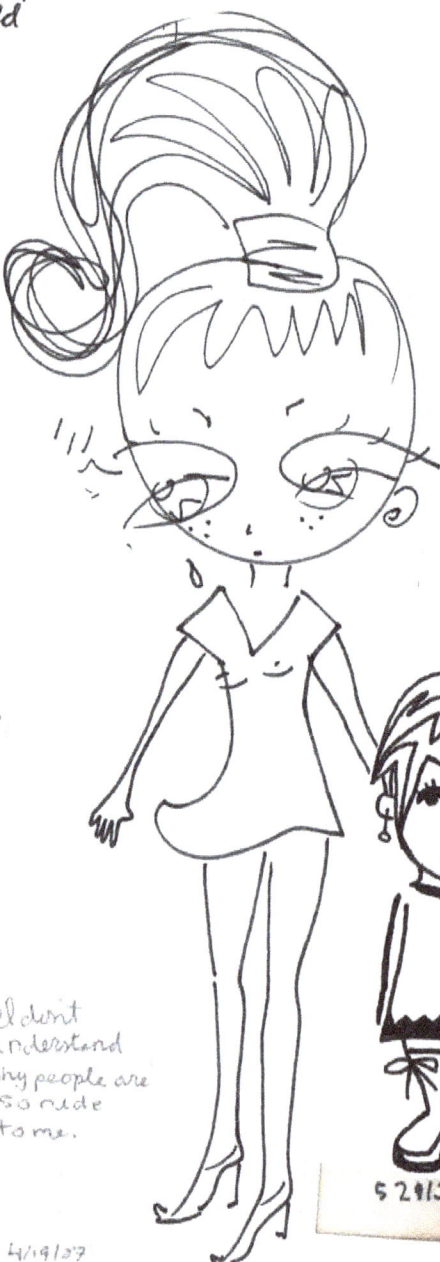

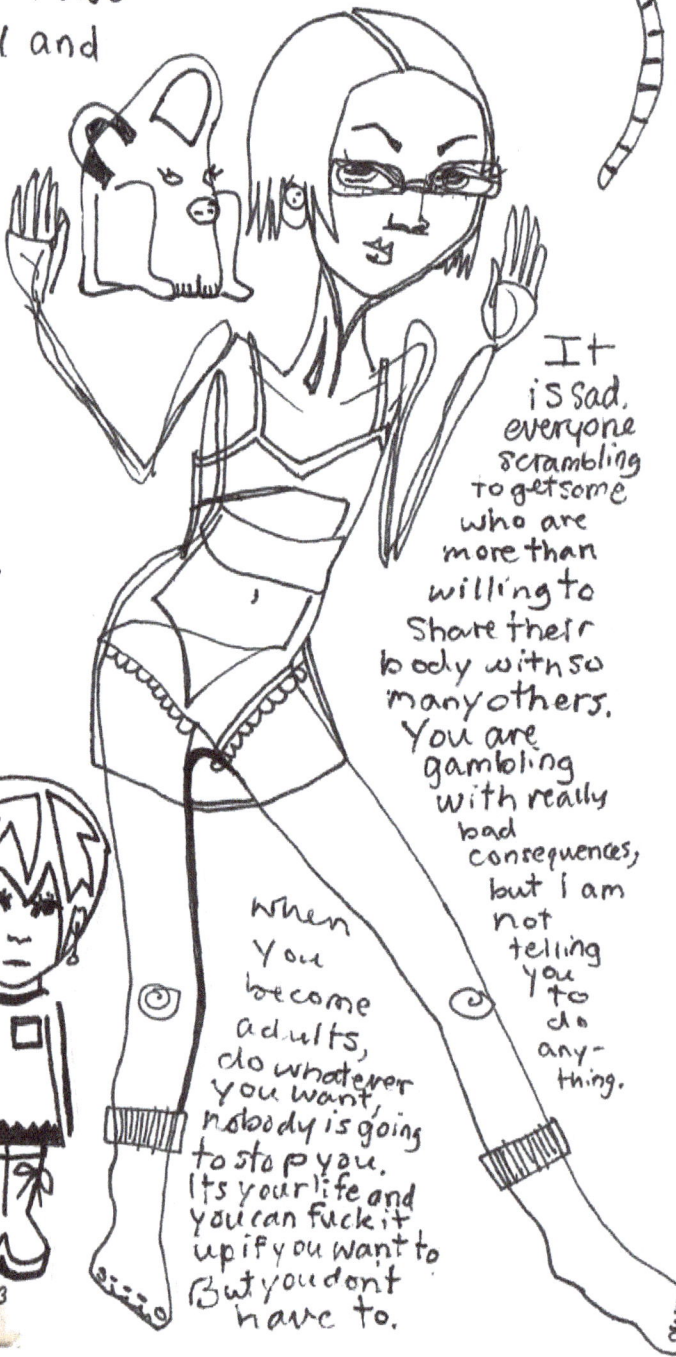

It is sad, everyone scrambling to get some who are more than willing to share their body with so many others. You are gambling with really bad consequences, but I am not telling you to do anything.

When you become adults, do whatever you want, nobody is going to stop you. Its your life and you can fuck it up if you want to. But you don't have to.

I don't understand why people are so rude to me.

5.2913

4/19/07

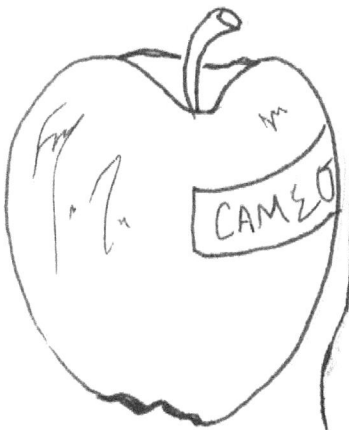

CAMEO

The Gateway

and

Addiction

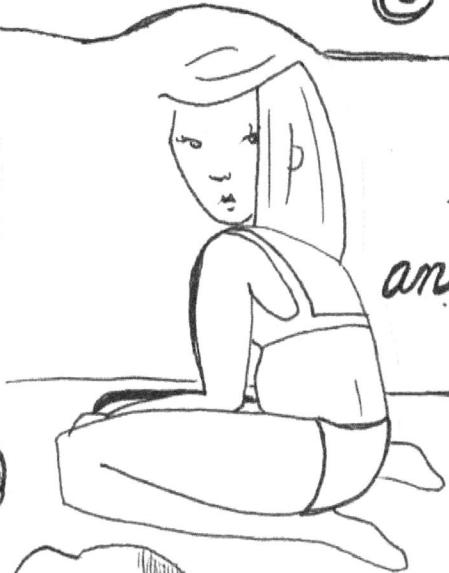

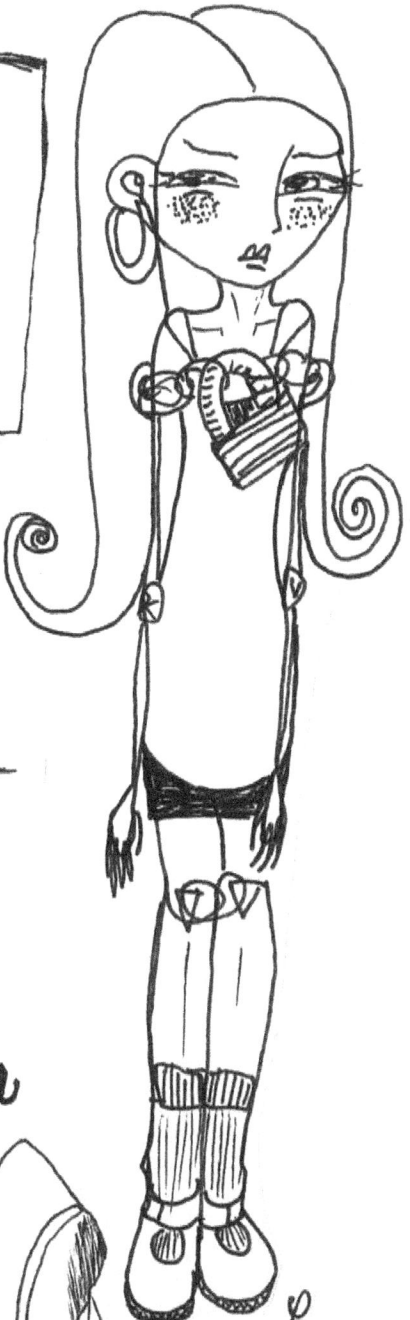

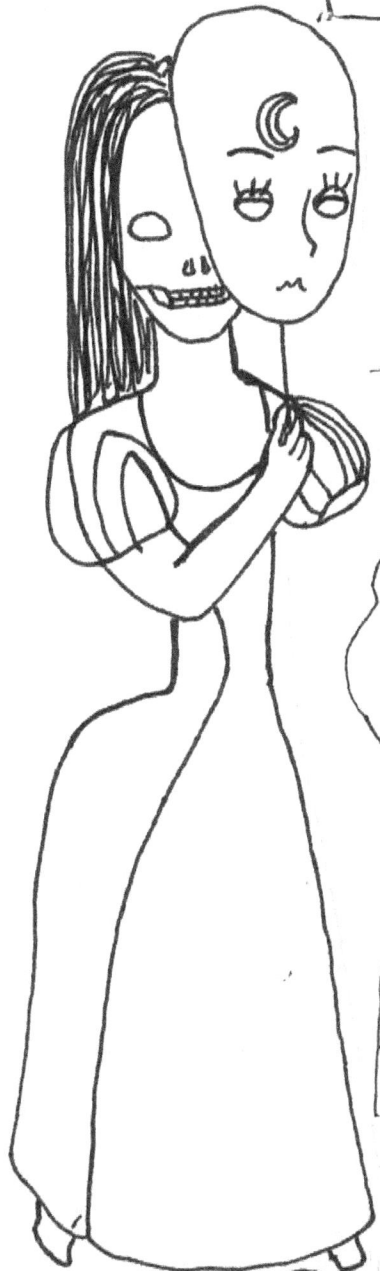

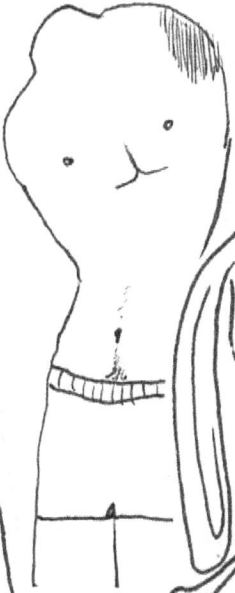

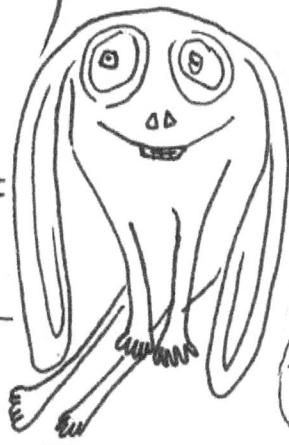

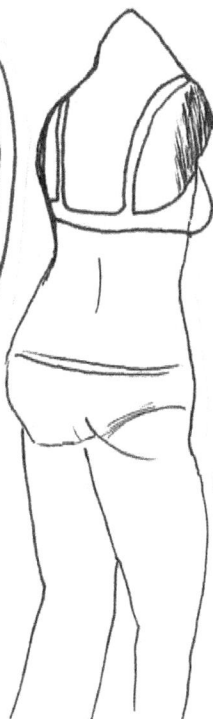

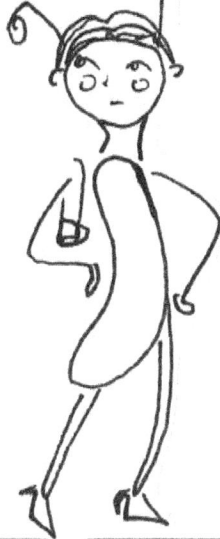

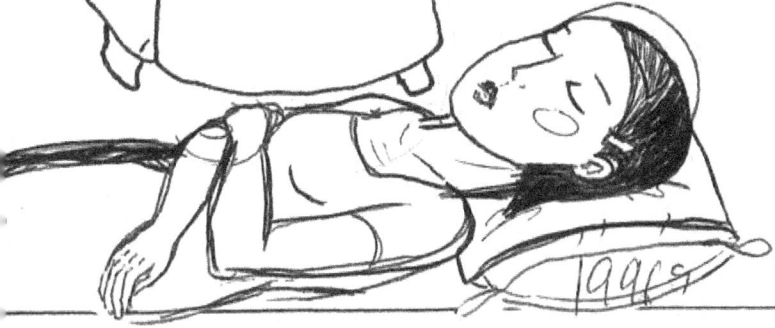

1996

Addiction is defined as a persons physical and psychological dependence on a substance that results in drug-seeking behavior despite the negative consequences in their life. The absence of an addictive substance results in Withdrawel. Opiate withdrawel can be so painful that death seems like a better option.

Alcohol and

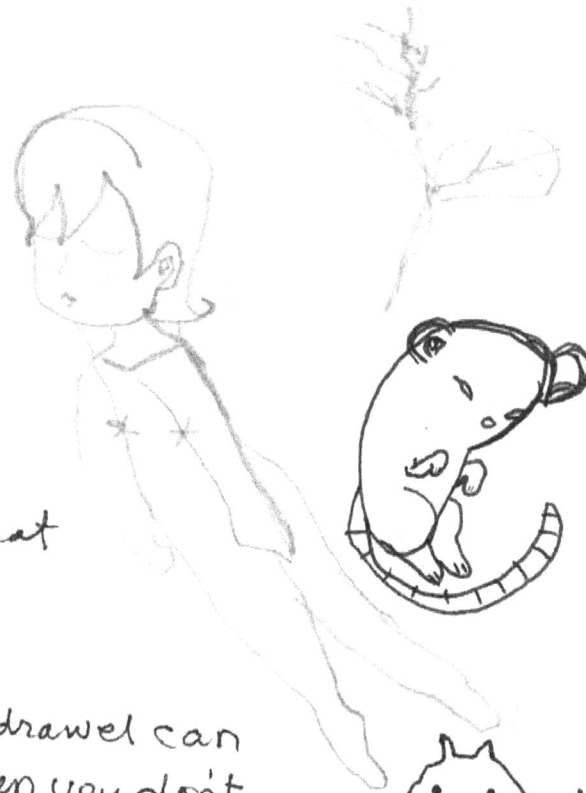

Benzodiazapine (anxiety meds) withdrawel can result in seizures and death. When you don't know your tolerance, or the purity of the drug, that can result in overdose. Your body either stresses itself to exhaustion or is depressed to the point where your heart heart stops, your lungs crap out or your brain dies. Addiction is a disease that is ruining the lives of our nations future, young adults.

Must Have
2.7.09 vc

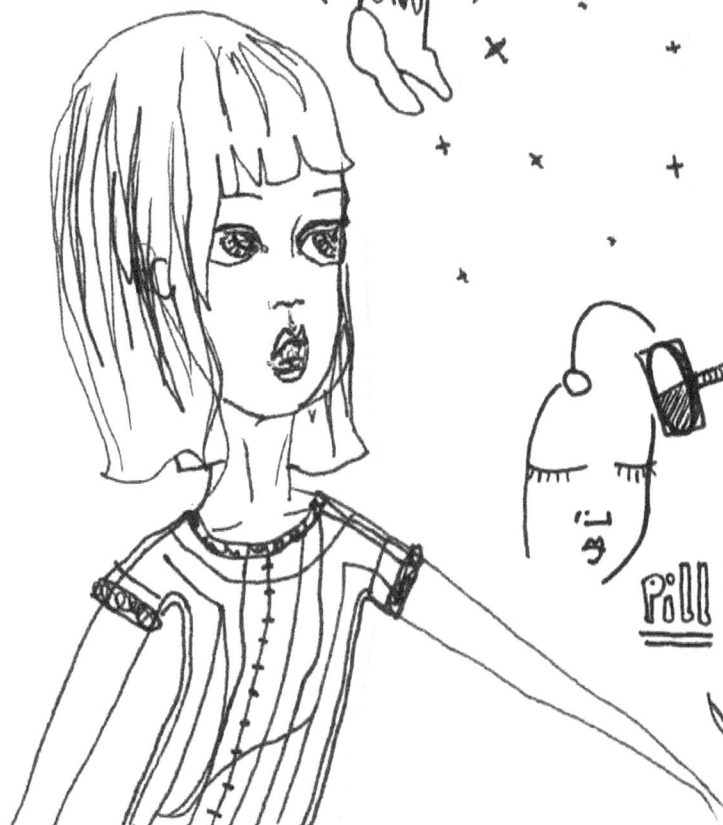

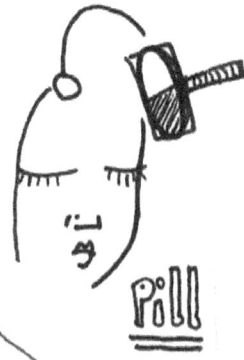

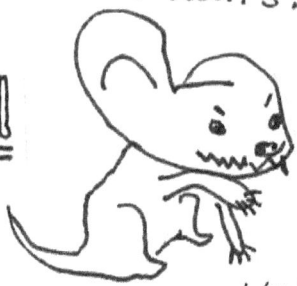

Pill

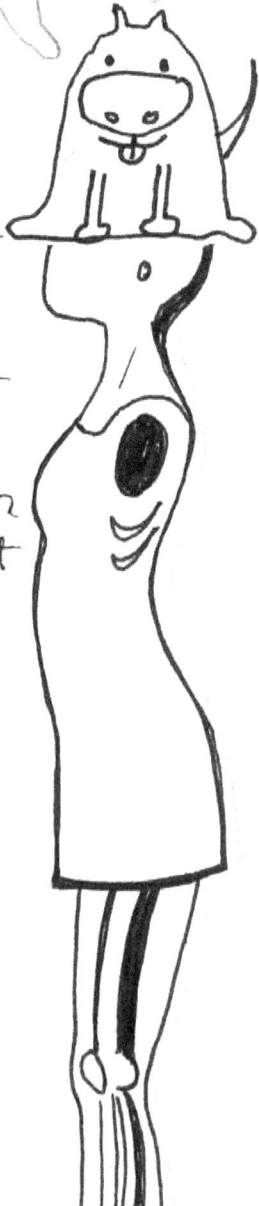

4/20/06 vc

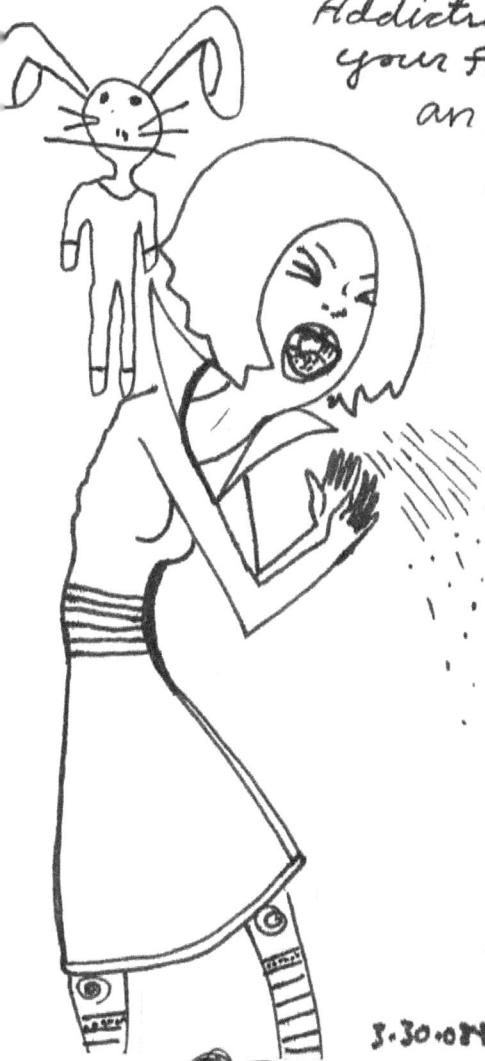

Addiction is genetic. If you have addiction in your family history, you are more likely to become an addict. It does not mean a person has to become one. I have addiction in my family history. I know this and I know myself. I become addicted very easily. In my brain, the reward system gives me a gold star. My brain just sucks up addictive substances and quickly builds tolerance.

☆ The reward systems' natural chemicals either die or slow to the point where your brain **cannot** generate them fast enough to make you feel normal-good. More please. Now damit. Now. When you flood your brain with feel-good that is instantaneous, your natural system is not needed, so your brain adapts to the outside introductions. The change is permanent. The severity of the damage depends on the length of

8.30.08 VL

time and the strength of the drug of choice. Early treatment increases the possibility that your brain may regenerate and repair some of the damage.

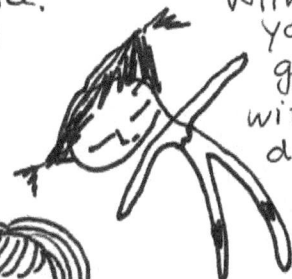

With addiction, you can't get motivated without your drug. Think coffee.

12.20.08 VL

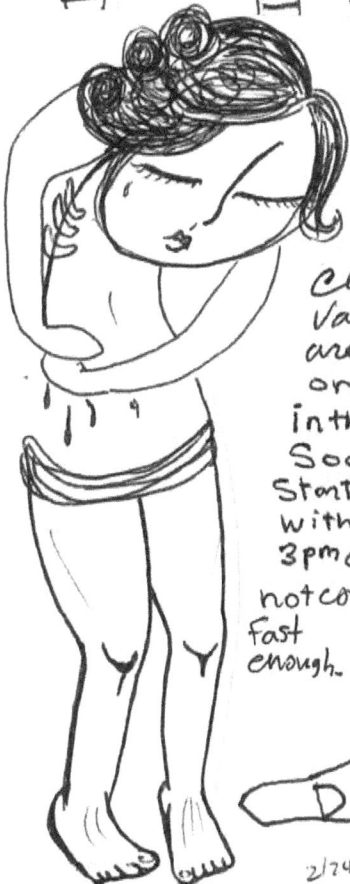

I almost got addicted to Valium, a benzodiazepine. They are used for mood swings. I was on a low low dose. I took 1 in the morning, 1 in the afternoon. Soon, I could not start my day without it, 3pm could not come fast enough.

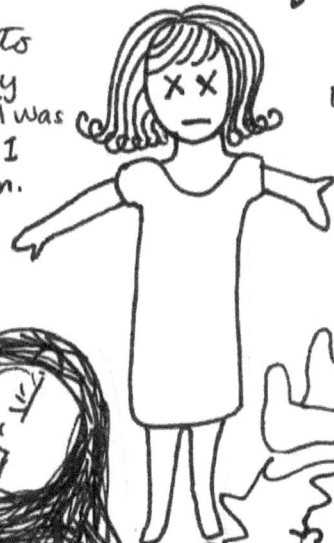

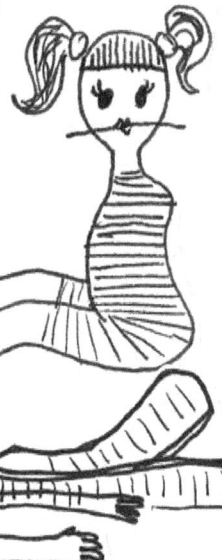

2/24/06 VL

The Gateway is made of two doors.
One side is alcohol,
the other is tobacco. They are legal,
cheap, and everywhere. They are also
EXTREMELY addictive. The less time that
you are addicted to anything, you can
potentially get out with minimal
damage. Once you are a legal age
to consume these product, drink
and smoke all you want. Our
government will love you. They
prey on addicts by taxing
the crap out what you
need. Everyone pays
taxes, addicts pay more
taxes by purchasing
alcohol and tobacco.
Marijuana has been
labeled as the gateway
drug and has been criminalized
for decades. In the 60's,
during the Vietnam war,
hippies were smokers, they
were also seen as social
deviants for
their
protest.

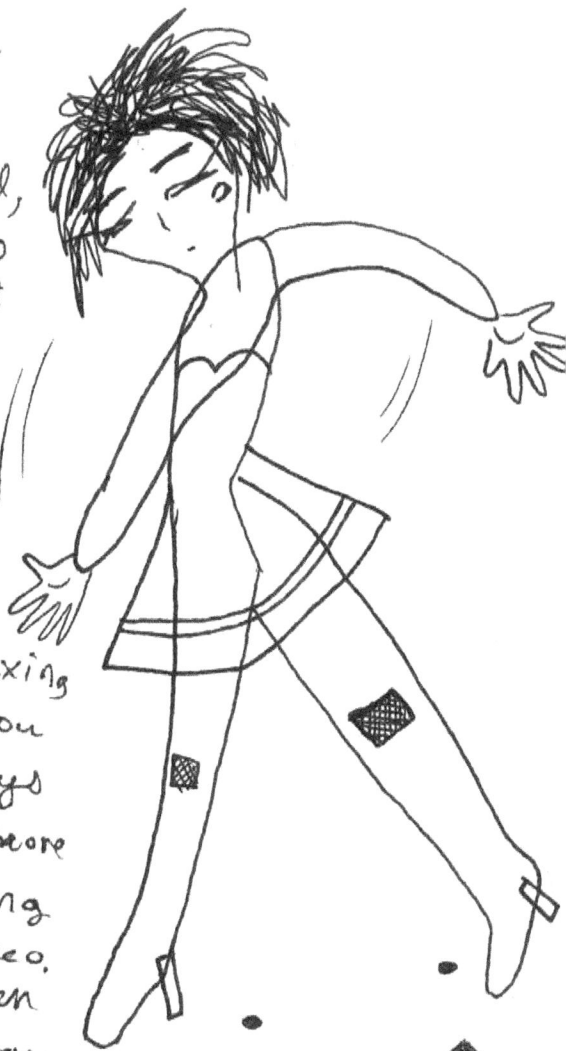

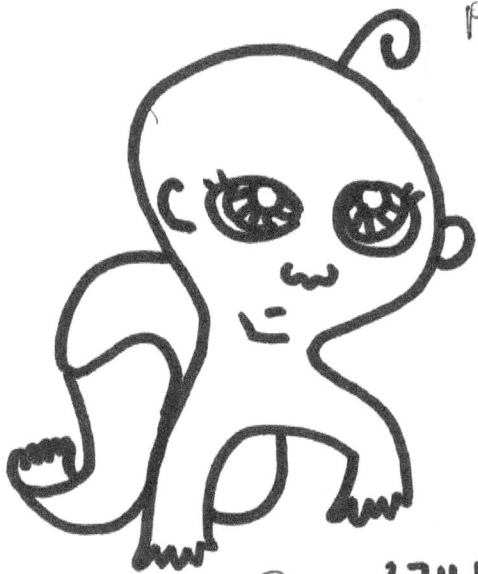

2711 VCD

Cannabis
users are
everywhere.
They are
not out
causing
mahem
like
drunks,
though.

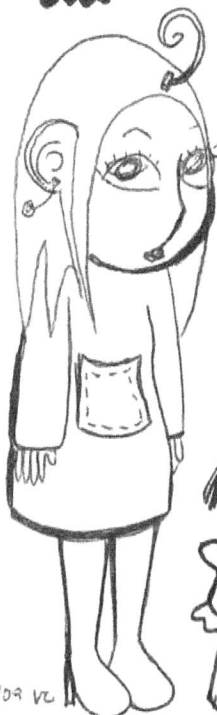

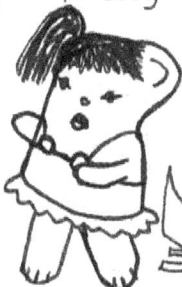

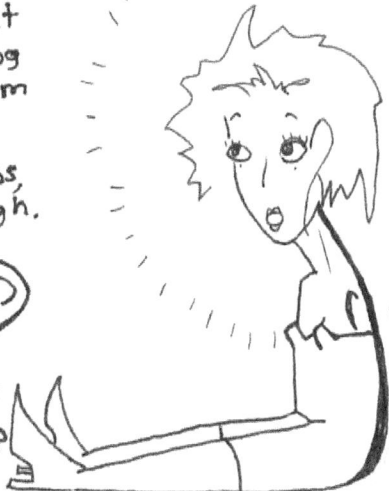

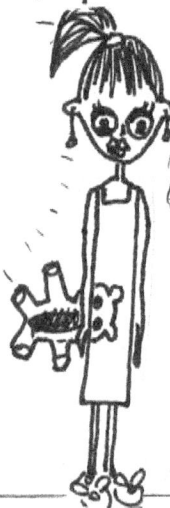

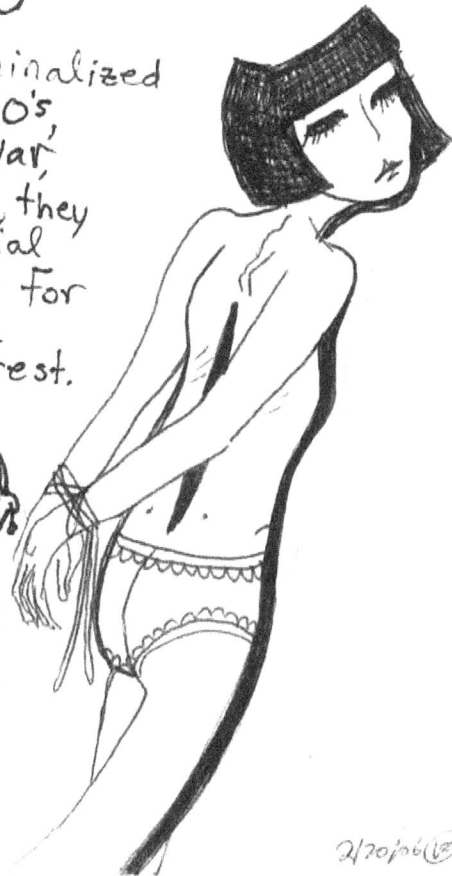

Commercialism and adults make an impression on young people. A lot of people use alcohol and tobacco. They all seem to be having FUN. For young adults, alcohol and tobacco are the first forbidden but legal substances. They are the shiny RED button that you are not supposed to press, no matter what. Both are very harmful to your health, but that doesn't matter if you learn at a young age that it is ok to do these things. If you took a second, you will notice all the alcohol and tobacco advertisements around you. They are EVERYWHERE, from magazines to commercials for BEER and Football.

skreeet?

aaaaargh!! run for your life!

Both introduce addiction to your growing brain. The younger you are, the easier it is for your growing body to integrate them INTO your normal brain chemistry.

So, where there are adults, there are often tobacco and alcohol around.

Alcohol is used to celebrate at holidays, functions, sports, parties and turning 21.

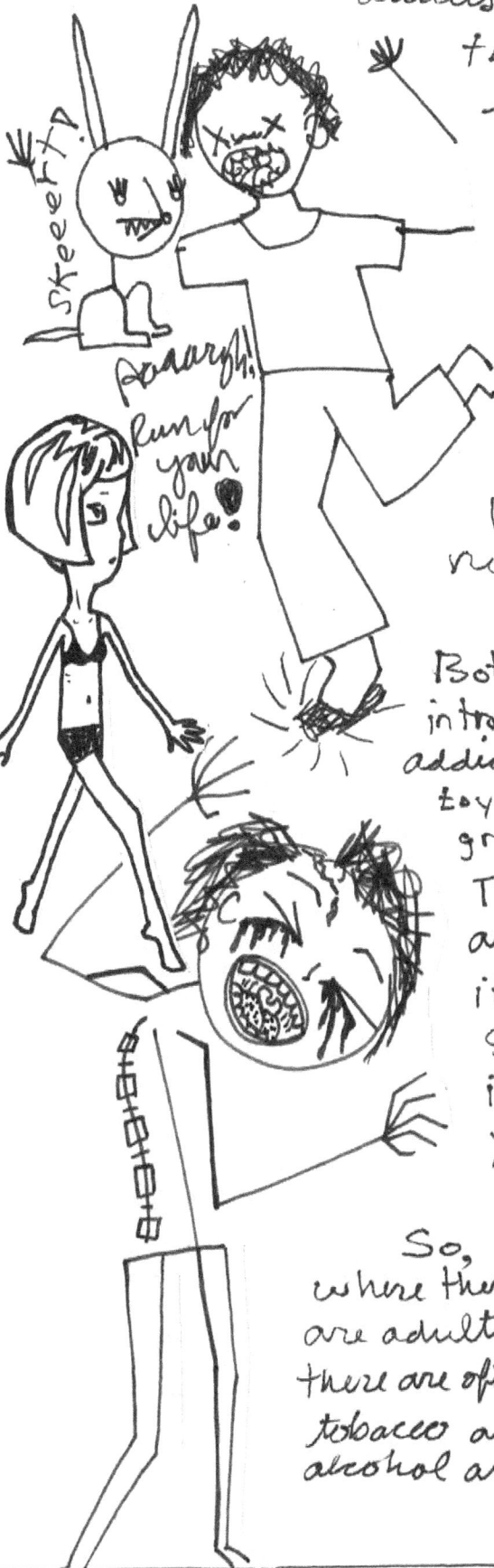

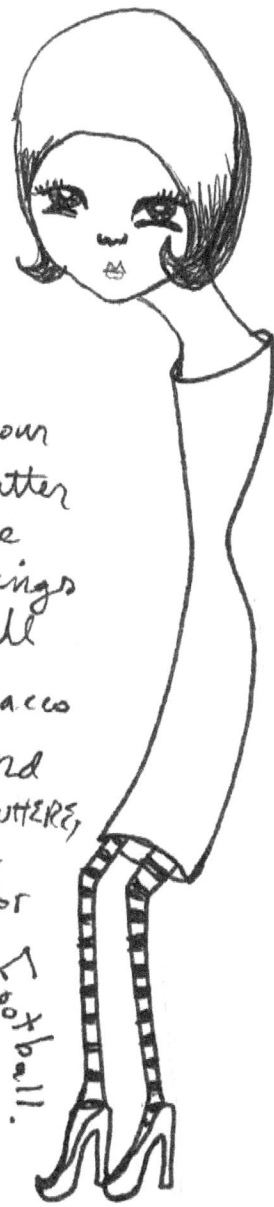

7502

I have been addicted to nicotine for over half my life. As a smoker, I know that the first one you try makes you feel pretty messed up and you will probably like it. You will probably "smoke when you drink", which can cause you to drink more often. Once you buy that first pack, you are IN. Alcohol and tobacco may as well be conjoined twins. Alcohol is a depressant, nicotine is a stimulant. Opposites attract.

The longer you stay in the alcohol scene, you are more likely to use other social, illicit drugs because your judgement is altered. Alcohol is used with every drug. It is cheap, so if people don't have drugs, they drink. Using alcohol with other drugs can easily result in death.

Sadly, I have known many young adults in my life who died this way.

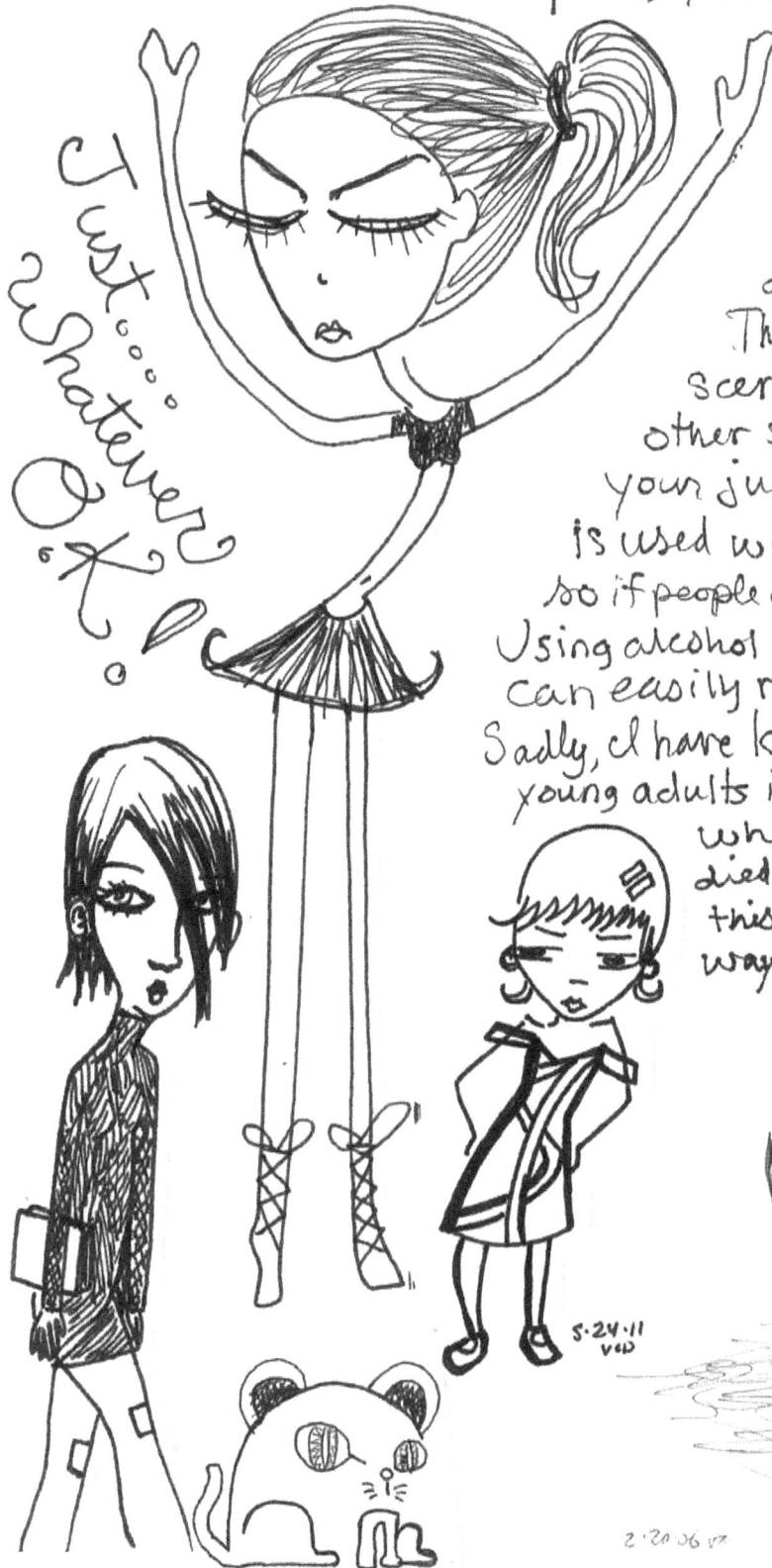

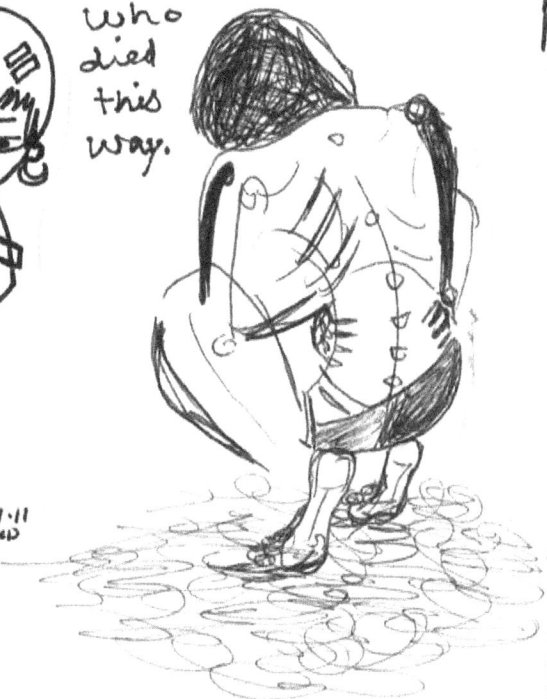

Just..... Whatever. OK?!

5.24.11
VCD

2.20.06

If you feel like crap all the time, just know that adding addiction makes you feel like more crap because your brain is constantly screaming at you to pleasure it.

When a person becomes an addict, they only slightly resemble themself.

Any bad or criminal behavior can be rationalized in order to get what they need. They will lie, scam, scheme, and break the law. You will hurt people you love, you will hurt innocent people. You will do ANYTHING

From rolling smokes from butts to prostitution and pawning moms jewelery and little brothers game console.

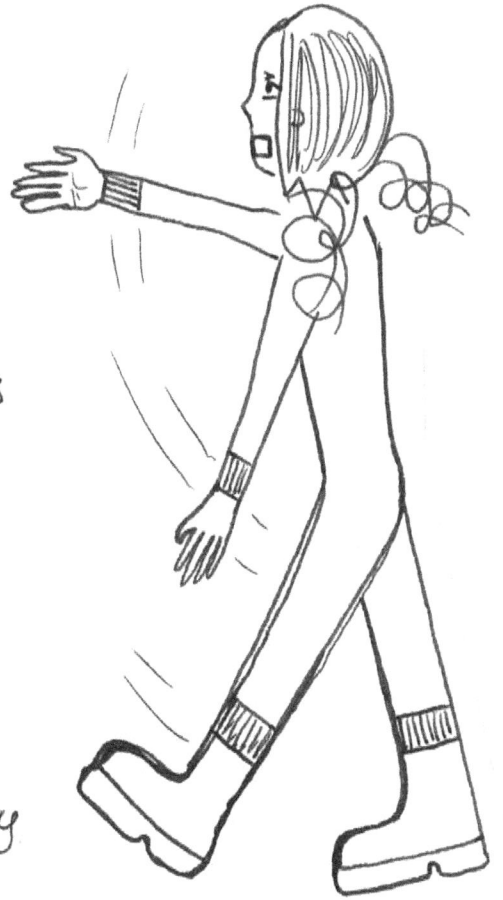

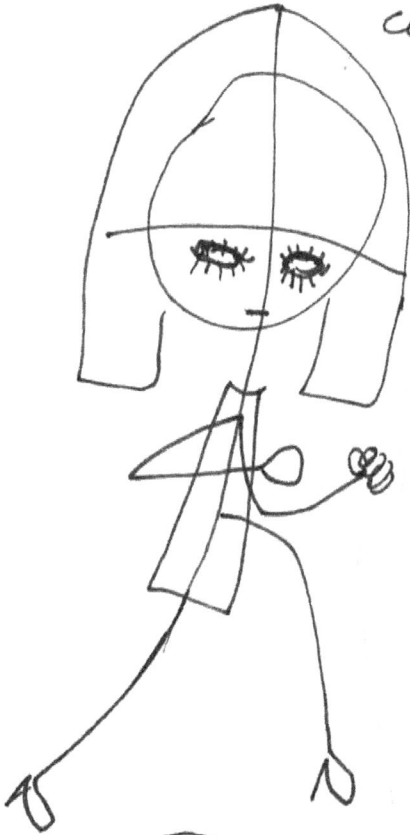

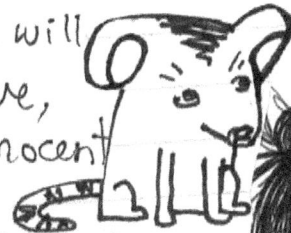

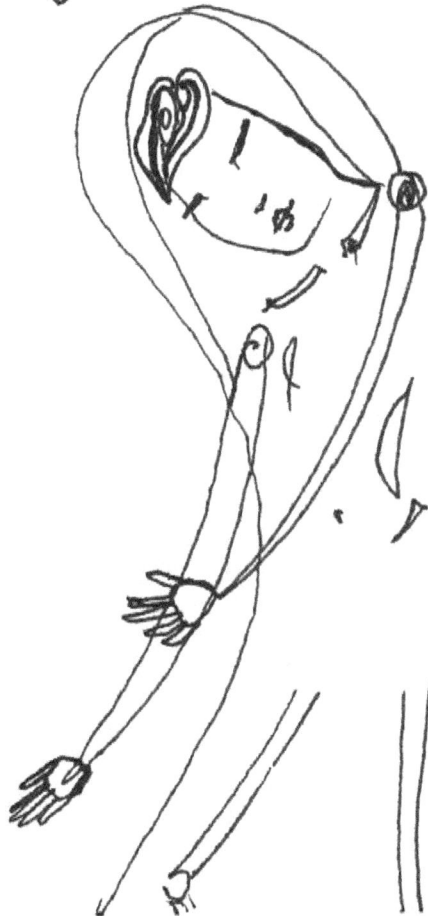

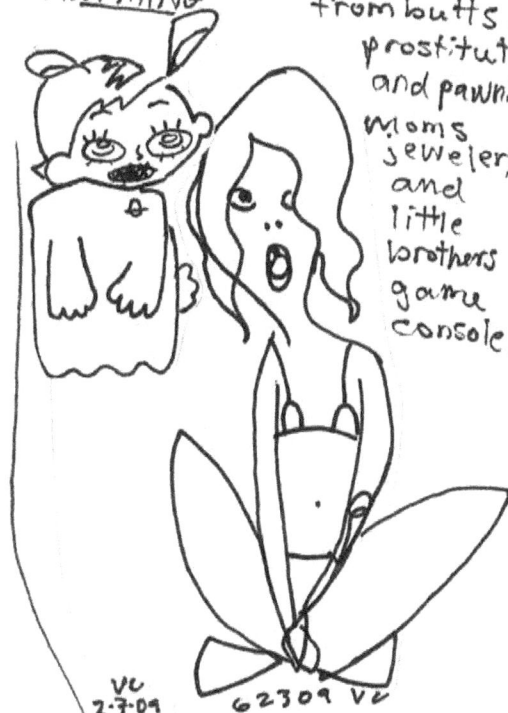

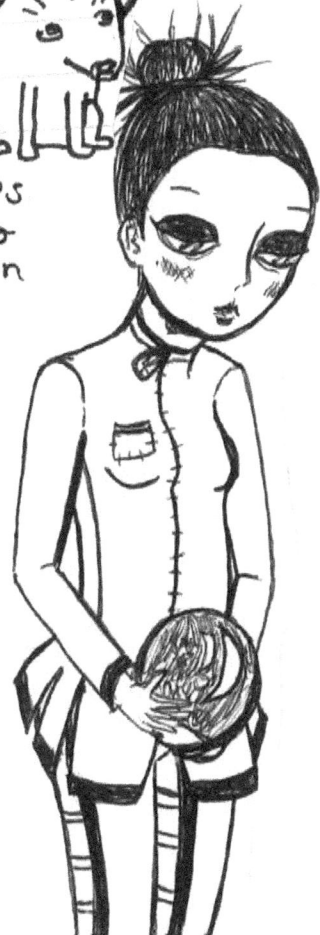

V.L
2-7-09

62309 V.L

2/20/25 V.L

Recovery for any addiction is not easy, fear can keep a person from getting treatment. The first issue you must deal with is guilt from your past. You must rebuild your life and relationships. Nobody wants to get hurt and trust is extremely hard to earn back once you have lost it. You have probably forgotten what it feels like to be loved because you feel like a rotten, worthless piece of garbage. You have to abandon your drug-using friends, places, and paraphanalia. You have to change your behaviors and be able to recognise your "triggers". You need to learn new ways to cope with normal emotions and learn to have fun again, naturally. Some people you hurt may never forgive you or have already made up their mind about you. This, you have to learn to accept. It is easy to Royally screw up again and again, but not realize it when you are an addict.

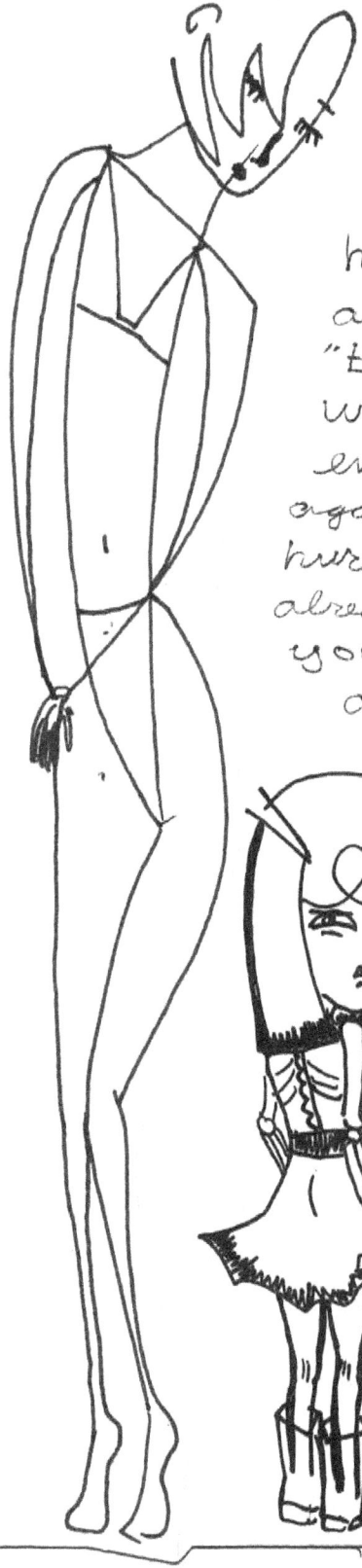

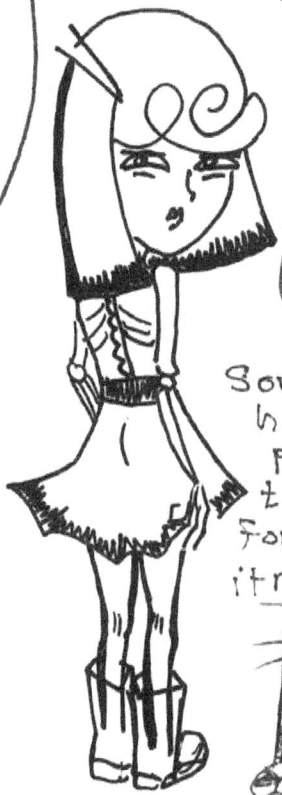

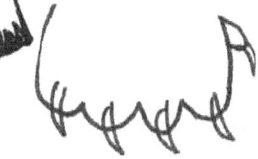

Sometimes, you have to leave people behind to move forward and it really hurts.

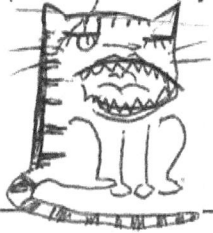

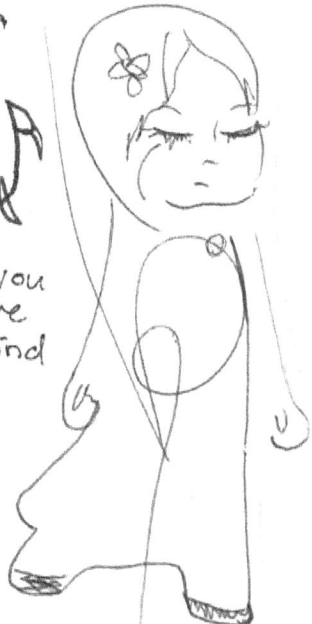

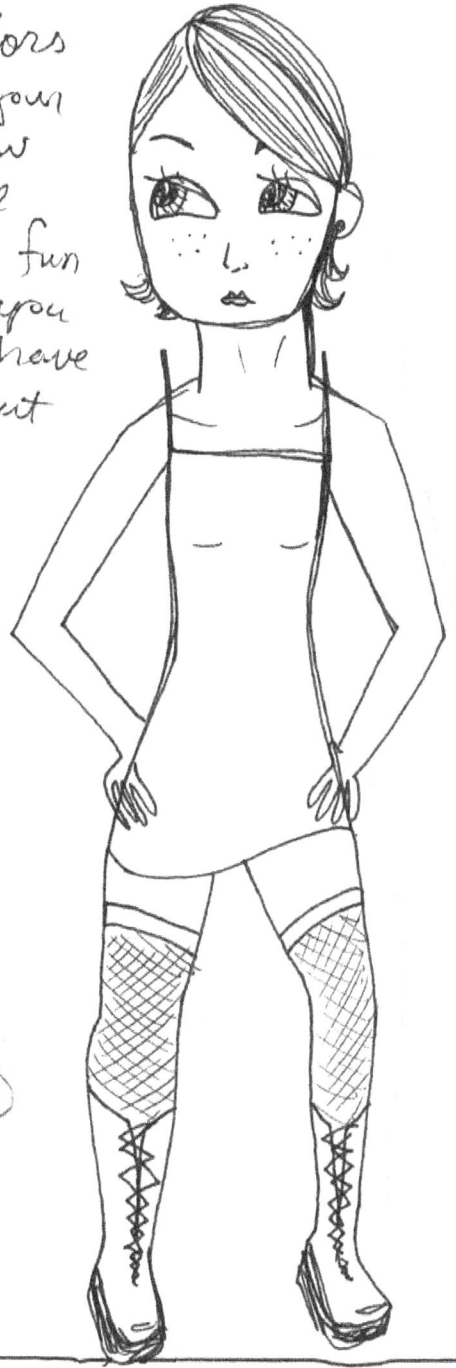

As a person in recovery, I know that people you know are either for you or against you. Some may understand what you may be going through, others can't even imagine it. Recovery requires a lot of support or it can be easy to have a relapse. When you have a relapse, people will gossip and see relapse as a shameful dirty word. They often don't understand

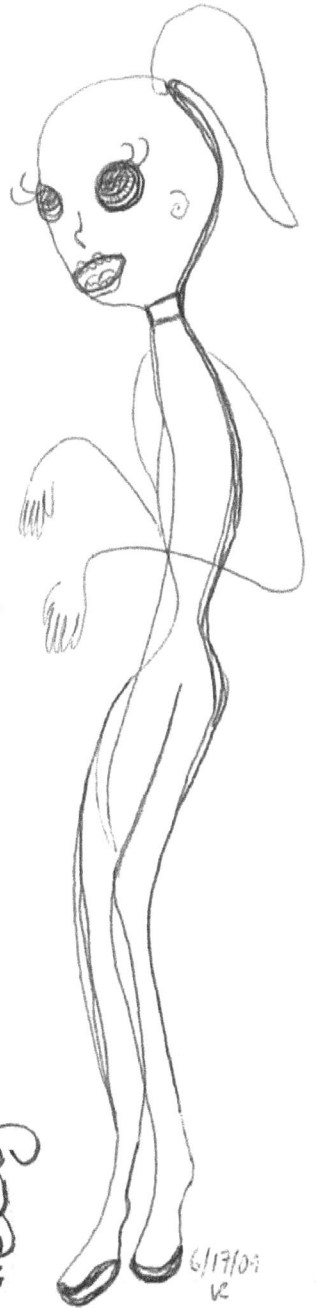

that addiction is a chronic brain disease. RELAPSE HAPPENS. i have quit smoking many times. When I start again after years of being quit, that is a relapse. Once I smoke 1, I am BACK IN. I know its a bad habit and that it can kill me, but I am an addict.

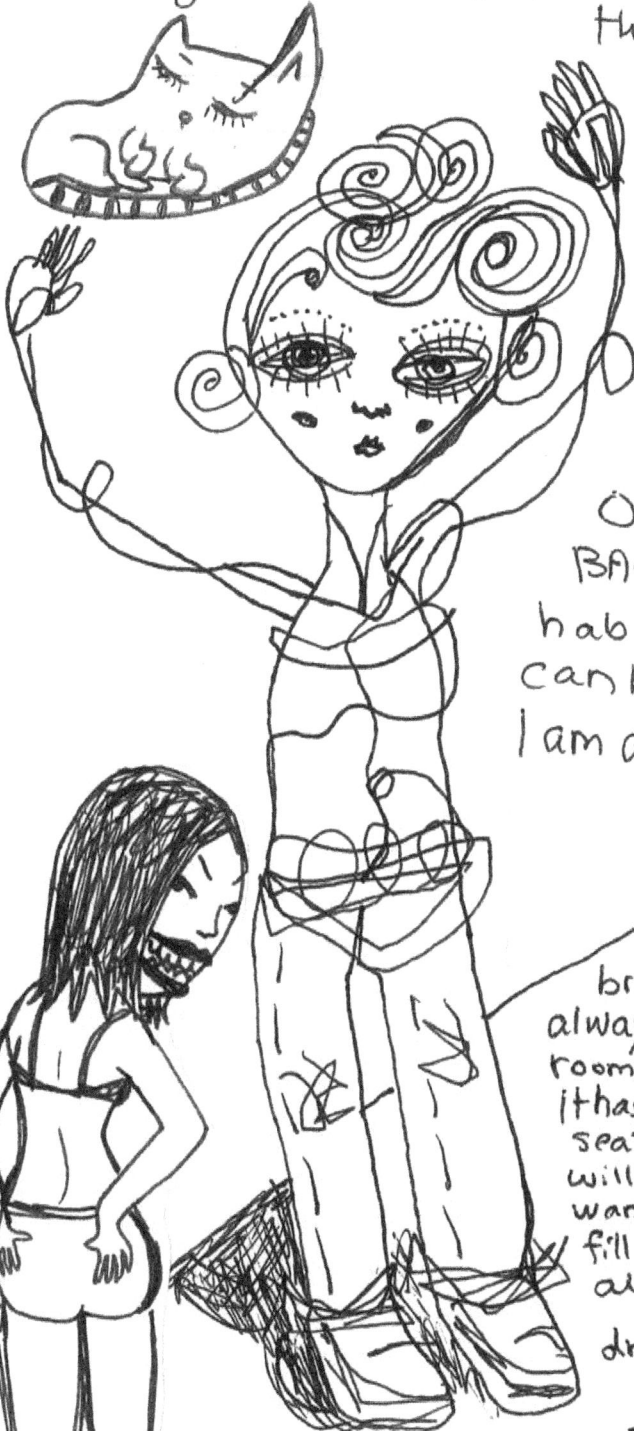

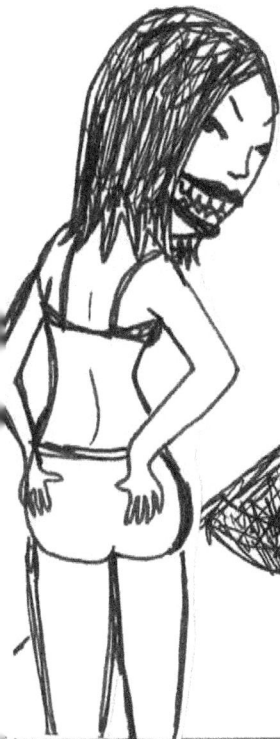

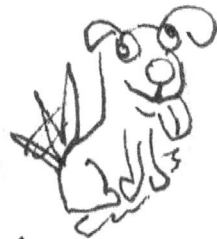

Your brain will always have room for an ex. it has a special seat that it will always want you to fill it with alcohol or drugs.

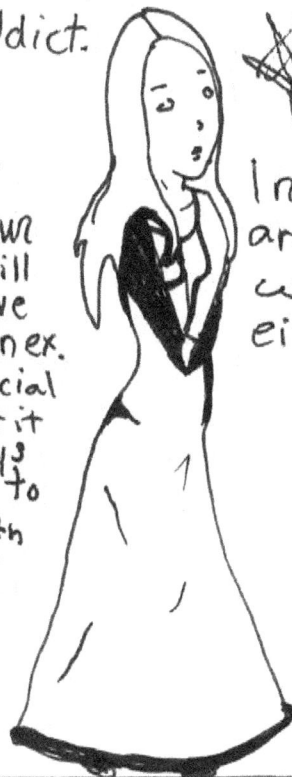

In recovery, there are no "once-in-a-whiles." You are either IN or OUT.

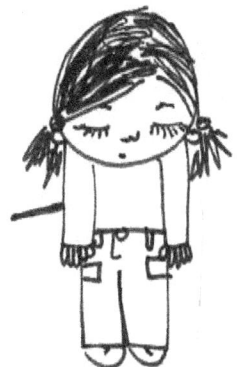

I'm Sorry.

6/17/09
vr

B 413

Imaginary scenario of what addiction is like:
The pond is the drug, the gatekeeper is your dealer.

Imagine a magical pond that you hear people talk about. They say it takes your problems away and makes everything painless. You find someone to take you there, the gatekeeper lets you in FREE the first time. What a great guy. There are a lot of people around and you are nervous, but you take a drink of the pond water anyway. It tastes like shit, but the next minute you feel painless, powerful, and invincible. You look in and see all of your dreams coming true, you have pond friends and they Love you. When it is over, you feel life drained out of you and you leave, stay, or come back. The price of pond time is money, money, money, aging your body and mind, and demolishing a part of your brain. You don't care. You will do anything for pond time, where you feel loved and good.

The dreams in the pond become your REALITY. Being away from the pond REALLY sucks.

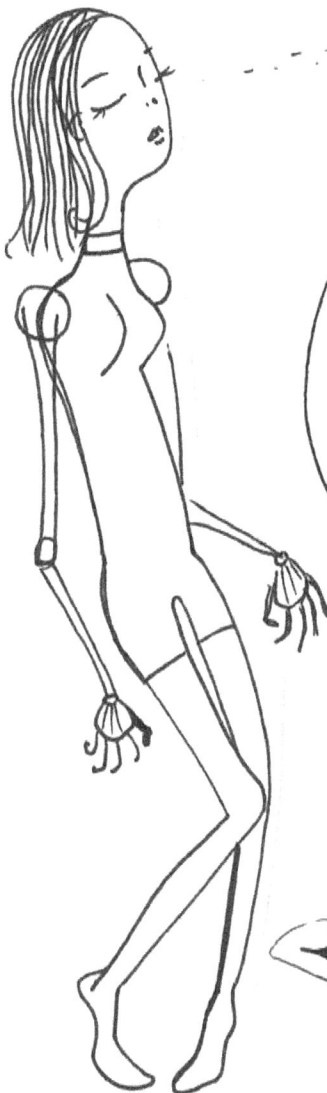

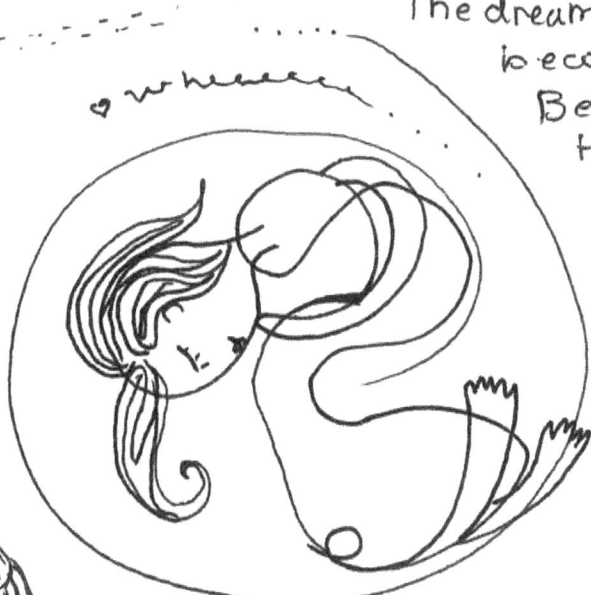

whheeeee

Your reflection in the pond doesn't look like what or who you remember. That doesn't matter as long as you can drink the magic.

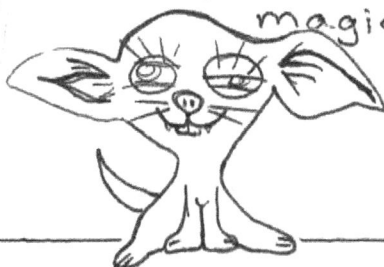

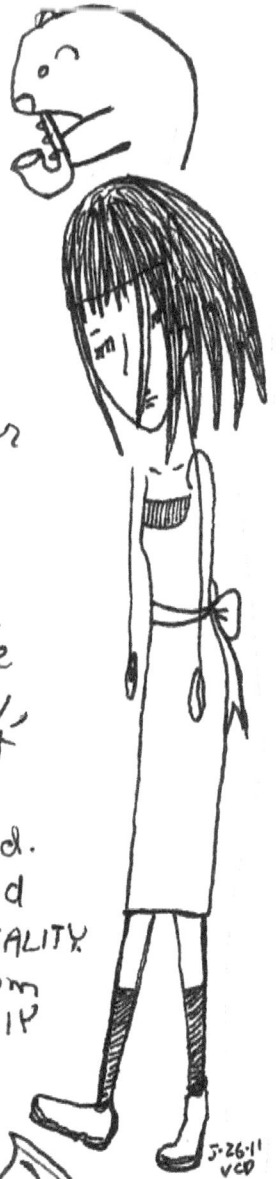

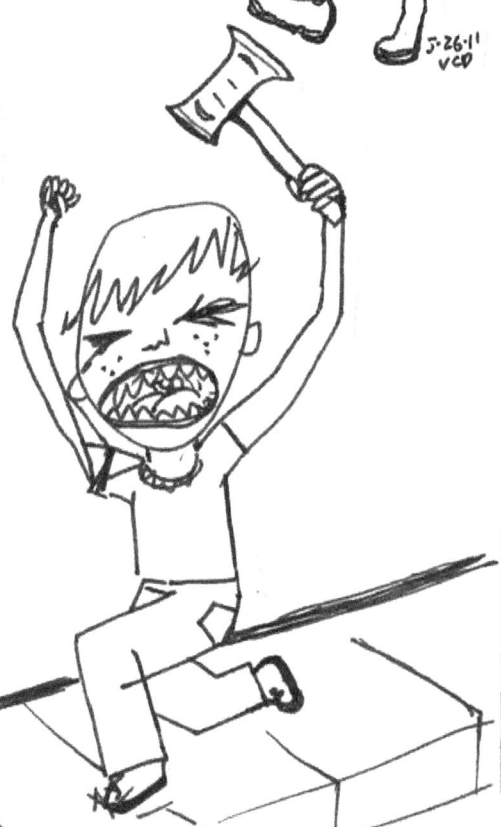

J-26-11
VCD

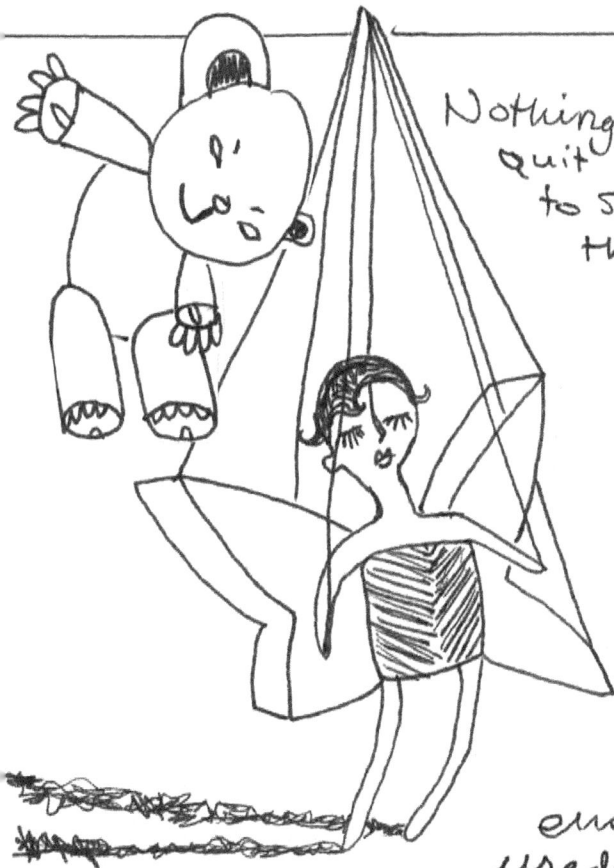

Nothing else matters to you so you quit your job or get fired, you tell your family to screw themselves. You tell yourself that you can find ways to get money. Those ideas eventually run out, all of your bridges are burnt. You give up sleeping, eating, bathing, and safety. Money runs out. You have no material posessions. You appeal to the gatekeeper, in pain. He does not care about you. If you got no money, valuables, or sex, Get The Fuck Outta Here. You turn to prostitution. You are his sexual slave. When he's had enough of you or you get too old and used-up, there is a new young kid who Just Got IN who he has his eye on.

You stand outside the gate, wishing you would die. You can work hard all day, feeling like shit and eventually end up in prison, killing yourself, or dying.
Or, you can seek help getting back to reality.

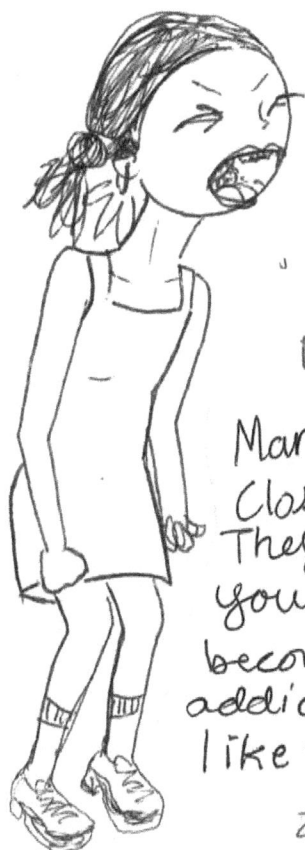

Waah!

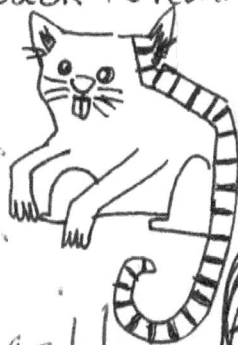

Many people are Closet Addicts. They never tell you not to become an addict like them.

2/15/06

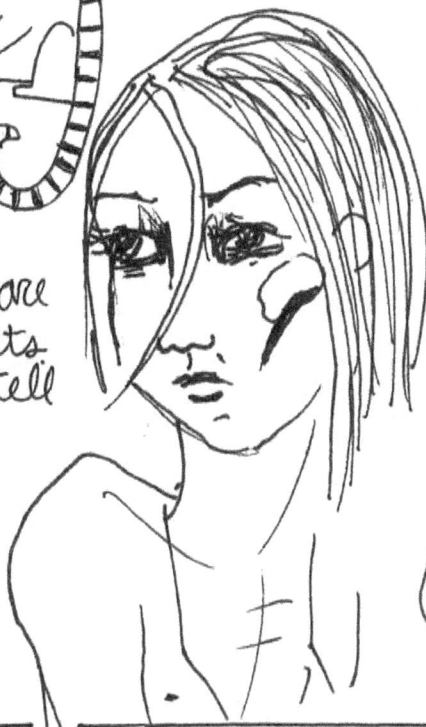

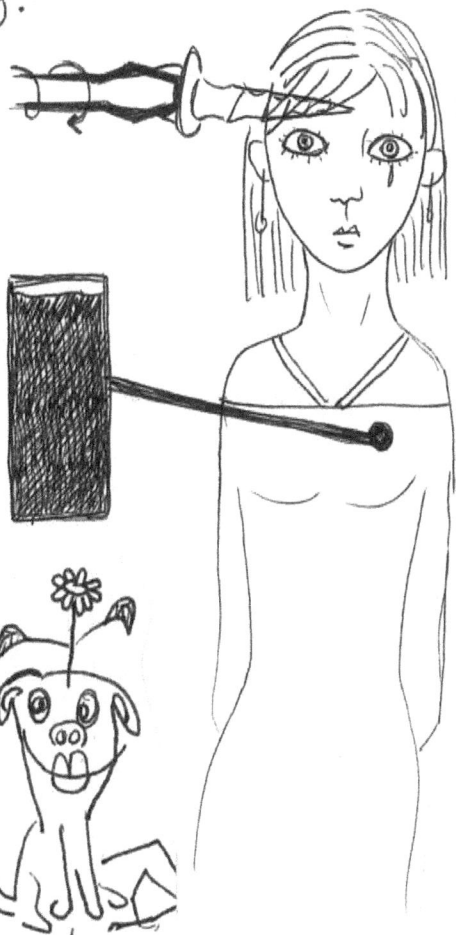

Life is not easy and can be really unfair, but it can be fulfilling. You can have your whole future planned out, but life can bring anyone down. What affects you, also affects those around you, wether you plan to or not. The "easy" way is to not get involved or try things that may cause addiction, but it is easier said than done.

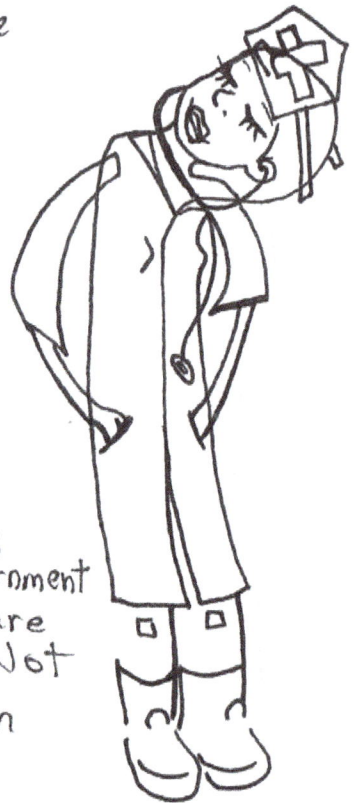

Doc Derr

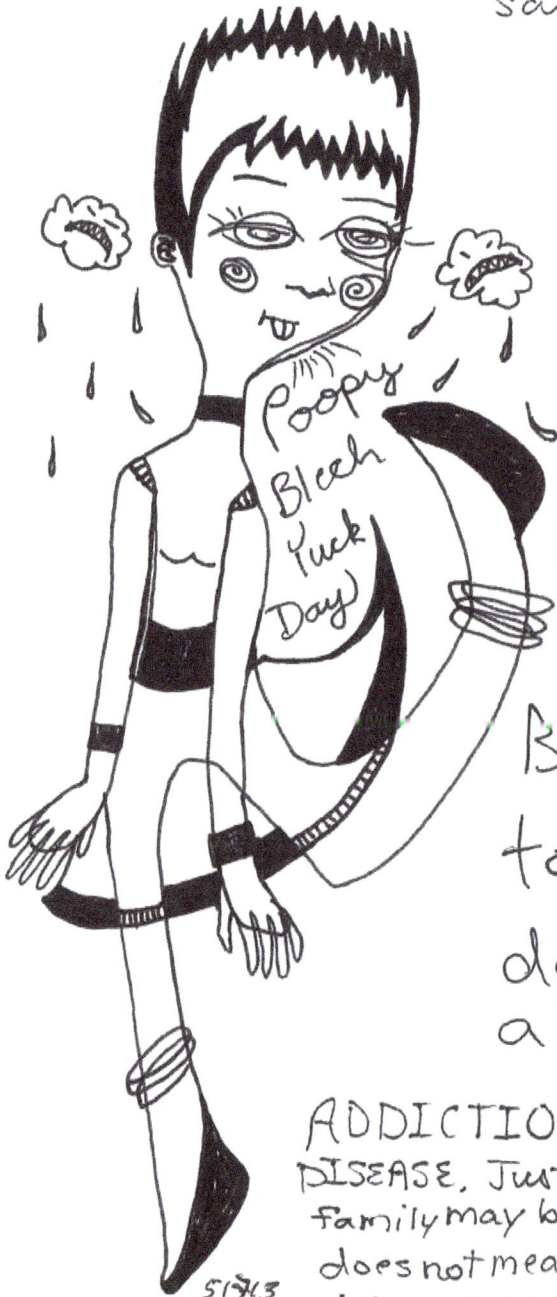

Poopy
Bleeh
(uck
Day)

Just say no is BS and government efforts are a joke. Not one person plans to be an addict when they grow up. Most get IN by messing around.

10·24·09

5/10/08

Bad things happen to good people who don't deserve it all the time.

ADDICTION IS A PREVENTABLE DISEASE. Just because your whole family may be alcoholic drunks, does not mean you must become one. It is your choice to gamble with.

5/9/13

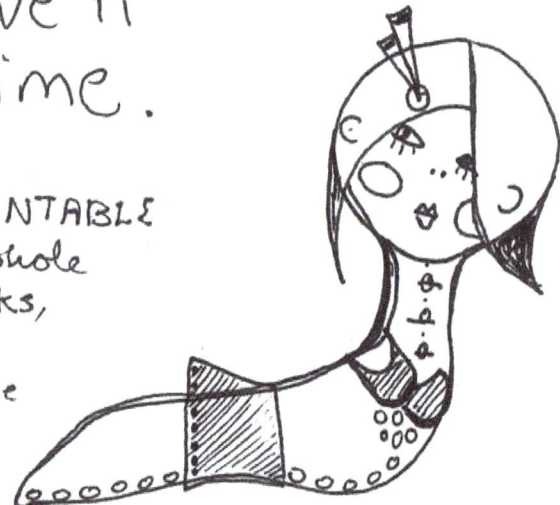

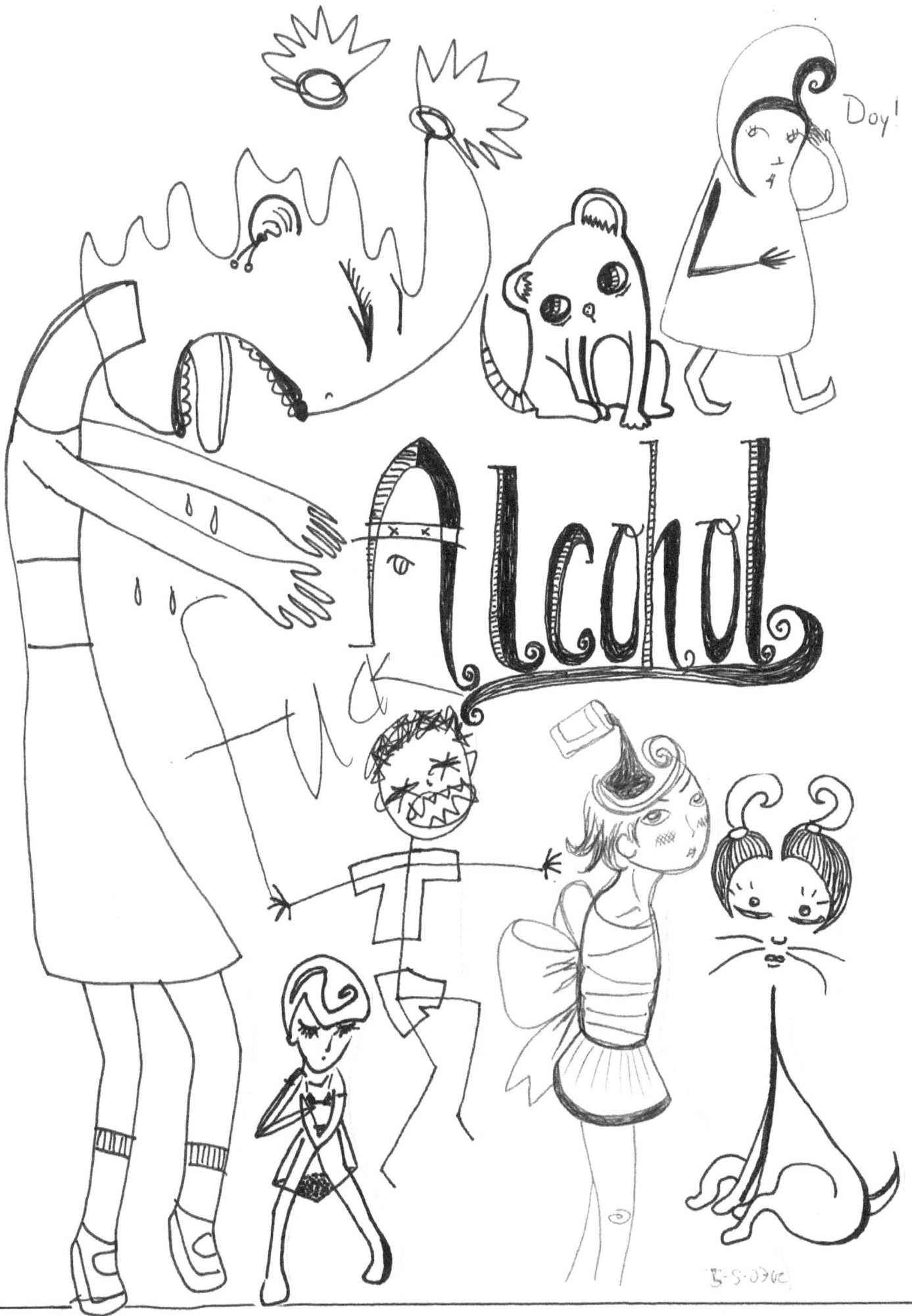

Alcohol

Doy!

The more appropriate warning label on alcohol products should be this:

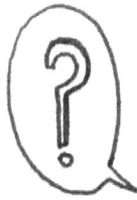

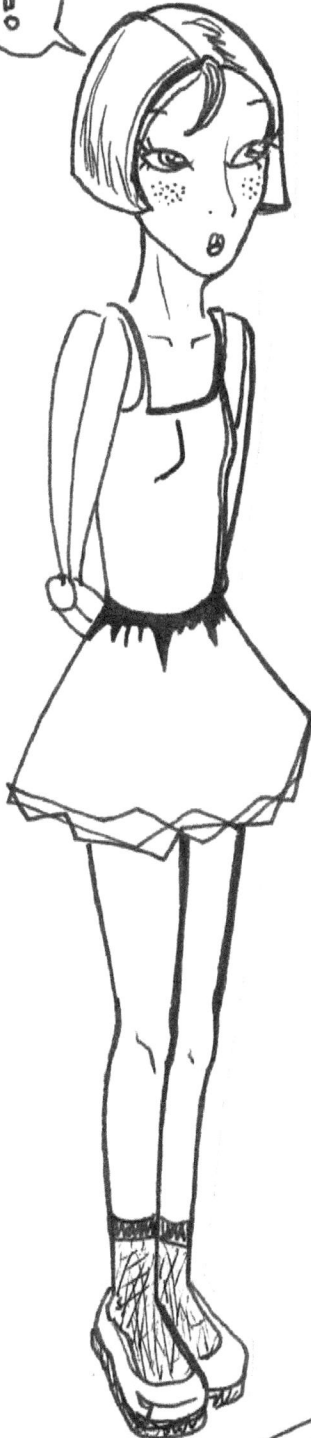

Warning Deliberate consumption of this product may cause serious harm to your health. Keep away from children and pets. Accidental ingestion can result in alcohol poisoning, dehydration, and death. Side effects possible. Side effects include, but are not limited to:

- Slurred speech
- Dizziness
- Loss of coordination
- Defattening of skin
- Premature aging
- Vasodialation (flushing)
- Rosacia (red nose)
- Personal neglect
- Impaired judgement
- Addiction (chronic brain disease)
- Overdose (poisoning)
- Vomiting
- Dry hearing
- Diarrhea
- Dehydration
- Gum/peridontal disease

- Cancer
- Heart disease
- Osteoporosis (Bone density loss)
- Infertility
- Incontinence
- Cirrohsis
- Hydrocephaly ("wet brain")
- Brain mass loss (shrinking brain)
- Brain density loss (spongy brain)
- Demensia
- Irrational behavior
- Exaggerated emotions

- Contraction of STI
- Spontaneous or assisted abortion.
- Birth Defects
- Fetal Alcohol Syndrome
- Intellectual disability
- Suicide
- Homicide
- Rape
- Crime
- Unintended pregnancy
- Child abuse
- Child neglect
- Child molestation/rape
- Incest
- Domestic violence
- Fatal/non-fatal accidents
- Property damage

- Promiscuity (slutty)
- Prostitution (whore)
- Divorce
- Poverty
- Bankruptcy
- Risk-taking
- Delusions of grandeur
- Lawsuits
- Law conviction and imprisonment
- Humiliation
- Depression
- Seizures
- Gossip
- Job loss
- Self-suffocation (choking on vomit)
- Brain damage
- Coma
- Death

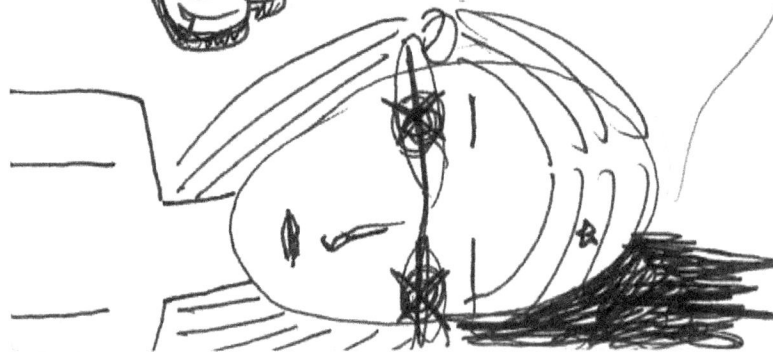

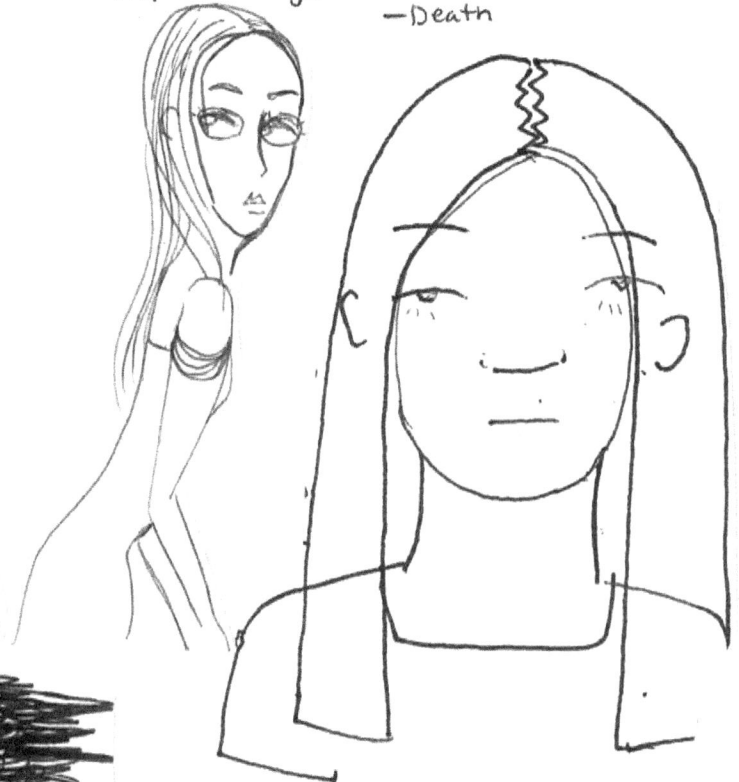

Alcohol. The technical name is ethanol, or ethyl alcohol. This is the same active ingredient in hand sanitizer. It has disinfectant qualities as well as flammability. Ethanol is what makes drag racers able to shoot flames, and it is also used for molton cocktails. Alcohol is a toxin. When a person ingests it, they become INT_OXIC_ated. It is one of the few freedoms people fought for, Prohibition Repeal. Alcohol is used to celebrate everything. Alcohol is portrayed as fun and sexy, relaxing and soothing: Pain free and Careless in a Bottle.

We grow up with alcohol advertisements and alcohol consumption. It also causes social blight, brain disease (addiction), and health problems. You might realize when you are older that the silly aunt or uncle was just drunk all the time.

The fancy explanation of what alcohol is that it is the product of fermentation of sugar starches and yeast.

In english: Alcohol is the byproduct, or waste, of yeast, whose diet is the sugar and starches from decomposing, or rotting produce.

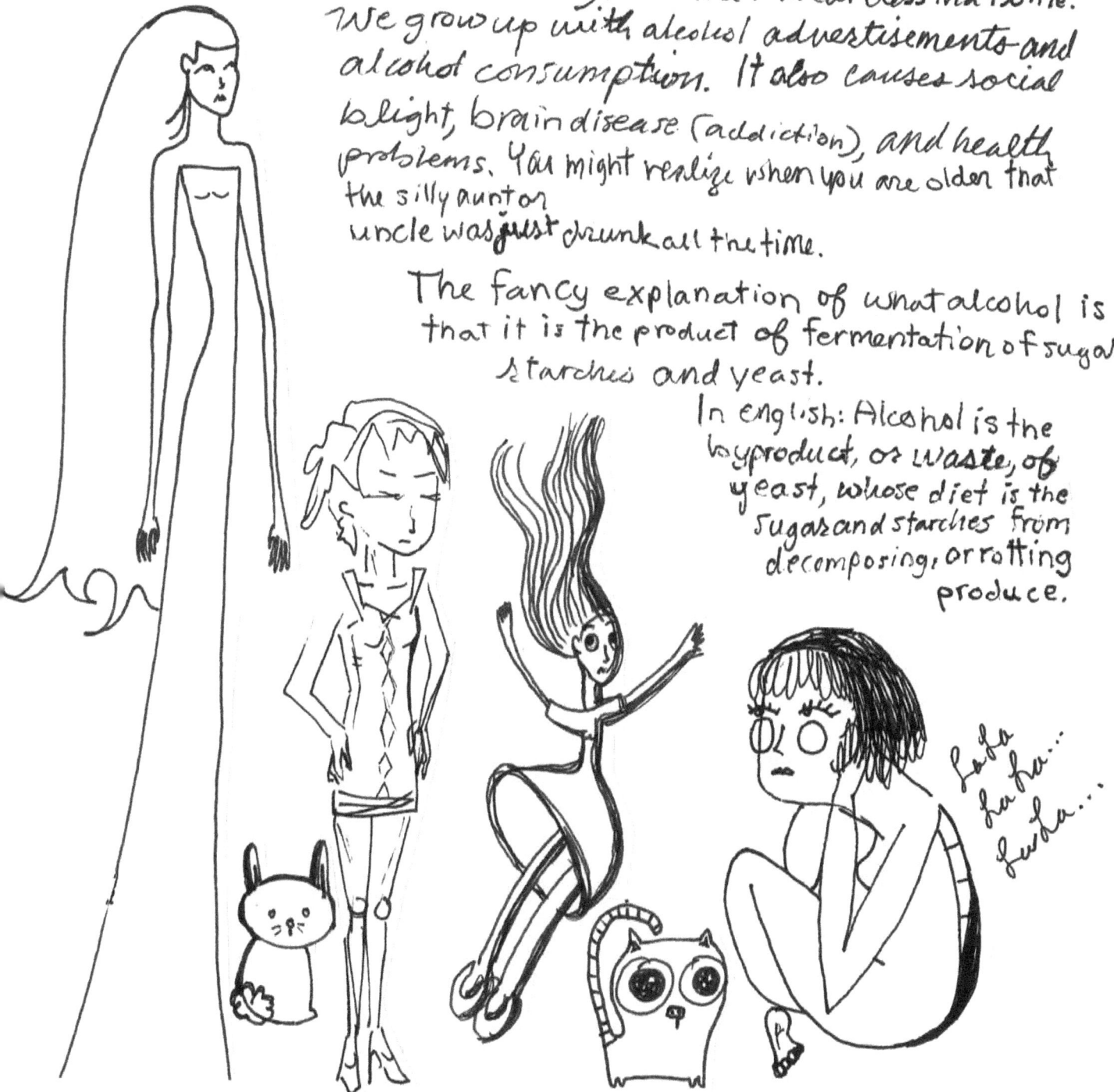

ha ha... ha ha ha ha...

When you turn 21, nobody gives a shit how much you drink. The information that is required to be on food and drink products pertaining to nutrative value and ingredients, is absent on alcohol containers. There are warning labels on tobacco products and second hand smoke is harmful. Effects from alcohol to yourself and others, is also harmful.

The cautions offered to adults is this:

- Do not drink while pregnant.
- Do not operate a vehicle under the influence of alcohol.
- Drink responsibly

Over the counter medications have more precautions than alcohol. Everybody is always bitching about underage drinking. Do as I say, not as I do. Read the news, read the police blotter. Read about womens' shelters, homeless perspectives, addiction perspectives, homes for sexually violated children, and the emergency room. Read about suicides and tragic alcohol-involved accidents and look back on your own life.

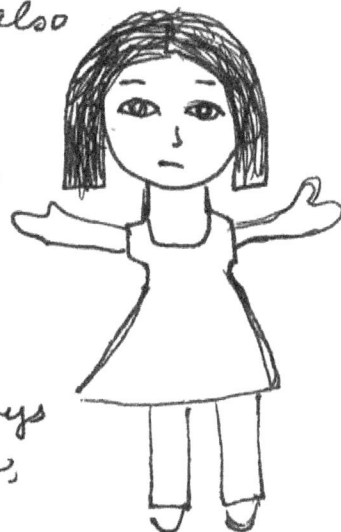

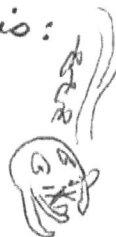

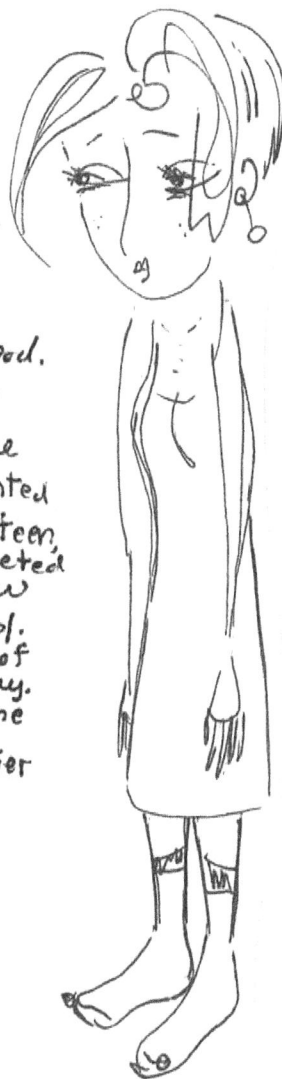

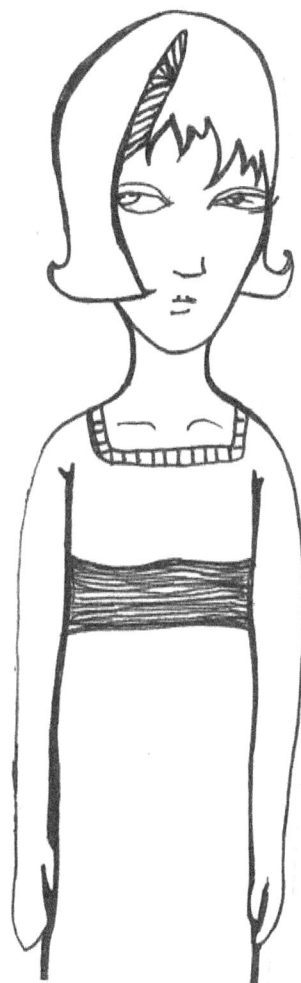

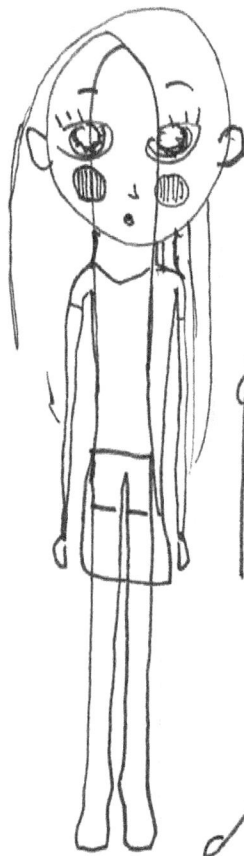

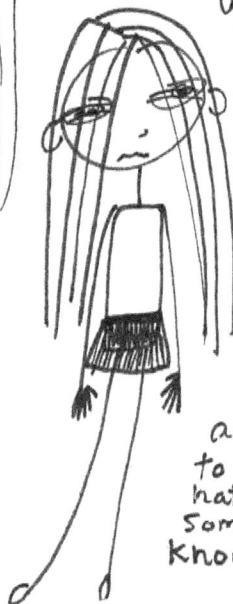

Alcohol ruined my childhood. I grew up in a village and my mother was an alcoholic. She was emotionally stunted so when I became a teen, we fought and competed like sisters. I grew up around alcohol. I saw the dark sides of people I saw everyday. I saw fuckedupshit, some of that was done to me. Mom always had a hangover on my birthday and that kinda ruined it for me. I was her dirty secret and she took that secret to her grave. I know she hated me somehow for something, I will never know what for.

Alcohol, From lips to Butthole.

— Alcohol kills helpful bacteria in your stomach and intestines. It wears down and desensitizes your mouth, throat, and stomach. Long-term use can cause ulcers and several kinds of cancer. Example: Alcoholics can stomach hard alcohol, light beer tastes like water.

— Alcohol is absorbed by the stomach immediately, delivering via bloodstream, to your entire body and brain. You become dehydrated.

— Alcohol causes vasodialation. Your blood vessels open wide and cause a person to have a flushed (red) look. Long-term use causes a red bulbous nose, think alcoholic cartoons. It causes rosacea also. Both are irreversible.

— Alcohol "defats" skin, causing a weathered or leathery look.

sssssssss ghhhh hh

sssssssssssshhh

Premature aging results because of the lack of skin lipids and the consistent drunk face. Overly happy, sad, suicidal, or angry. Cosmetics can not help once the damage is done, too late Jack. The crag stays.

Brain. The brain is covered by a thick layer of tissue. Between that and the skull is the blood—brain barrier. The barrier is thin or absent over some parts of the brain. One of these is the back part, your motor (movement) control center.

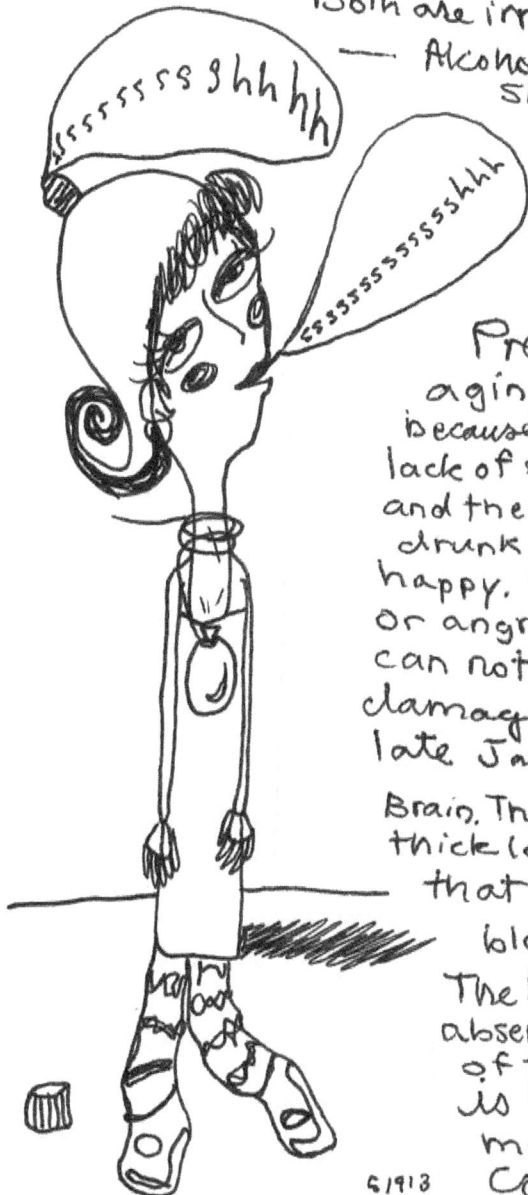

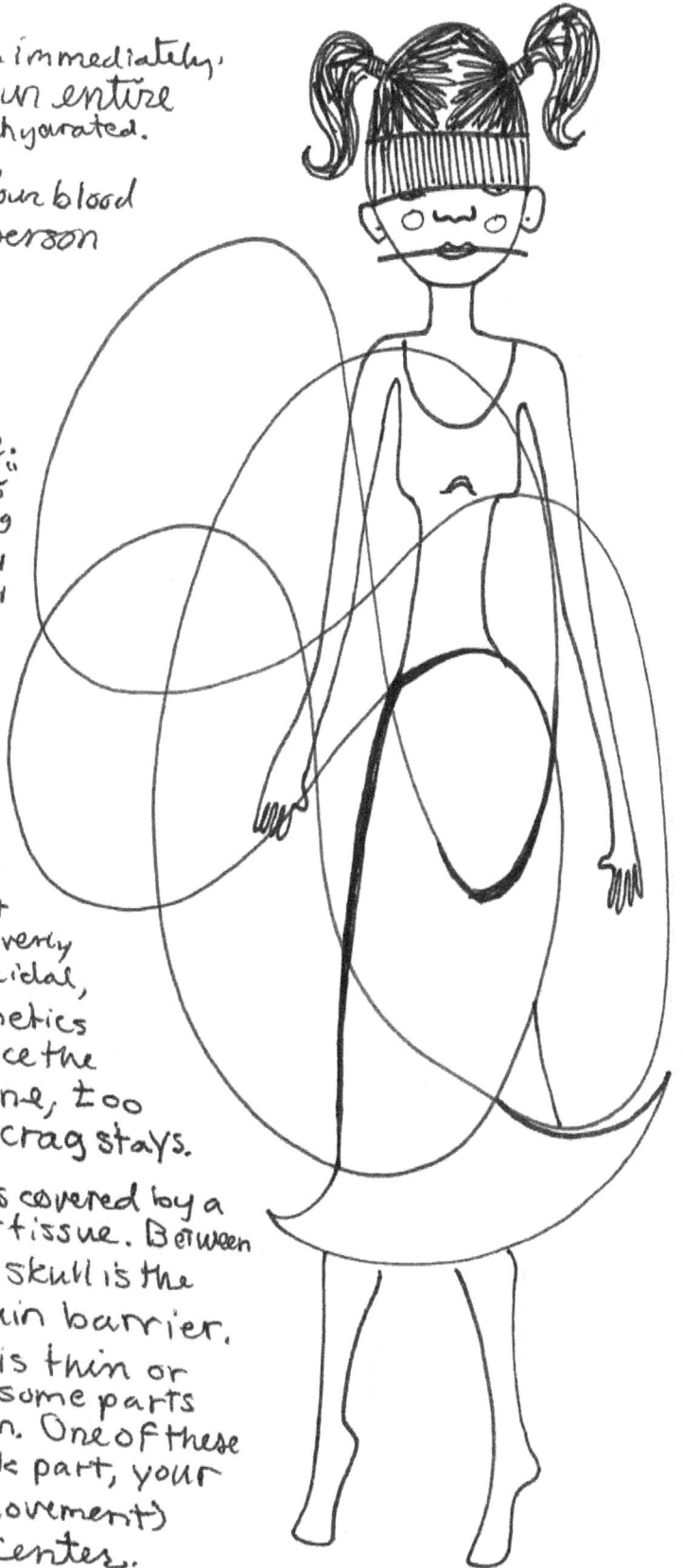

61913

— Balance and spacial perception are affected first. This is why police officers give you a spacial and balance test when you are drunk driving.

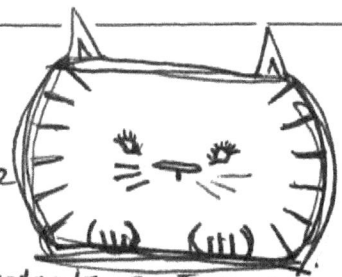

— You vomit profusely. The midbrain controls autonomic functions like breathing, heart rate and systems management. Your primitive survivalist brain is detecting a **foreign** contaminant in your bloodstream. When you vomit, that is your brains first response, to expel contaminate poison. Every consumer of alcohol has vomited at least once. People who don't puke have usually built up tolerance. They need more to get to the level of intoxication they want.

— Alcohol is a nervous system depressant. Any time you move or feel anything, your brain is transmitting sensations, controlled movement, and spacial perception to your conscious brain. When your nervous system is depressed, sensations are numb and painless. The more you drink the more judgement you lose. Judgement is knowing consequences and right from wrong.

This, plus numbness makes people feel invincible, which they are not. They are just a drunk dumbass.

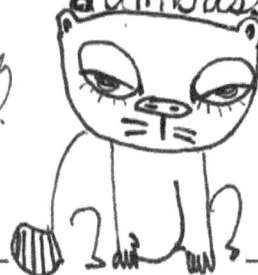

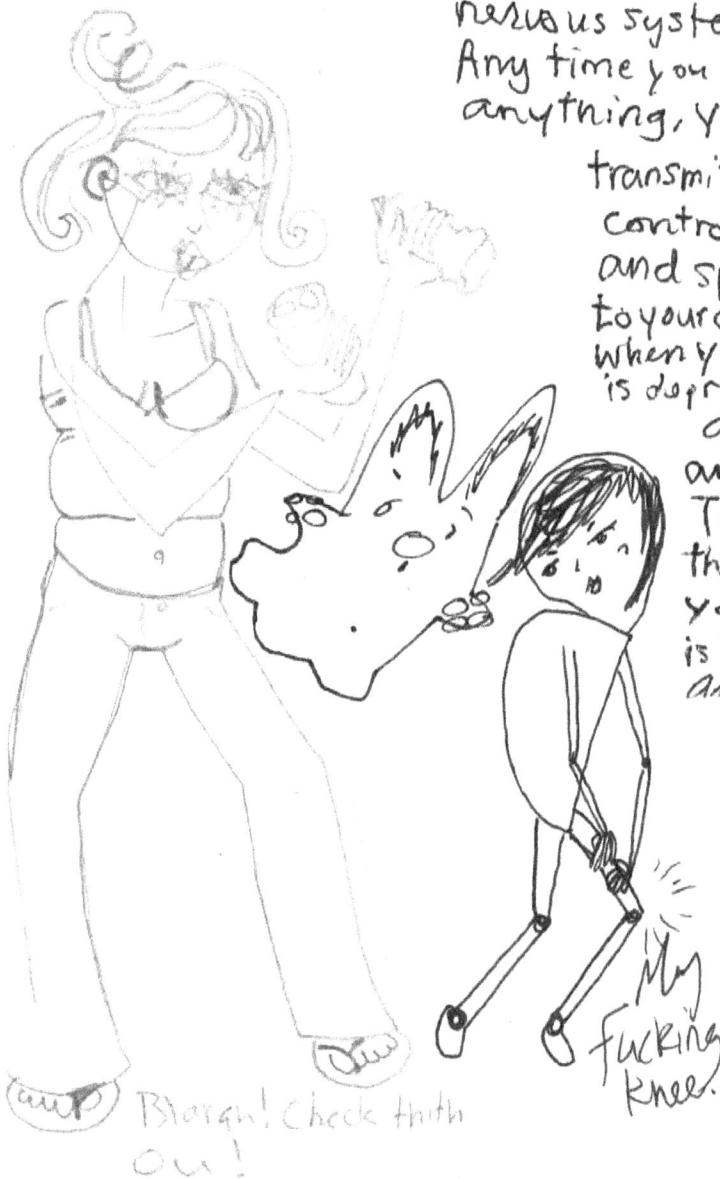

My fucking knee.

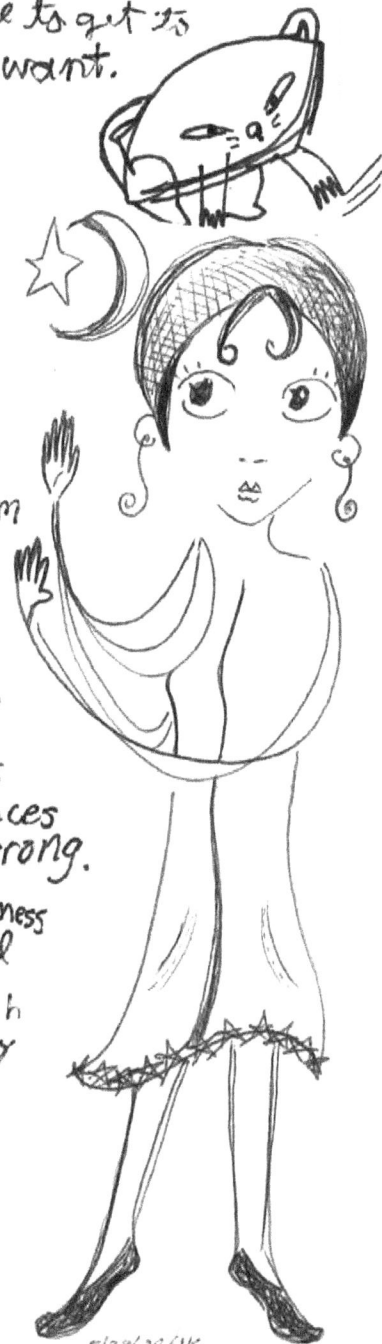

Blargh! Check this out!

Balance

5/28/09/UC

— Losing judgement and physical strength is the ideal situation for a rapist to victimize a person. Rapists single drunk-people out. All they have to do is go over and talke to you, then their foot is in the door; All they have to do is act like a nice guy or Good Girl. They might tell you after that it was not their fault because they were drunk and they would "never do that when they are sober." B.S.B.S.B.S.
Sorry to break it to you, but there is no excuse for rape..

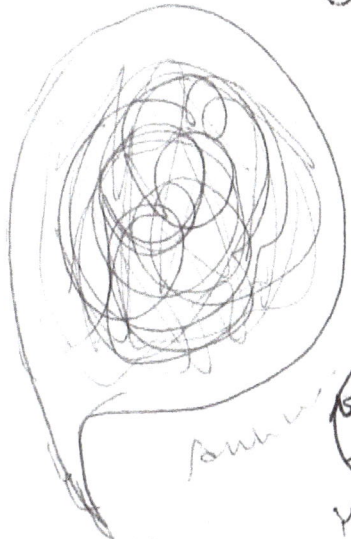

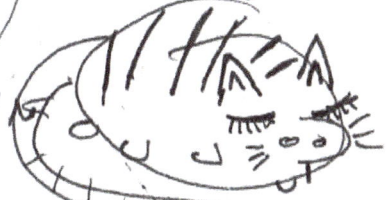

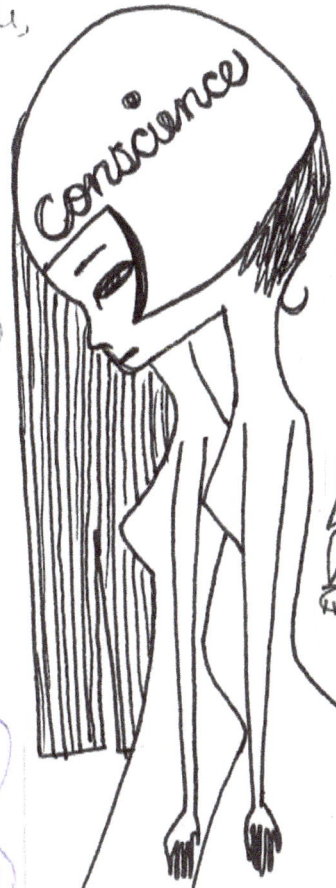

You + alcohol (- judgement + other drug)
= Coma or overdose or death.
You + alcohol (- judgement + physical strength)
= Rape

You + alcohol (depression + depressant)
= Suicide
You + alcohol (- judgement + sensation)
= Broken body

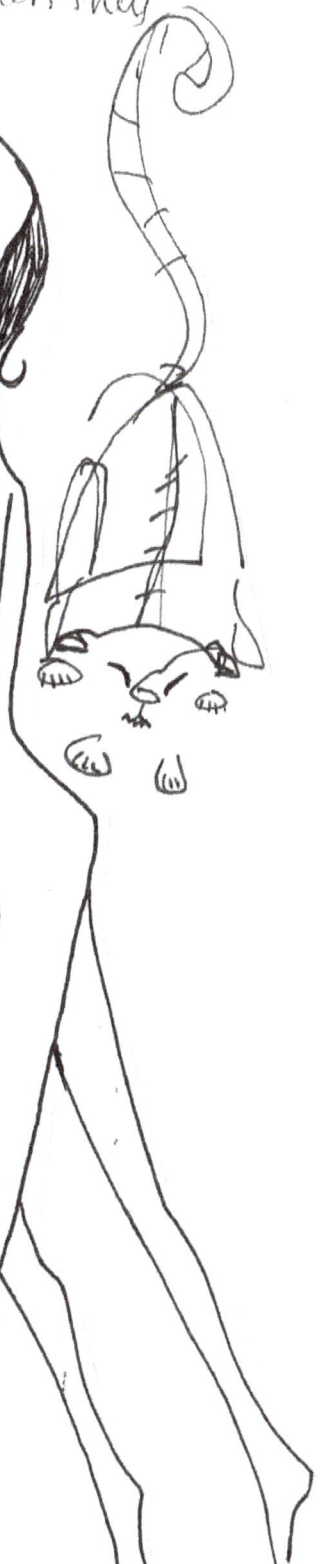

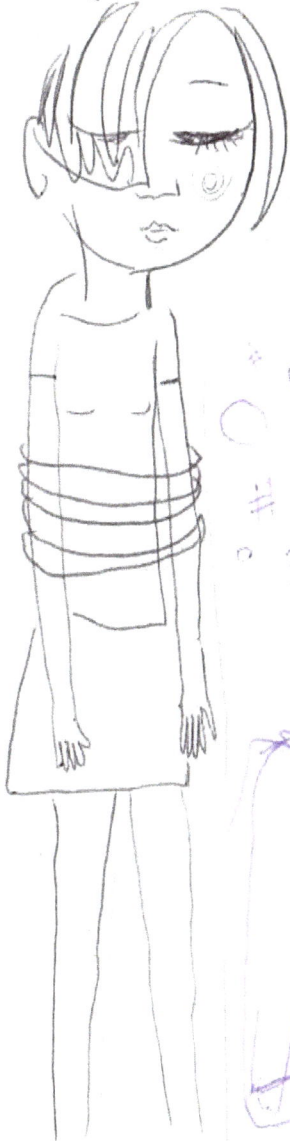

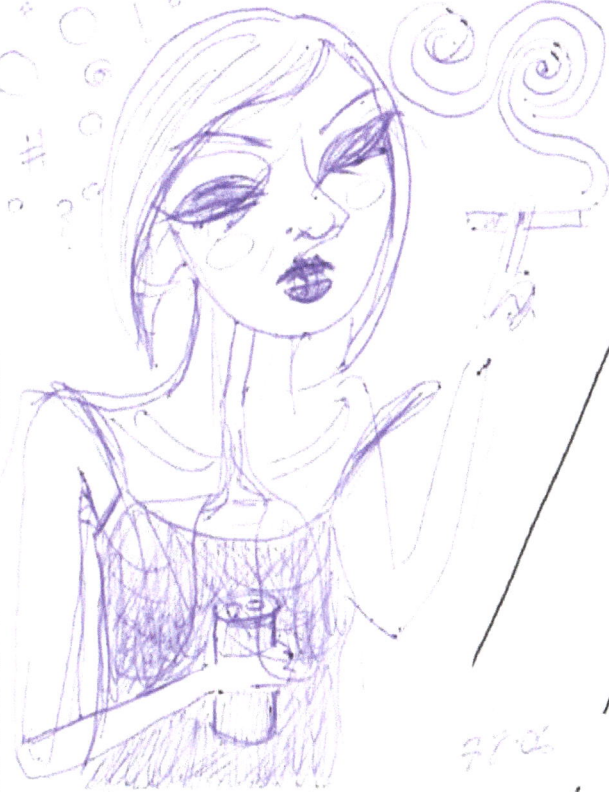

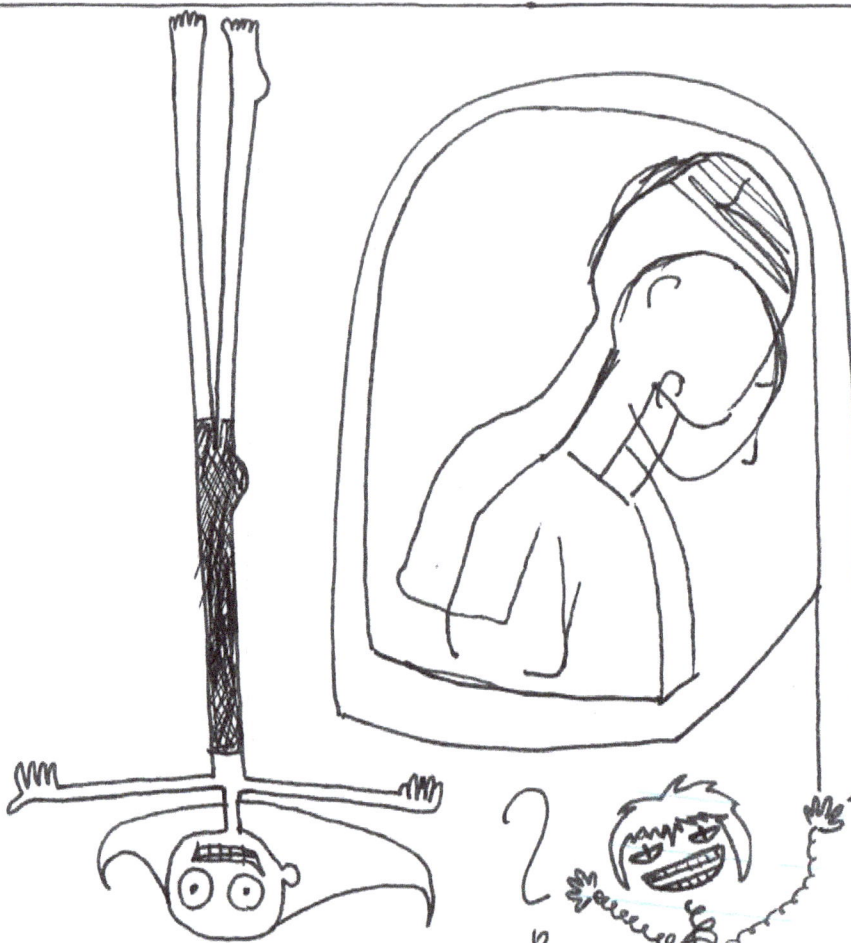

Blackout Memorybanks shut down. Alcohol also makes it easy for people to drug you. You hear the next day that you were crazy last night. You might wake up in jail, in the hospital, or next to your Rapist♡ You pray for evidence of a condom, at least, as you sneak out. Everyone knows you and whoever did whatever; Some tried to stop you. You might wake up Alone and naked, with no idea how you ended up there in the First place. It has Happened to me, and happened to people I have known.

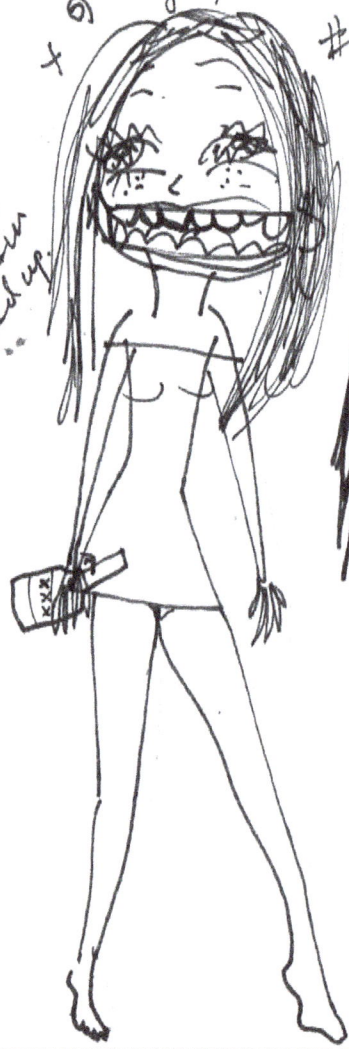

Daaah i'm fucked up

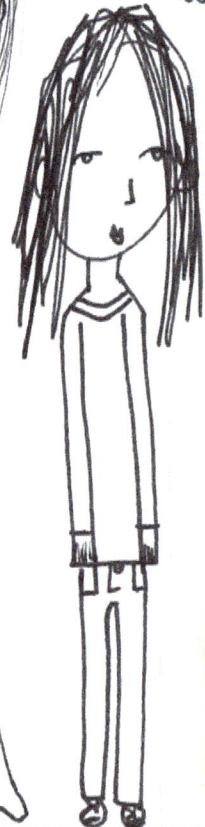

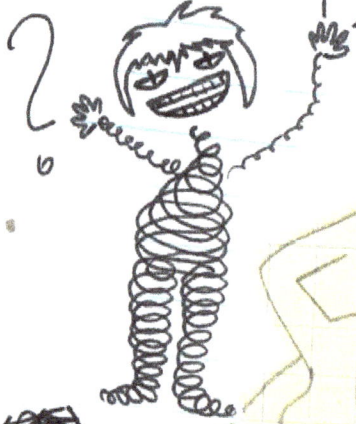

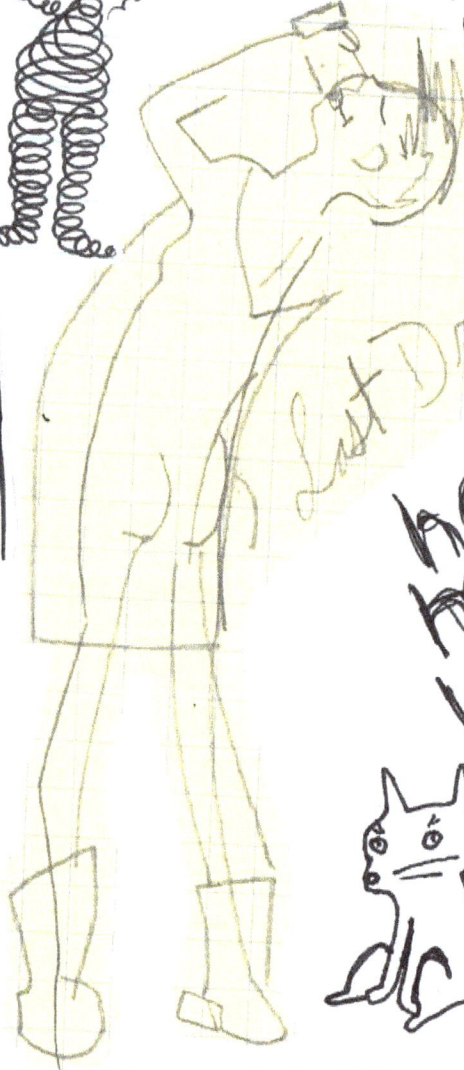

Last Drop

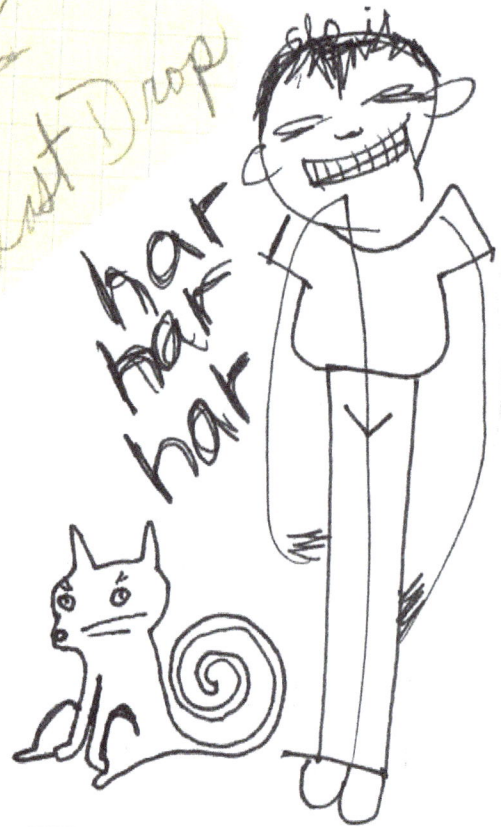

har har har

Passing Out Your body shuts down, people rape you and humiliate you. You can lose consciousness anywhere. People pass-out in drive-thrus, on the lawn, or while taking a pee. They die in water, they die by hypothermia, they die by suffocating to death by sleeping, passing-O-U-T and choking on their own vomit. Turkeys drown in the rain. They are facinated by raindrops and they stare transfixed with their mouths open. Turkeys are stupid. Alcohol takes away a persons survival instincts. If you are drunk in the forest, you will probably be mauled by a bear because you are easy prey. The Next Day: Hangover. This means your body is dehydrated to shit. Too much caffeine causes the same symptoms as an alcohol hangover.

People wake up still drunk and drive home or go to work, where they are slow and unproductive because they legally poisoned themselves the night before.

Some drunk more. This works by allieviating the acute alcohol withdrawel symptoms.

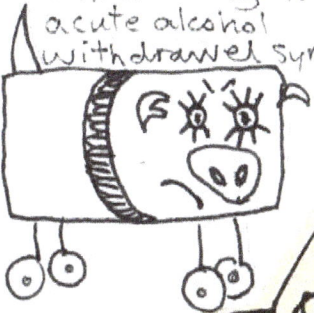

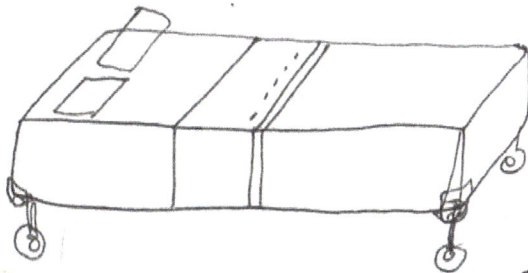

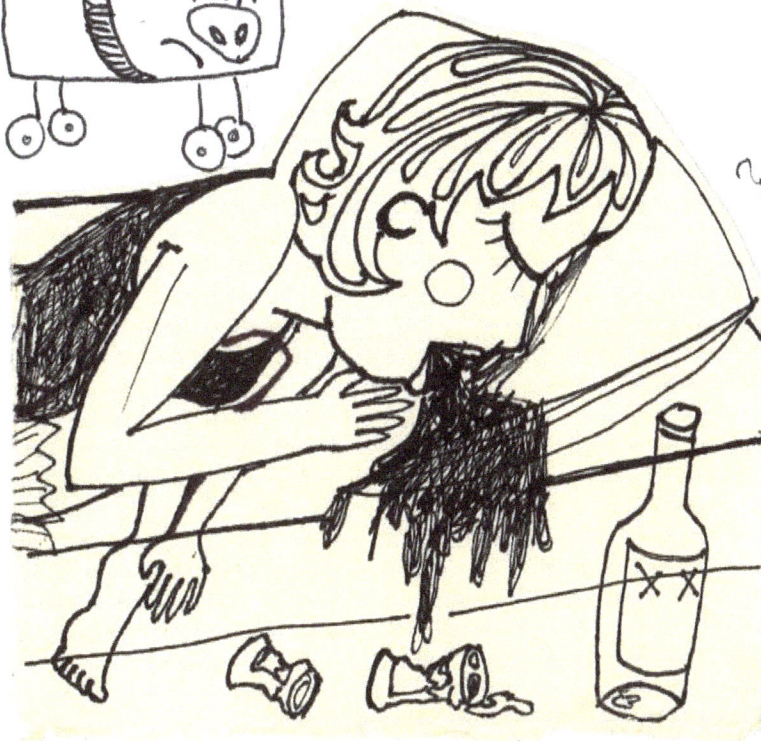

You feel like SHIT.... bleeech.
And you reek. I will never forget the smell of Day Old Drunk.

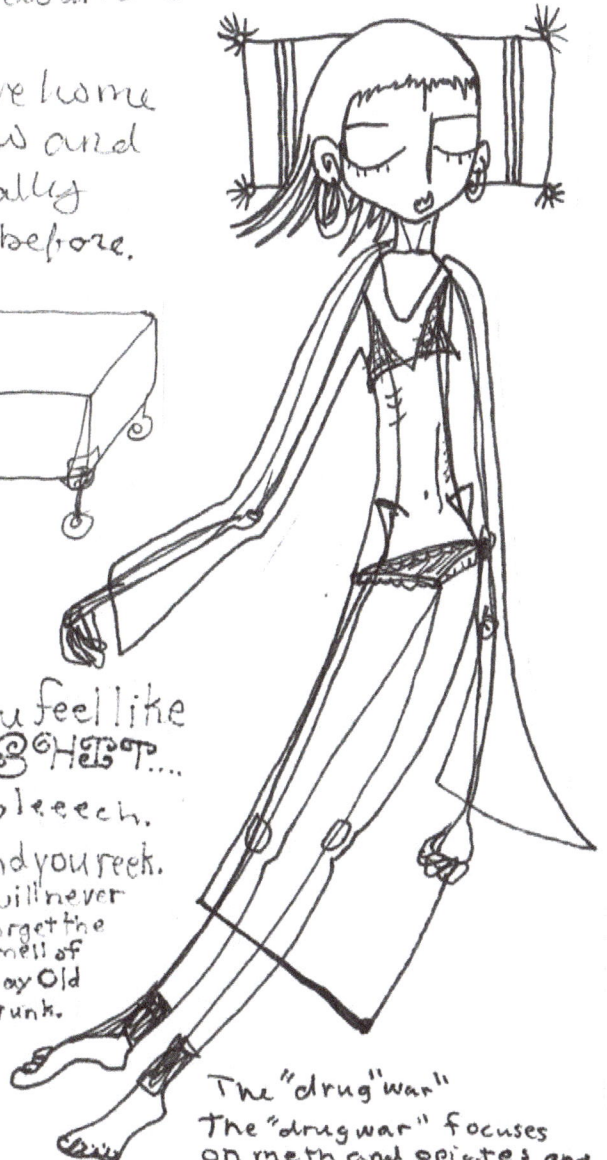

The "drug war" The "drug war" focuses on meth and opiates and marijuana. Not so much for alcohol, peoples best friend.

52913

The next morning, or whenever, when you regain
consciousness, you have a head-splitting headache. Sounds
are amplified, lights are blinding. You have not slept well
so you are slowed down and in pain, your mind and
body are exhausted from
processing alcohol. Your stomach is sour, raw, and
empty-feeling. Don't forget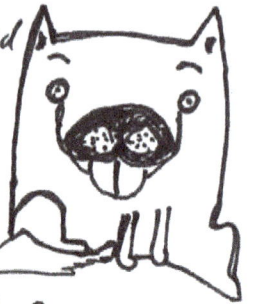
        the easy poops!
Greasy food coats and soothes your stomach,
like the pink stuff. More poop.
— If you drink often, you are prone to alcohol addiction,
    especially if you come from a family of alcoholics.
I never became an alcoholic. It tastes like shit,
and I don't enjoy being literally stupid and useless.
    Alcohol killed a lot of my family, but
    alcoholism is a problem where I grew up, to this day.
    I also don't enjoy knowing or not knowing if I
    was raped or why I have a black bruise
    on my face.
    Things are the same, if not worse, all over every
    state. Alcohol is the bottom line but people don't want
    to hear that. Efforts to educate people about
    alcohol are rediculous, they have given up.
    It went from Quitting Drinking information
        to Cutting Down on Your
        Drinking. People who stop,
        or never start, are out there,
        but not so much here.

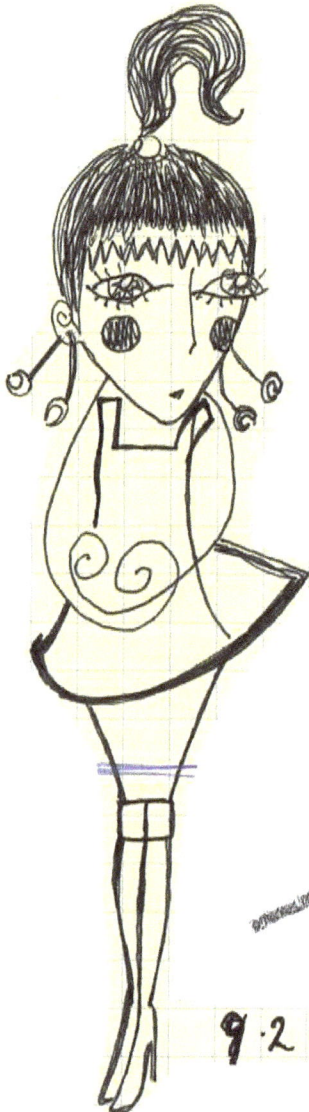

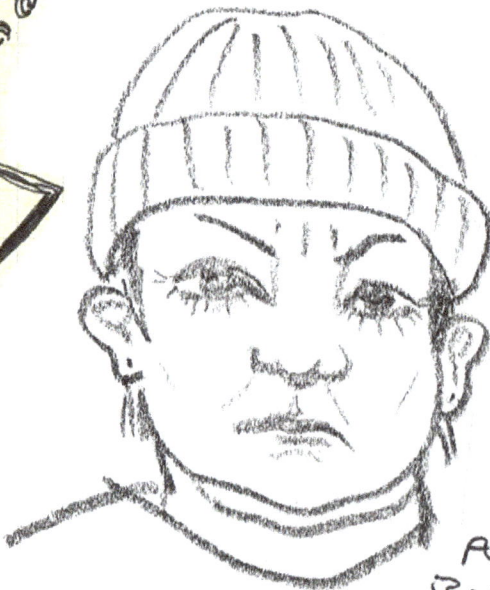

We have
the highest
rates of
terrible
things in
our
state.
Alcohol is the
Root Cause of
all of these.

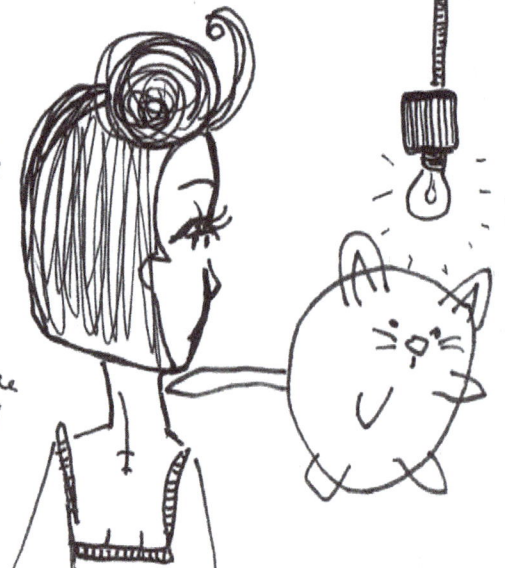

9·29·09

People love their alcohol and they won't stop drinking it. People get angry and say "YOU GUYS need to do something about this." What needs to happen may never happen. It is not any races' fault for introducing it to their culture. Nobody actually FORCES anyone else to drink. Drinking is a choice and devastating devient, tragedies happen, and keep on happening because of it. If they quit, they might actually have to deal with their emotions and care about themselves and others. They might have to grow up and have responsibilities.

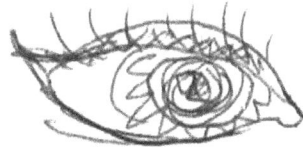

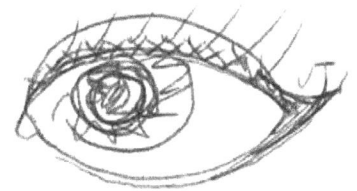

Crimes committed under the influence of alcohol are the consequences of CHOOSING to drink alcohol.

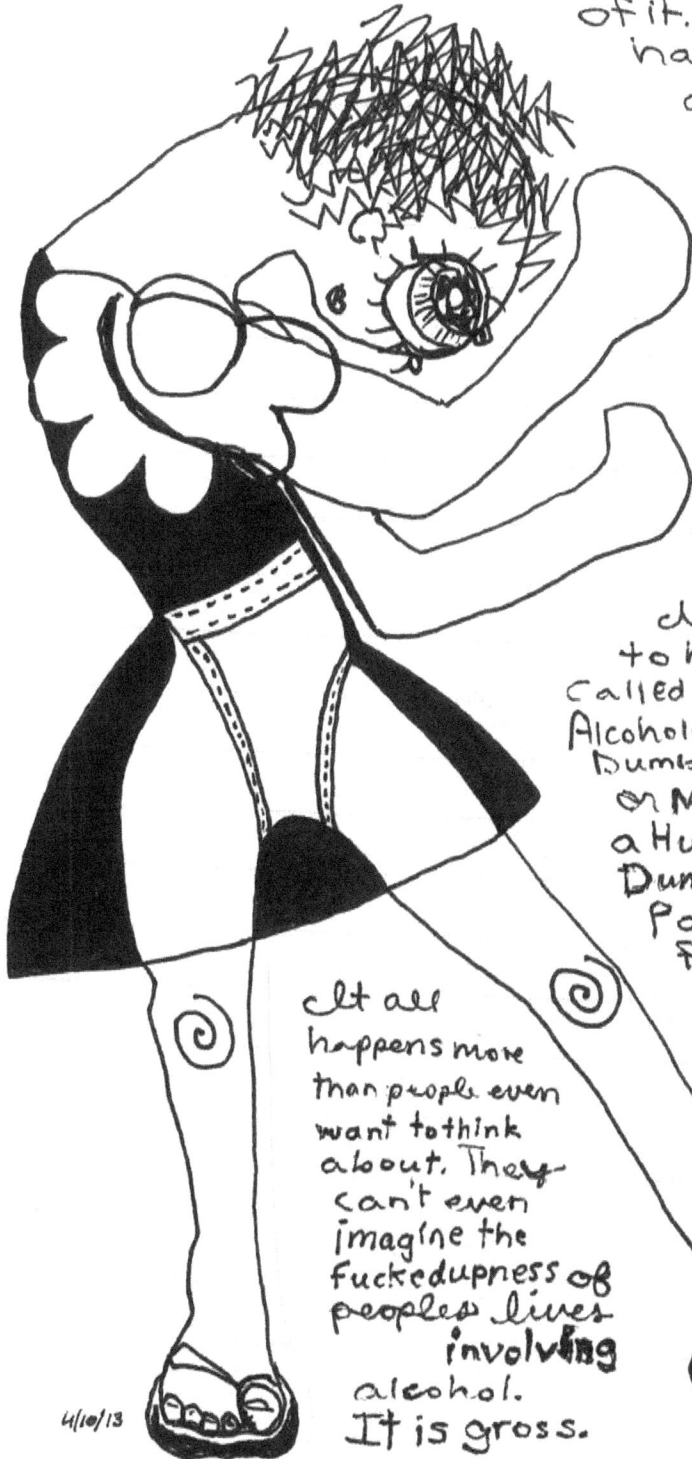

Daaah...

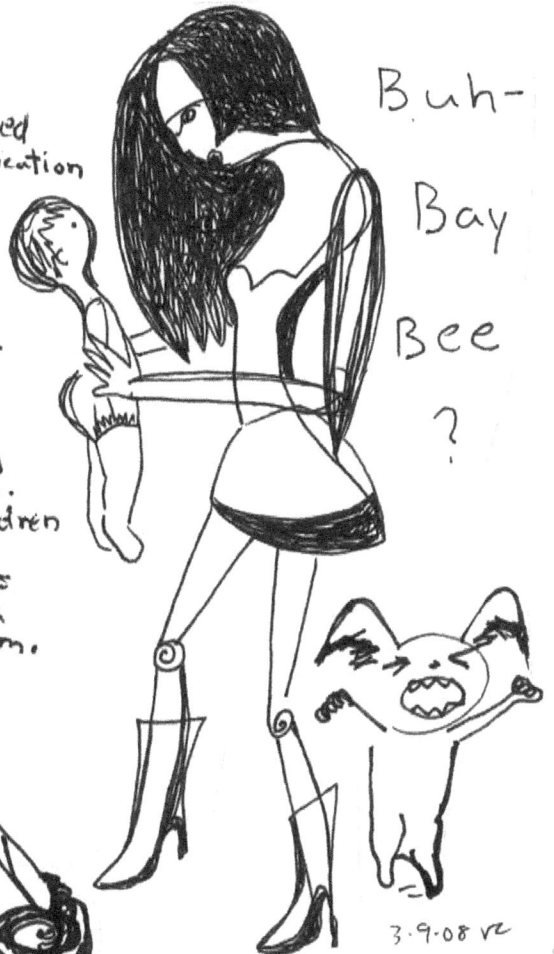

It all happens more than people even want to think about. They can't even imagine the fuckedupness of peoples lives involving alcohol. It is gross.

There doesn't need to be a publication called Alcoholism for Dumbasses or Making a Human for Dumbasses. Poor Fatherless Children. Poor children whos fathers fuck them.

Buh-Bay Bee ?

4/10/13

3.9.08 VZ

I do not drink alcohol. I am ashamed at my drunk incidents. I don't fuck people I just met or call my friend an effing-biotch. I was acting like a trashy drunk whore. I know I can feel horrible but I was being a bad person when I am usually a good person. I've been raped-blacked-out and passed-out. I will never know who, in one case. I have driven drunk, I have hurt peoples' feelings, and ralphed my guts out. The few times were too many for me. I am a "Light Weight" and always get made fun of.

Yuck Yuck Yuck NASTY Yuck. I will never forget the image and disgust when I saw my mother take a 5-second drink of pure whisky at 7a.m. We said eeeeeeew. She said What? It tastes sweet. I am getting treated for anxiety, depression, and Post Traumatic Stress Disorder, PTSD. The fact that I didn't get treated early, is why I have these at the severity level I have.

People on antidepressants are not supposed to drink alcohol. This can stop people from getting mental health treatment.

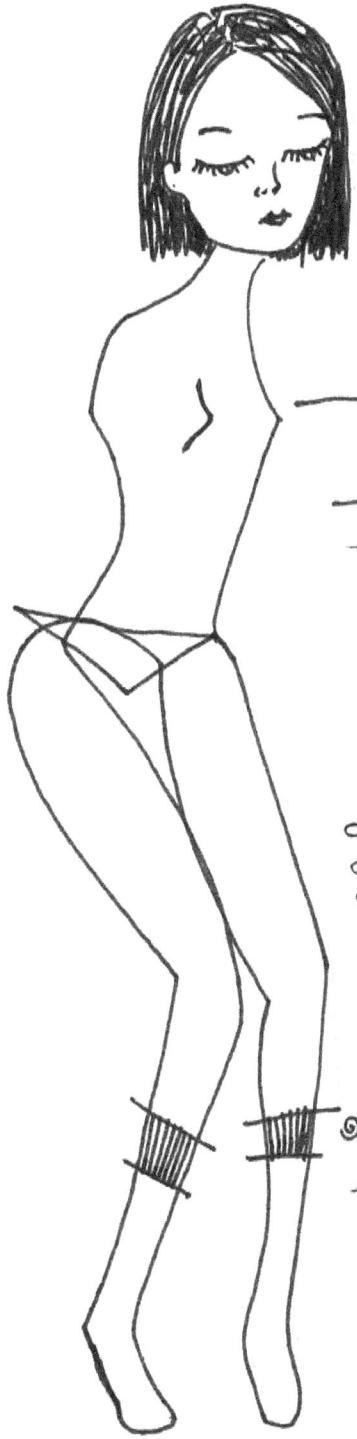

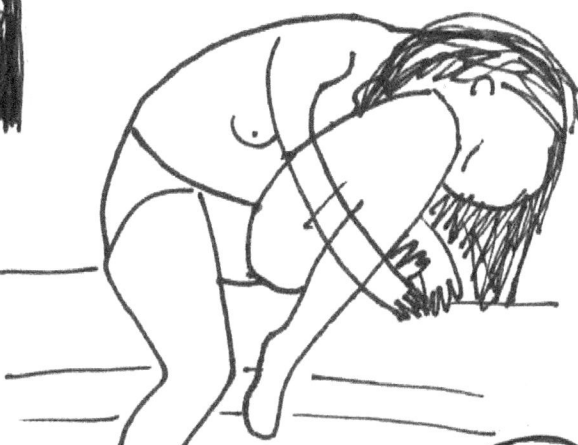

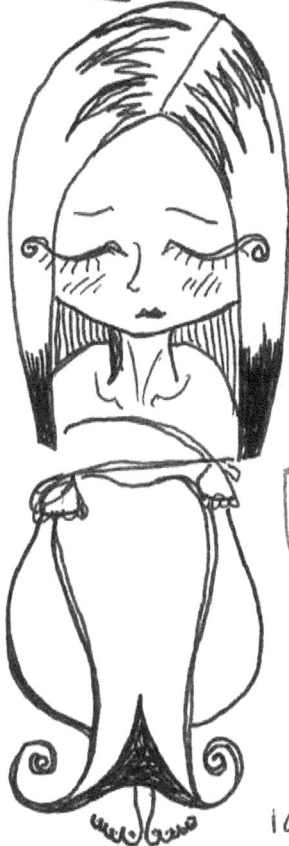

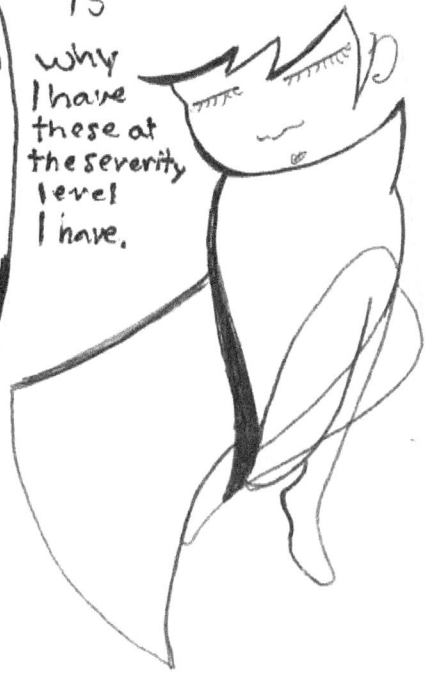

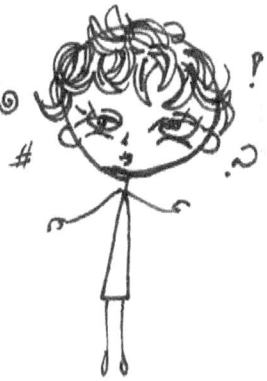

10/3/13

4/10/06

You
wanna
go get a
drink?

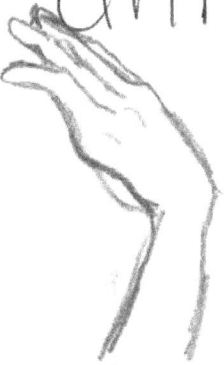

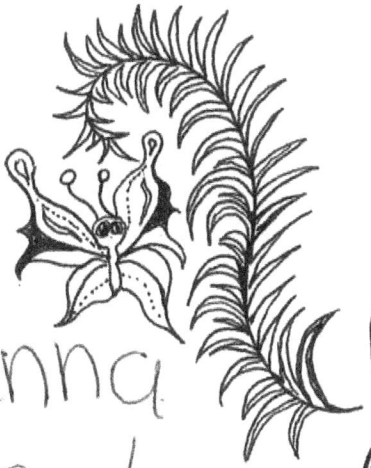

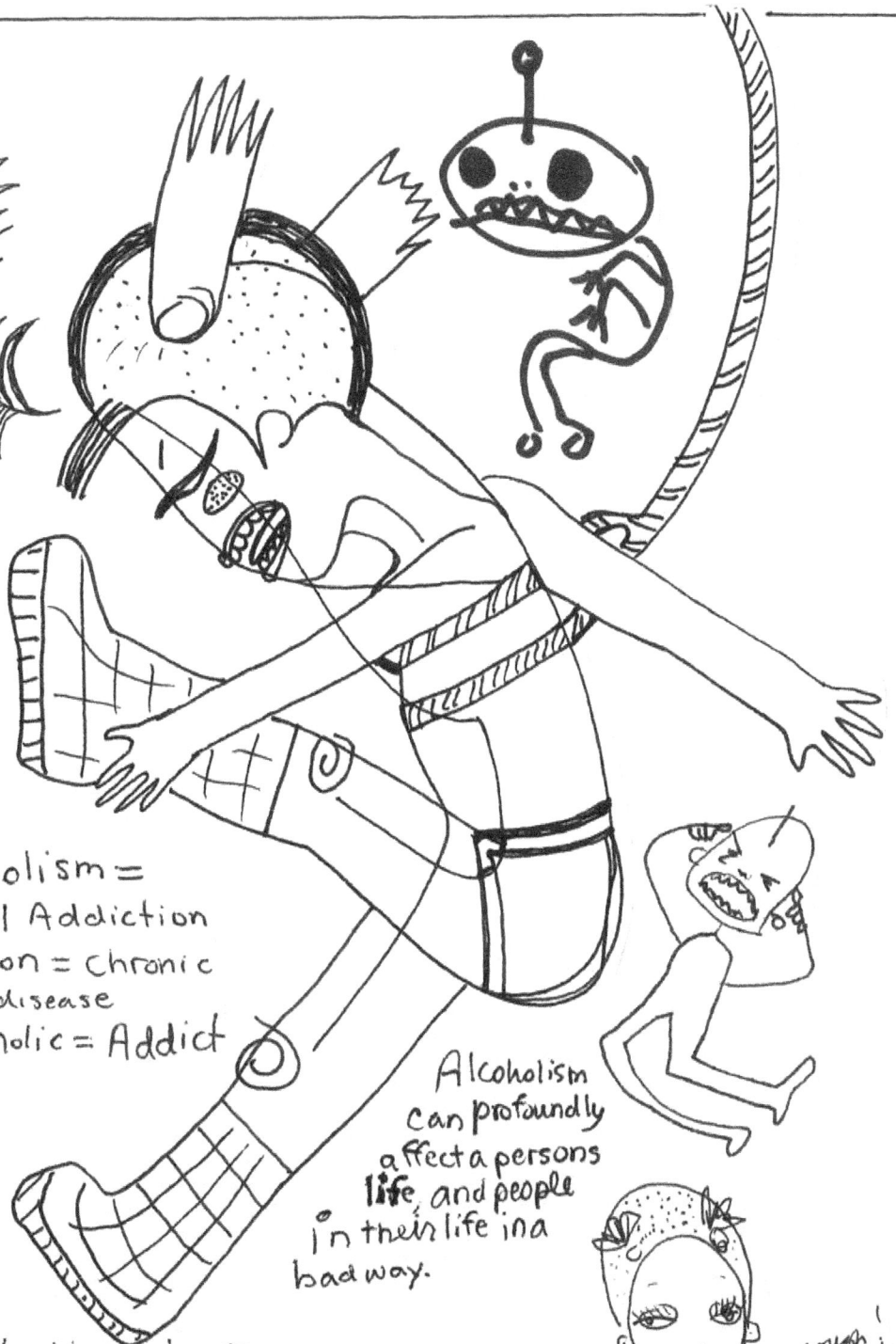

Alcoholism =
alcohol Addiction
Addiction = chronic
brain disease
Alcoholic = Addict

Alcoholism
can profoundly
affect a persons
life and people
in their life in a
bad way.

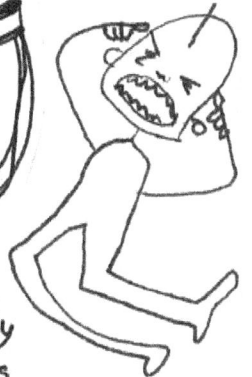

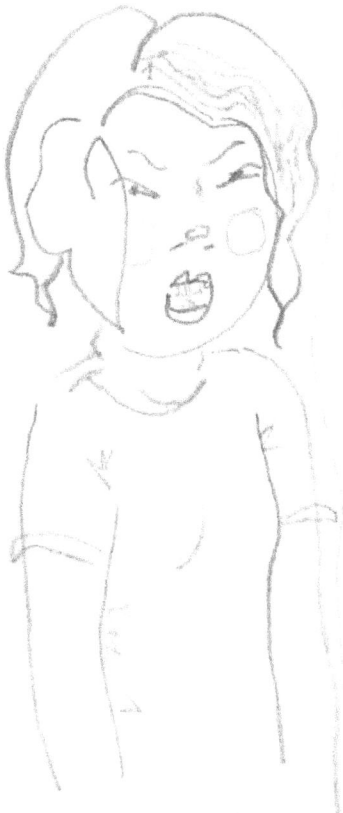

— Alcoholism starts as a
a pattern of abuse. Alcohol
makes a person numb to the world.
— It starts with weekends.
"Partying" makes you feel good.
you have friends that **love**
you. After some time, the
weekend couldn't come soon
enough so you come up with
more reasons, or ex<u>cuses</u>
to escape.
— Soon, you need it to relax
or sleep and getting motivated.
— Then, you start needing it to feel
physically and mentally "normal!"

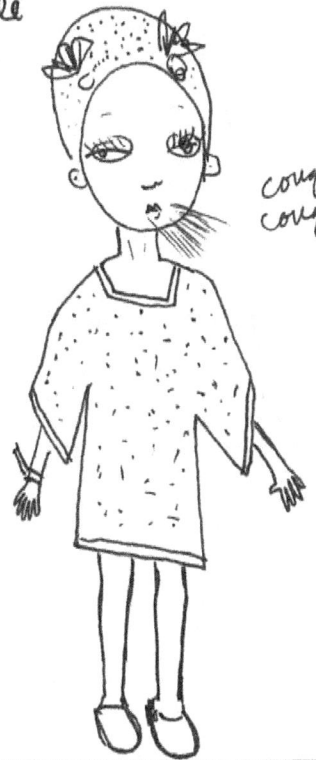

cough!
cough!

Long-term alcoholism can lead to health problems. Health problems leat to complications, then premature death. My mother died this way. She slowly poisoned herself to death at 41. A brain can break. Hydrocephaly (water on the brain) is when the mechanism for flushing cerebrospinal fluid out of the brain cavity, breaks. Fluid builds up in the brain cavity, causing brain damage. Boxing head injuries can this too. Hydrocephalic adults and "punch drunk" boxers have similar irrational behavior that is caused by pressure-induced damage.

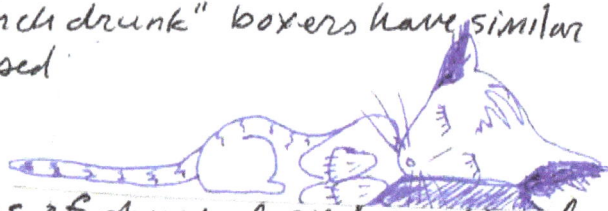

* Effects on **children** *
Children are innocent victims of physical and emotional abuse and neglect. They are victims of domestic violence. They see it, they experience it. This is the groundwork for many children who grow up to be fucked-up adults, like me. Two-parent homes are rare, divorce rates are high and single motherhood is rising. Children become timid and distrustful. They know when they are not loved. They grow up feeling empty, many commit suicide.

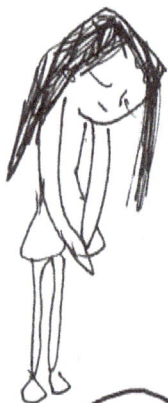

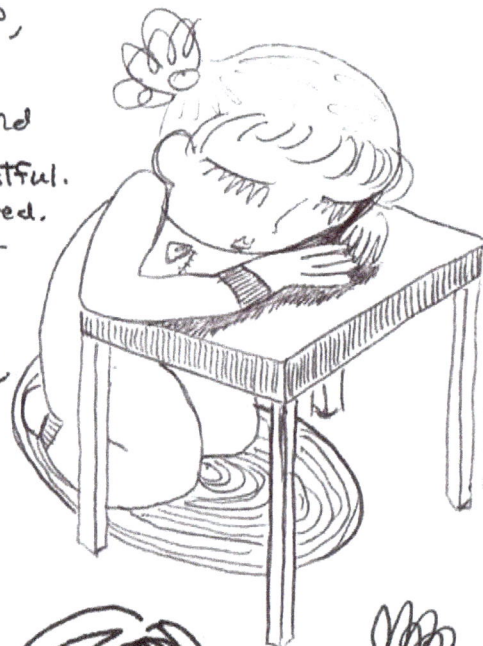

When a parent is an alcoholic, children suffer from alcohols' secondhand effects. They learn that drinking is ok to use when they are sad or to celebrate or when they are bored. Efforts against "underage" drinking are useless if a person learns at a young age that is ok to do what their parents do. Parents should be good examples but a lot of parents just suck.

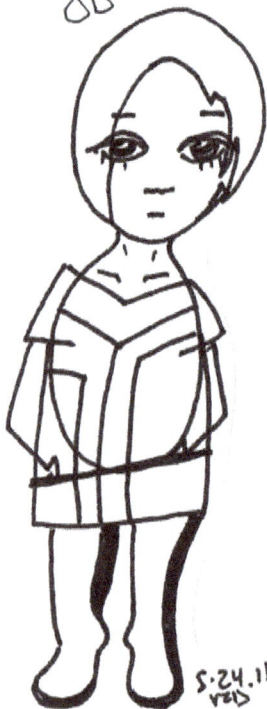

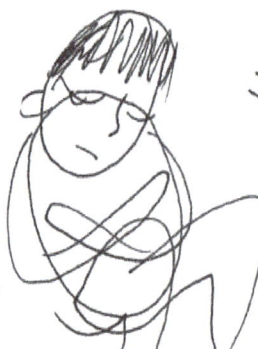

Huh?

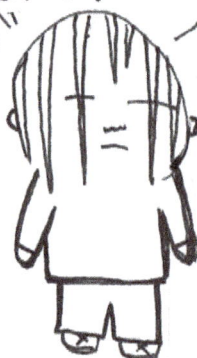

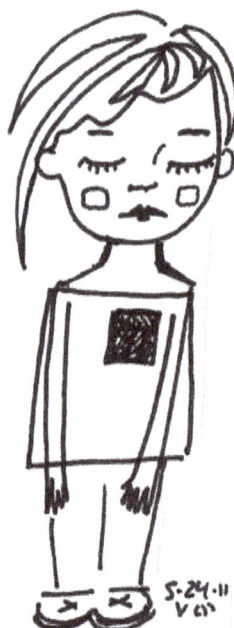

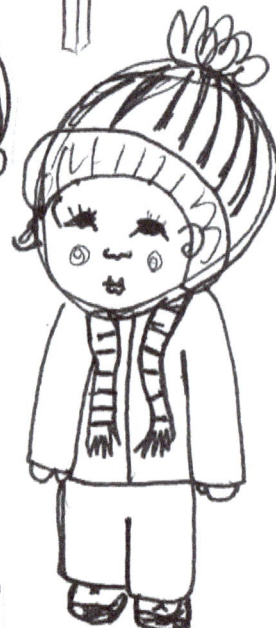

5·24·11
V613

5·24·11
V613

Children who are unsupervised around "partying" adults are in danger of being sexually-violated or raped. When I was 8, I was woken up in the middle of the night by a drunk man on top of me. He was forcing a french kiss on me and feeling up my body. I was terrified and had nowhere to turn. Dad was out of town and mom was passed-out. I saw this man 20 years later at the soup kitchen. He hugged me before I recognized him.

I was an isolated introvert and I got made fun of by adults. I felt alone up until that night, but that night I was alone. My parents were a disappointment in confrontations and affection. When I was a child, I got scared at night. There were so many times I snuck in their room at night and slept at the foot of their bed on the pile of dirty laundry, on the floor. I never got invited into the bed for a snuggle. I was a leader, a Teachers Pet, and very kind and non-judgemental. I learned that is called compassion. I didn't feel loved, so I loved others. I didn't want them to feel alone like me. I still don't.

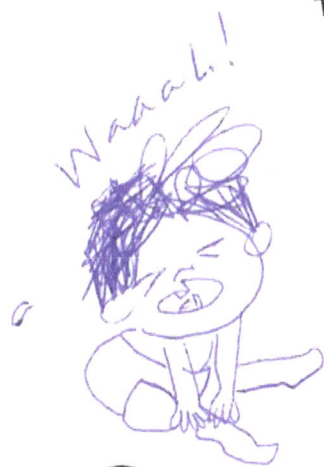

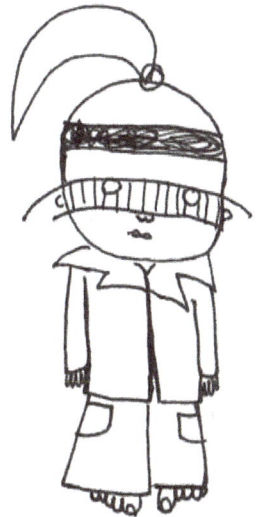

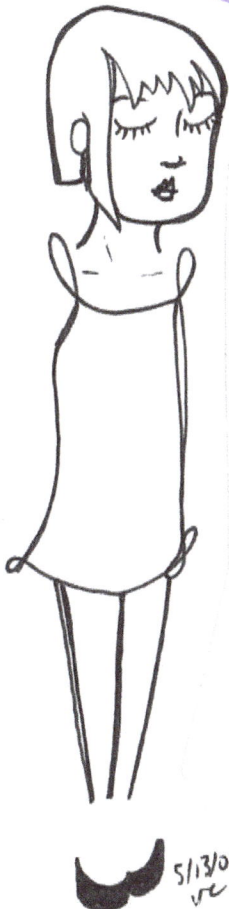

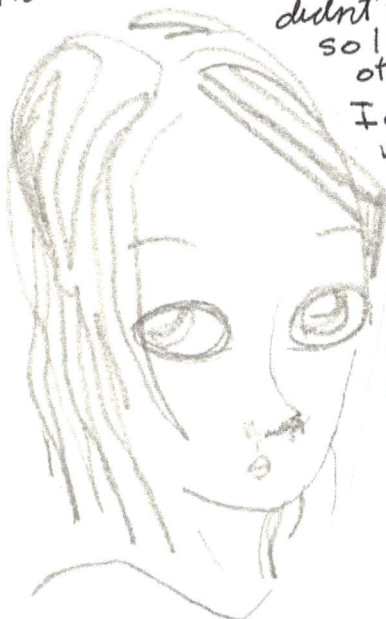

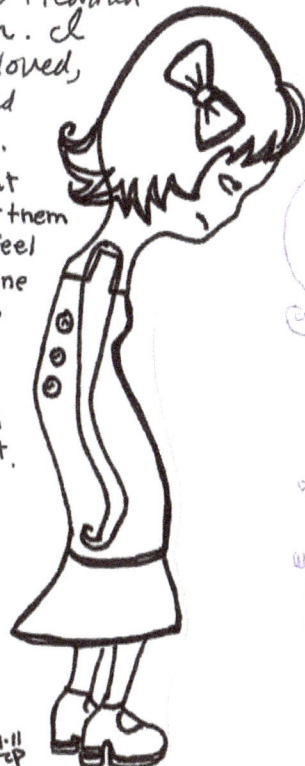

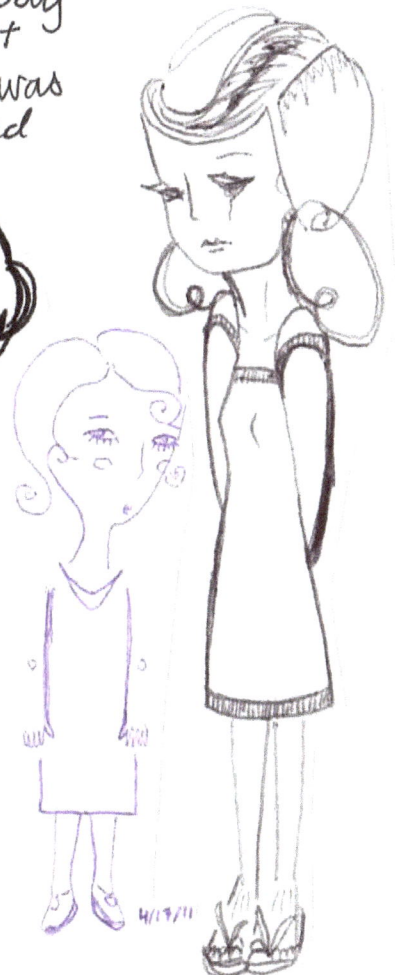

Waaah!

5/13/09 vc

5.24.11 vcp

4/19/11

Alcohol is usually a factor in everything bad that can happen to a child, from an angry cold-shoulder to rape. Addict parents are a factor too. Addicts carry their pain very close. They live in the past and are oblivious to the present and future. They obliterate their problems by blasting it with toxic waste. The poison affects everyone in their life. If you were affected, you might not know how it feels to be loved and cared for, but you don't know that. You just know your mind is racing or depressed. You can't control it, the only power you have is anger. You feel crazy if you let your bad mind suck you in. You might hate your life because you have to raise your siblings because your parents are not responsible enough to take care of themselves. When all you become is a babysitter for your fucked-up mom and/or dad is what causes damage that catches up sooner or later. The result is usually suicide ideology. (soo-ah-cide)(eye-dee-ology), the idea of suicide as an option or answer to problems. When a person grows up as NOTHING, and the only coping technique they have when they feel bad or sad is to drink alcohol, they don't know they can feel better, and that alcohol causes suicide.

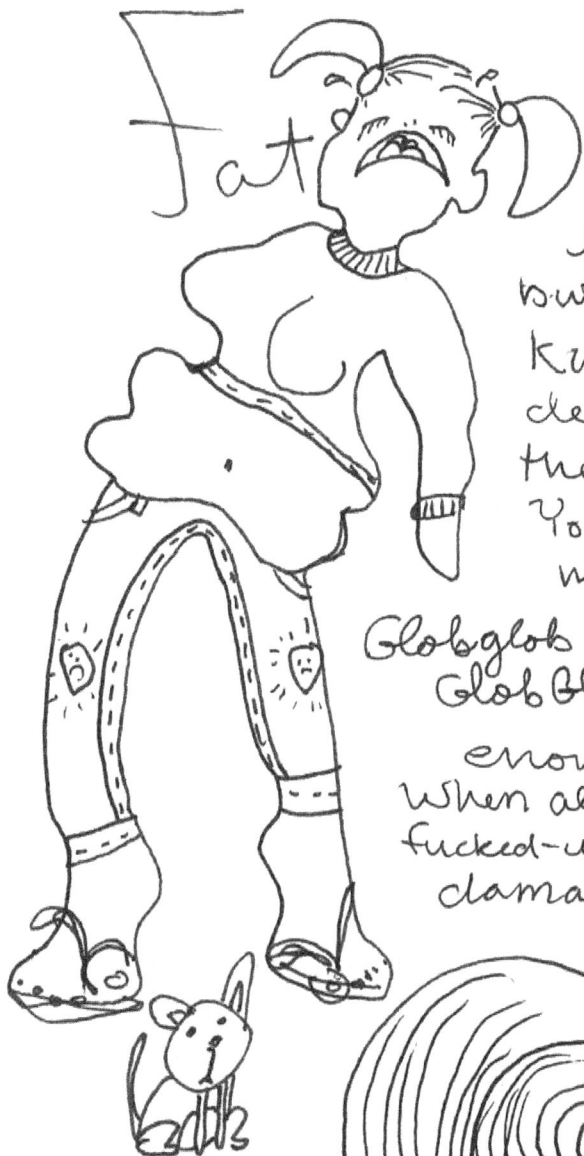

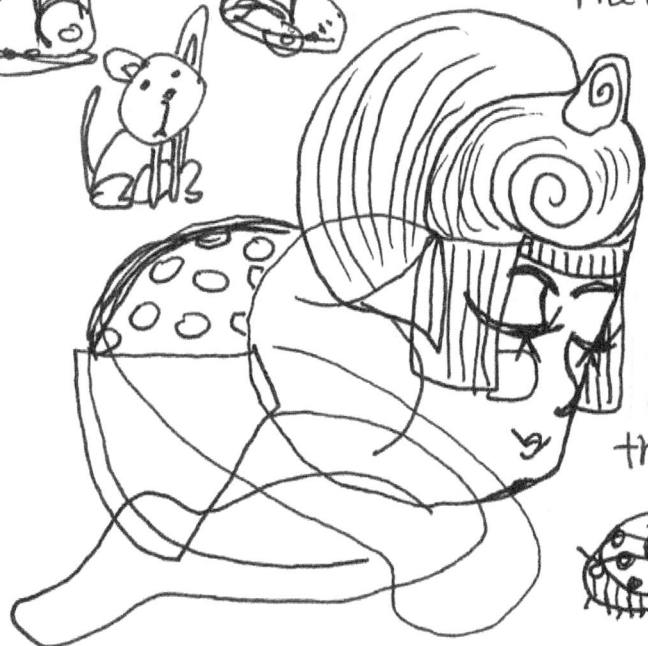

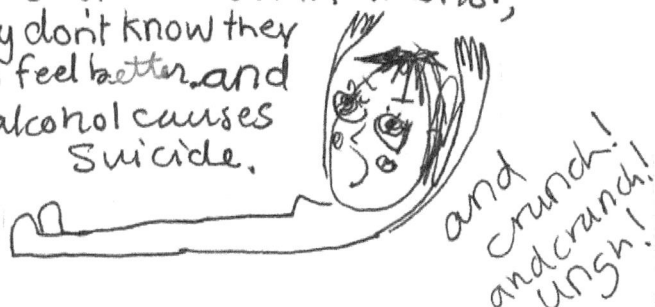

Globular

Fat

Globglob
Glob Glob

and crunch! and crunch! ungh!

Home is a child's world. If that world is good or bad, either affects the rest of their life. If this cycle is not broken by drug or alcohol abstinence, the alcoholic-parent-abuse-neglect-suicide, pattern will continue for generations. If a parents childhood sucked, you are likely to get a crappy childhood too if it involves alcohol or other addiction. I escaped this cycle by not drinking alcohol and not killing myself. I can see this cycle happening still and it breaks my heart. I know what it feels like to be voiceless and brushed aside. You can fight back. Addiction and Bad, or Non-parenting, and under diagnosis and treatment of mental health, are the causes of most suicide. In a place with an alcohol problem, the saying "It takes a village to raise".... a child" is not true. Instead, It takes every child to raise another child.

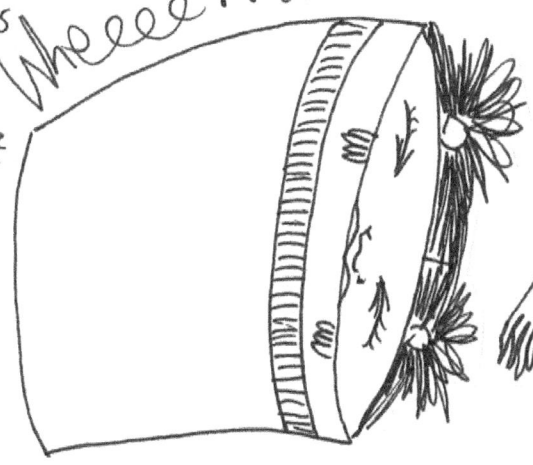

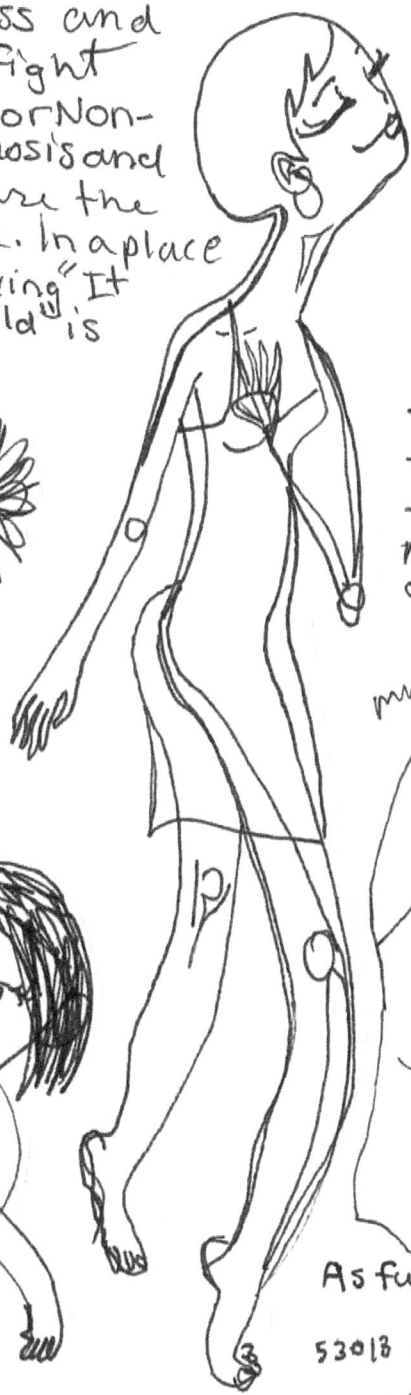

wheee!...

I'm old. Things were bad when I was a kid, they keep

getting worse. They are starting to get angry that councils can't magically stop suicide or other bad shit.

mmmmmm.... meditate

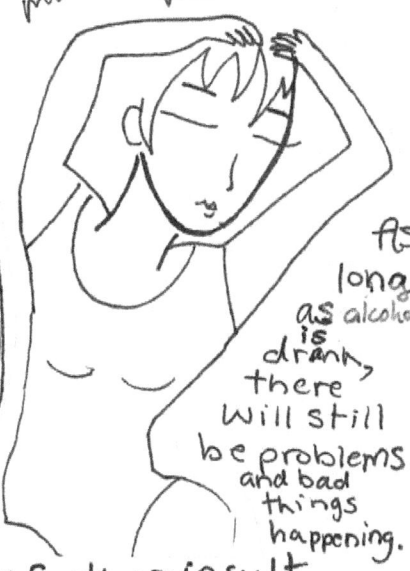

All mine.

As long as alcohol is drank, there will still be problems. and bad things happening.

As further insult, intoxicated people rant about it.

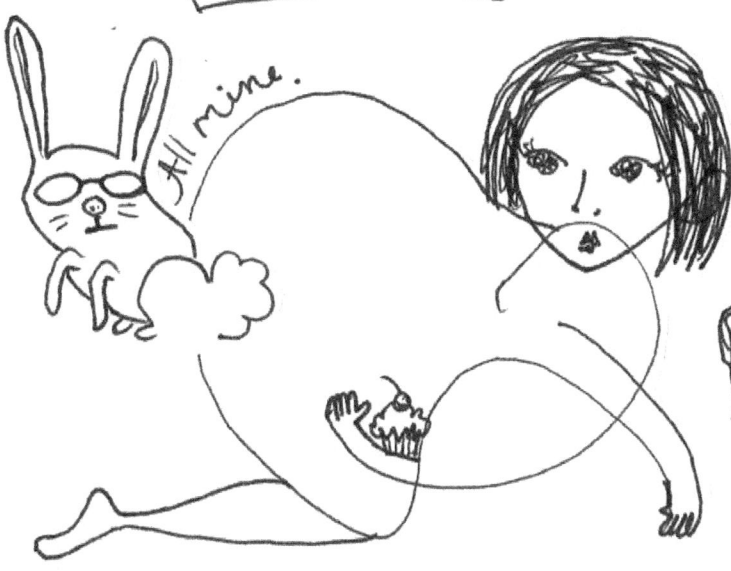

53018

Children should never be subjected to social devients that may hang out with their parents. They should not witness and experience people who "are not themselves." They should not see hysterically sad or angry drunks.

When it comes to mental health treatment, a lot of people just don't understand. The same goes for addiction. It is hard to explain and difficult to understand for someone who has not had the experience or been close to it. If you need help for mental health, there is nothing to be ashamed of. Nobody needs to know and nobody needs to know what you talk about in therapy. When you are in Talk Therapy, that time is all about you. It is hard to talk at first because nobody ever wanted to know about you and how you feel about things. It is hard work learning to love yourself and letting yourself be loved. It is difficult because you don't want to get hurt again. People who love you won't give up on you. They know you are strong but need patience and support. If you have to leave someone you love behind, hope for good outcomes on both sides. It is not the end of The World, only the end of A World that was hurting you.

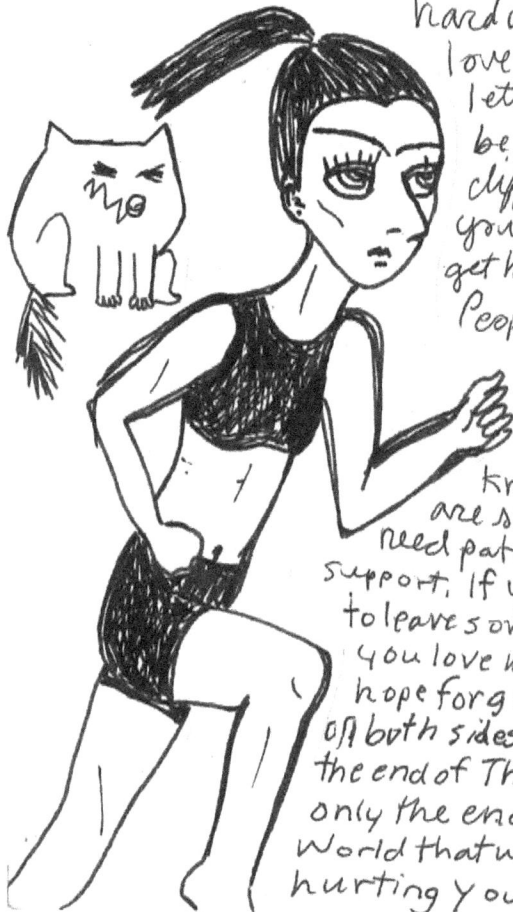

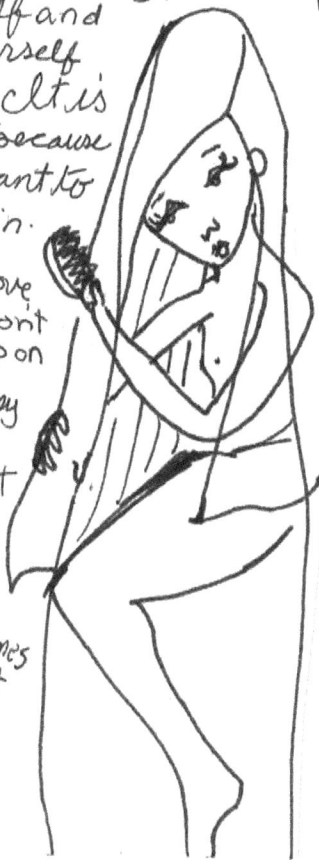

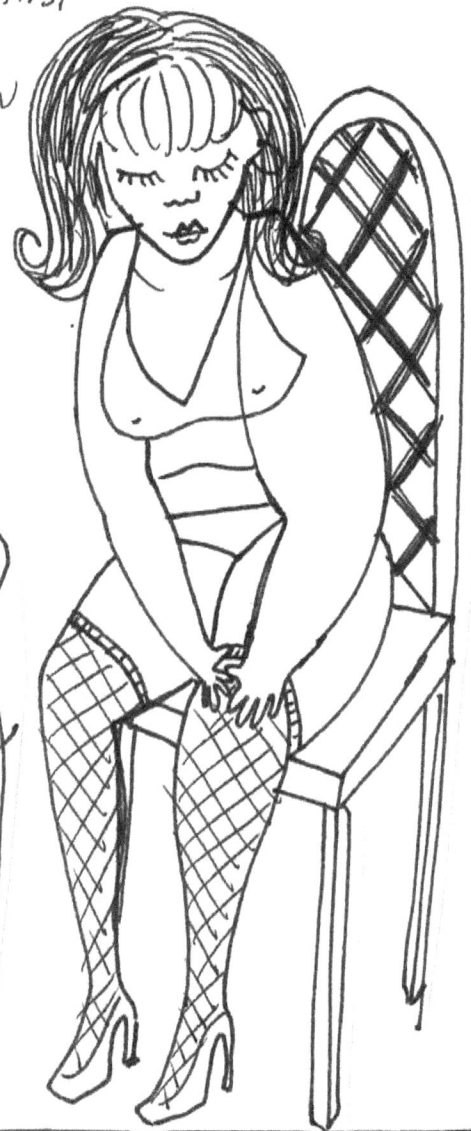

The Sadness is coming back.

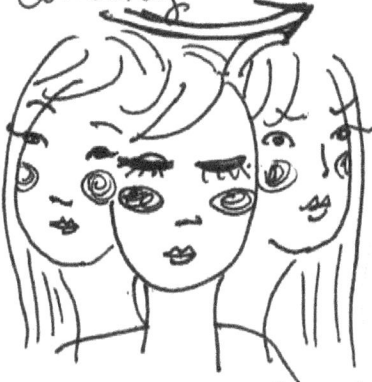

Just 1 Blink and I want to die... again.

Alcohol + Sex = RAPE or Sexual Assault.
Rape is the forced entry onto an unwilling victim.
Rape is also having sex with someone who is Blacked-out
or passed out.
Alcohol is involved in 65% of REPORTED sexual assault
incidents in Alaska.

- Alcohol intoxication makes it easy
for a rapist to overpower or threaten
a victim. Loss of judgement will
let you fuck anyone, any Shmo.
- Rapists look for the drunk ones
who need love. No Game idiotistic
Idiotic Morons are good at getting
someone
Pregnant.

Rape → Part of the Good ol'
College Experience. Get drunk today!

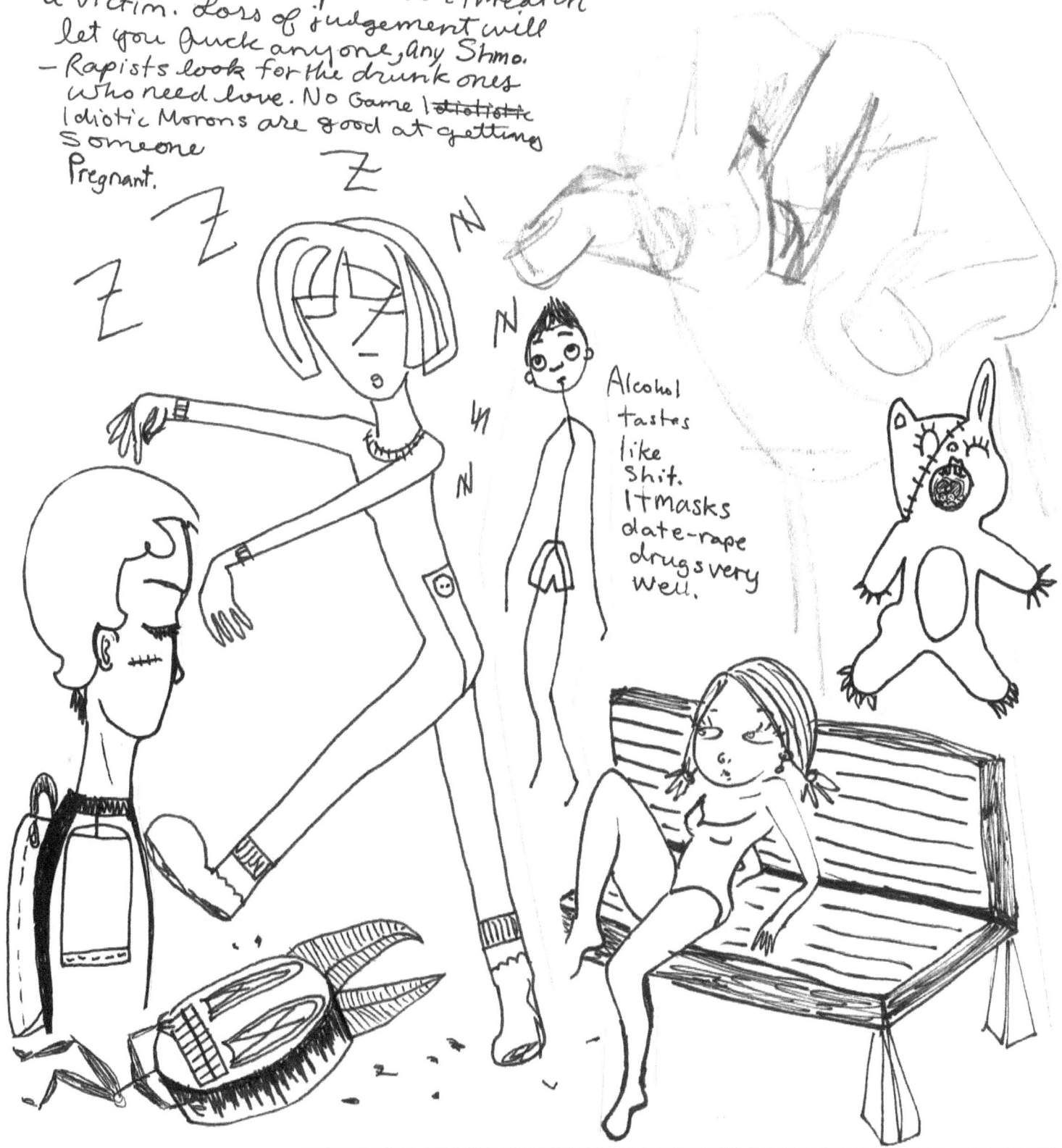

Alcohol
tastes
like
shit.
It masks
date-rape
drugs very
well.

Ladies get in FREE! Have a rape, I mean great night, hehe!
Hey Guys! Lets go get wasted and rape some chicks!
When the party is over, it's raping time. Yay! Hot passed out
drunk girl, score. Rapists may try to say their victim
was sending them "obvious sexual interest" signals all night.
BS. Rapists know who they want and they don't care who
you are. There are NO excuses to rape someone.
Drunk sex is Rape, Buzzed Driving is Drunk Driving.
Getting drunk socially allows everyone to
unleash Lil' Rapey. People let rape happen
to them all the time. The least you can do
is try to make your rapist wear a condom.
Good luck, oh wait, you got drunk too.
Their nerves are numb. They are violent
and they can't feel anything so using
protection is below them, they are too
good for that.
If you are gonna drink anyway,
don't go alone and carry protection.
Don't have sex with people you just met,
don't let them have sex with you.
    Friends don't let friends get raped, ♡
        unless they are getting
        raped themselves.

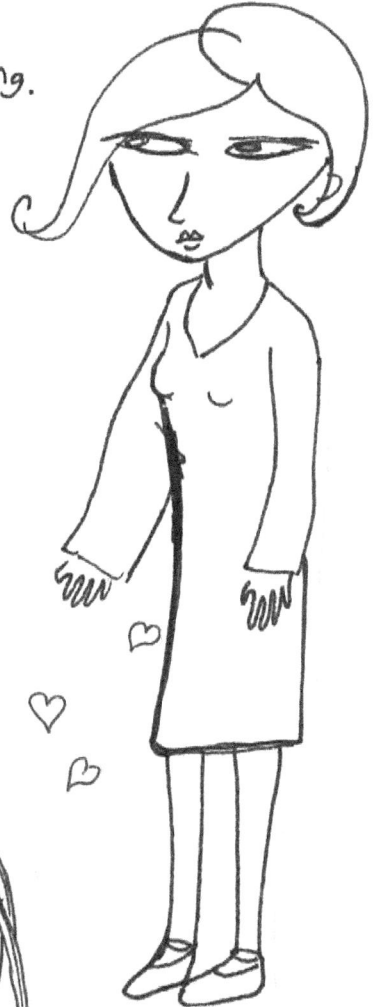

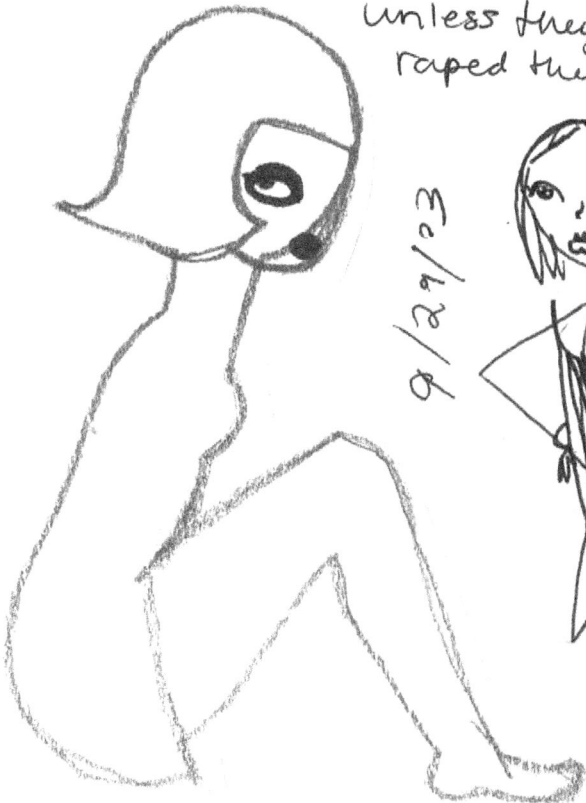

9/29/23

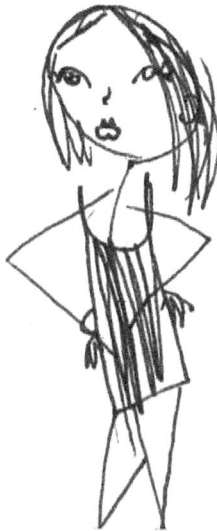

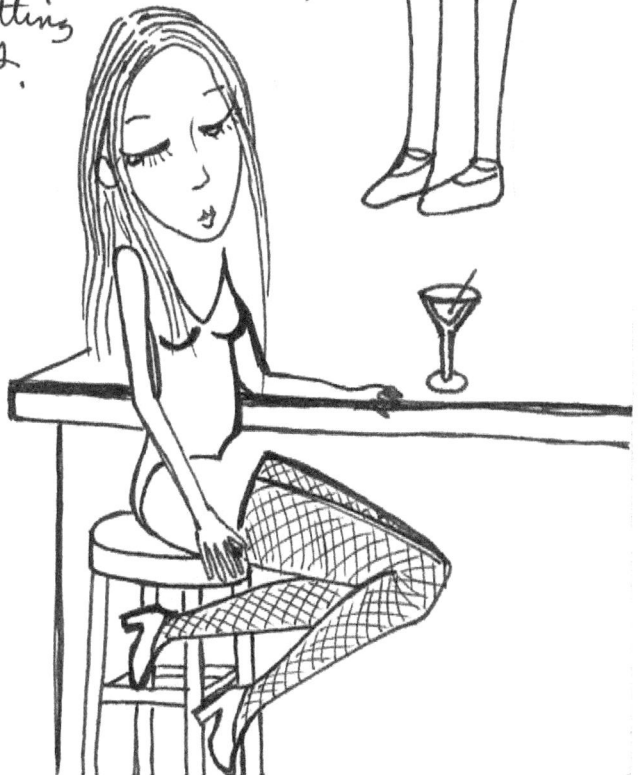

Alcohol & Suicide ♥ To kill ones' self

People who commit suicide are usually victims of depression, anxiety, mental illness and addiction

Anyone can become any of these.

Alcohol is a depressant.

When a person is depressed and feels worthless, adding alcohol makes your feelings feel REAL.

When you Black-Out, you don't know what you are doing.

You sob and slobber. Then you feel sorry for ~~themselves~~ yourself. Has anyone ever heard of a sad drunk? Ha. They get angry next. "Poor them, Ohhh, everything is soooo bad, the world is out to get Me, but no one cares about me. <Contradictive much?>

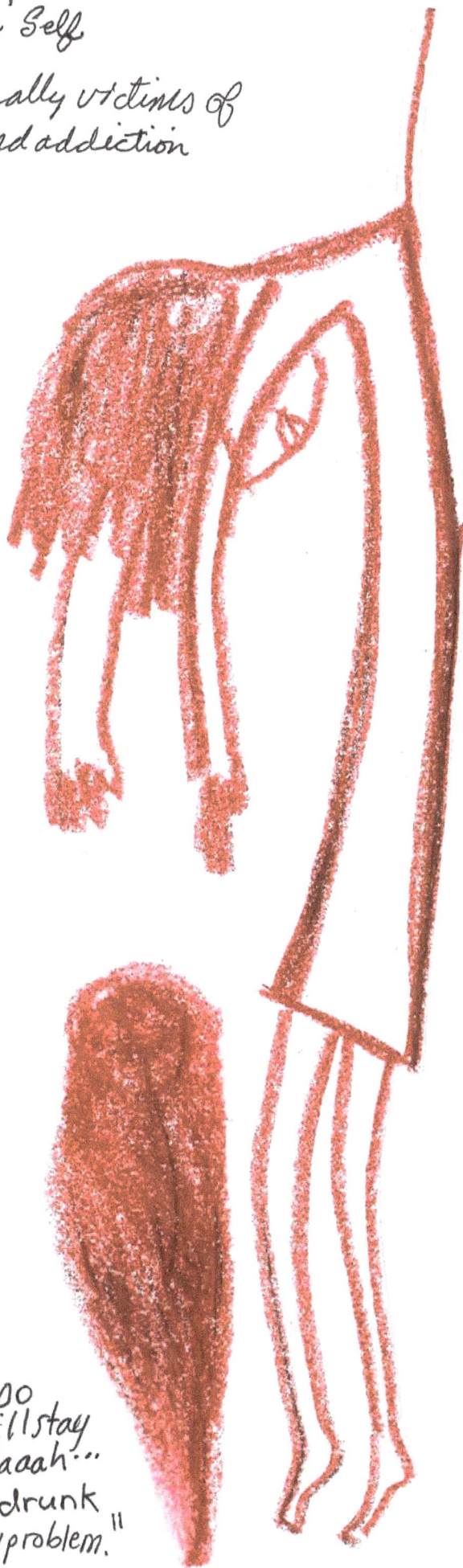

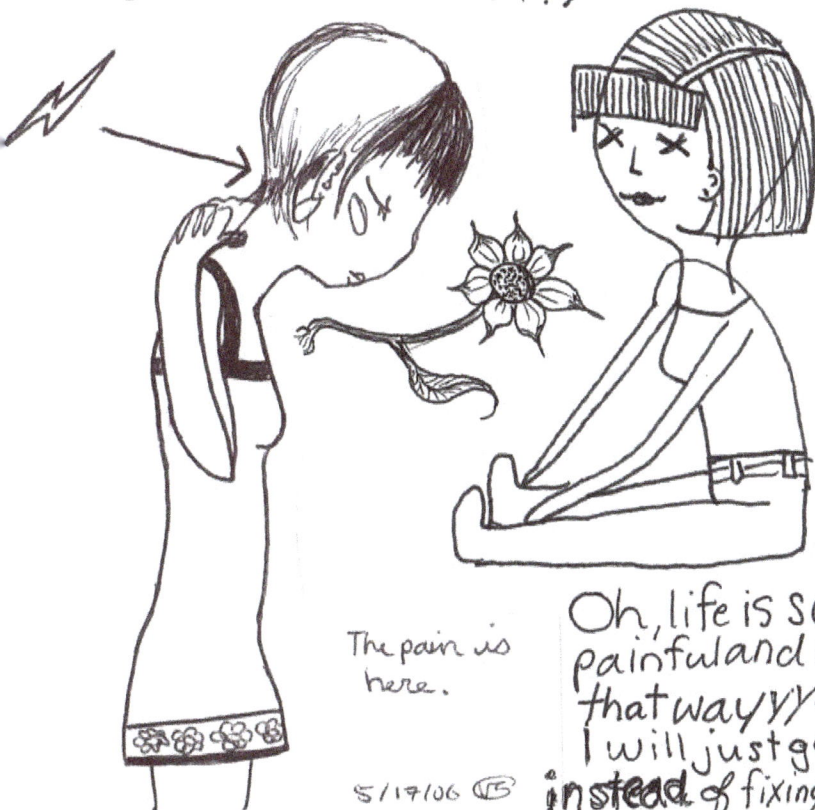

The pain is here.

5/17/06

Oh, life is soooo painful and will stay that wayyy. Waaah... I will just get drunk instead of fixing my problem."

If you need proof, go to an Alcoholics Anonymous. Recovering addicts don't make shit up. There are groups for friends and families of alcoholics. There are groups for suicide survivors, for the people who are left behind when a family member or friend kills themself.

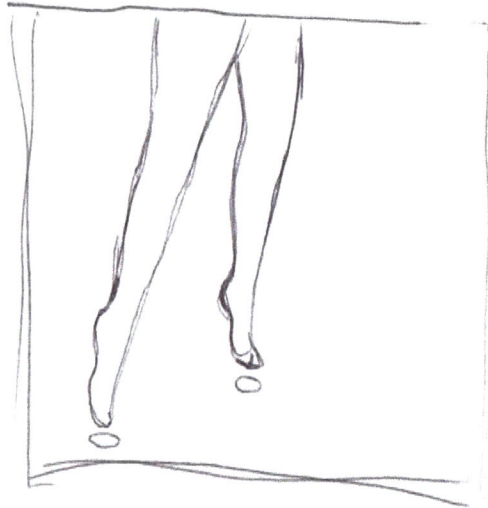

My mother was an alcoholic. My childhood sucked ass and that fucked up my brain and life.

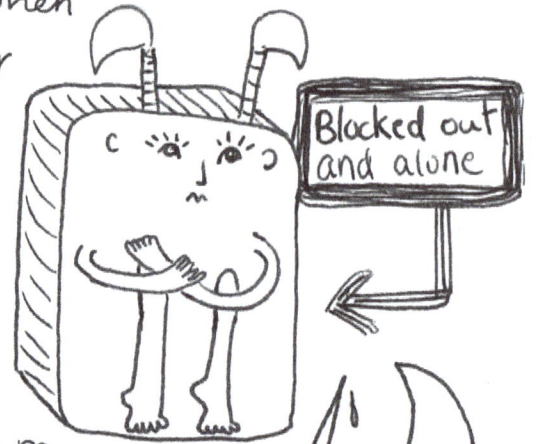

I was a loner and anxious. I never got into alcohol or hard drugs because of this. I have been suicidal for 17 years, and I am here because of that. That is how I survived my suicidality. No alcohol or hard drugs. I lived in my own created reality. One became the other when I was in college; the worse most pointless years of my life. I had toxic relationships toxic thoughs and feelings. I thought things would be better without me.

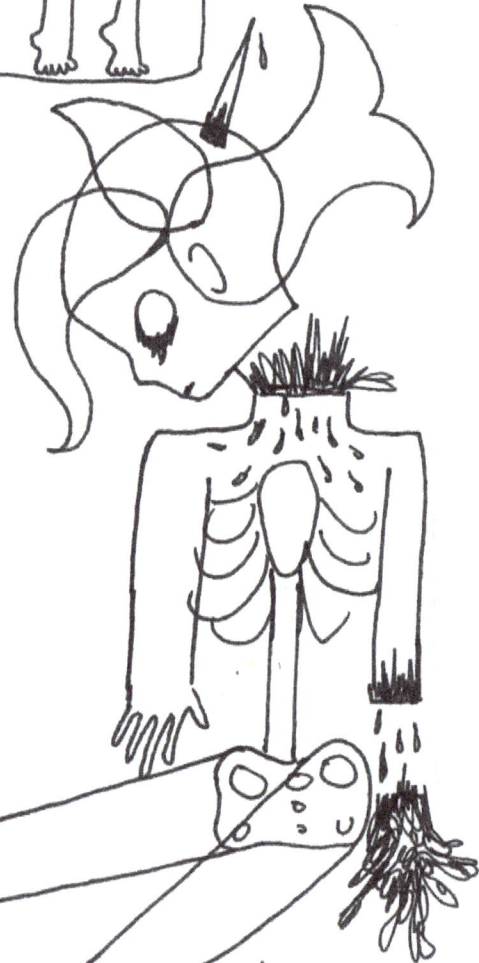

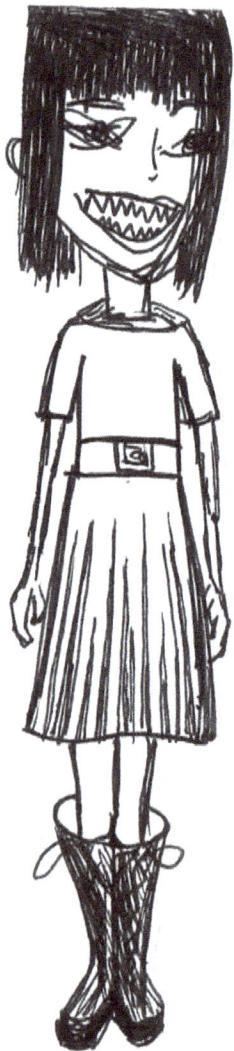

Blocked out and alone

eeew.

NOT TRUE

When a person kills themself they are killing a part of everyone they know.

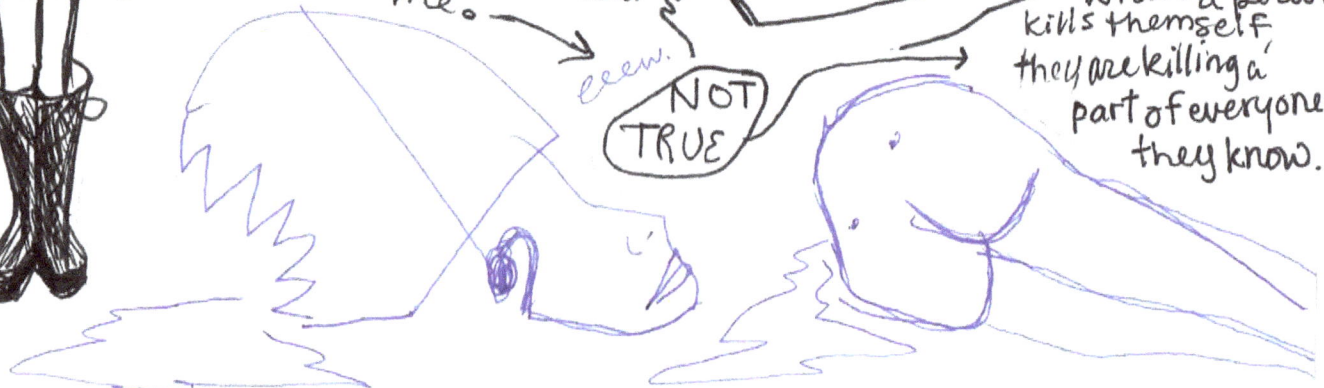

Alcohol + Stupid = ♡ 4EVER

The possibilities for doing stupid shit when you are drunk is endless. People get in accidents and people die. Emergency rooms are full on weekends and so is the mental health floor.

People commit physical and emotional damage by: — Drunk...

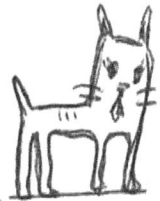

* Moving
* Talking
* Sex (Rape)
* Filming
* Photographing
* Dialing
* Text/sexting
* Social networking

When a person is drunk, they are _not_ themselves. People say and do devastating things that they "would _never_ do if they were sober." That excuse is BS. You can't say sorry for raping someone or committing suicide. Emotional damage takes a long time to heal. What is said is said, what is done is done. You cannot undo these. The _earlier_ you realize that alcohol is Extremely addictive and can easily ruin lives, you can stop drinking or never start.

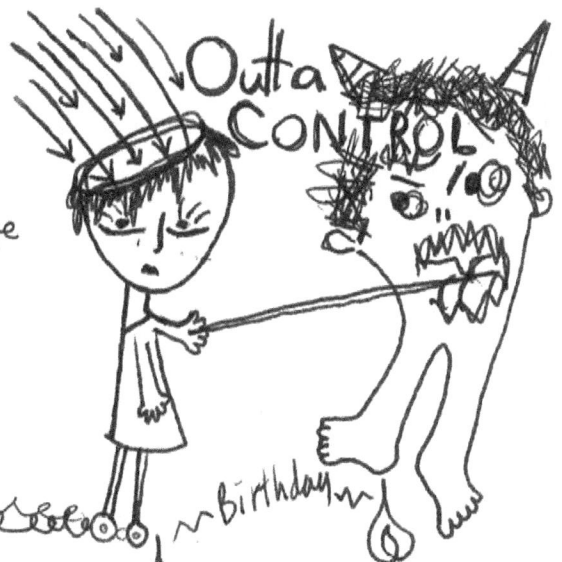

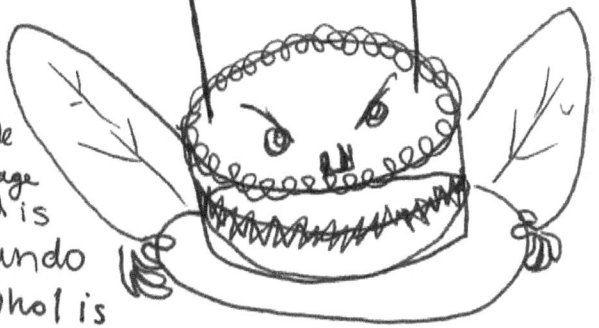

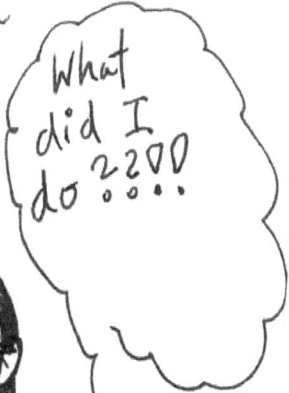

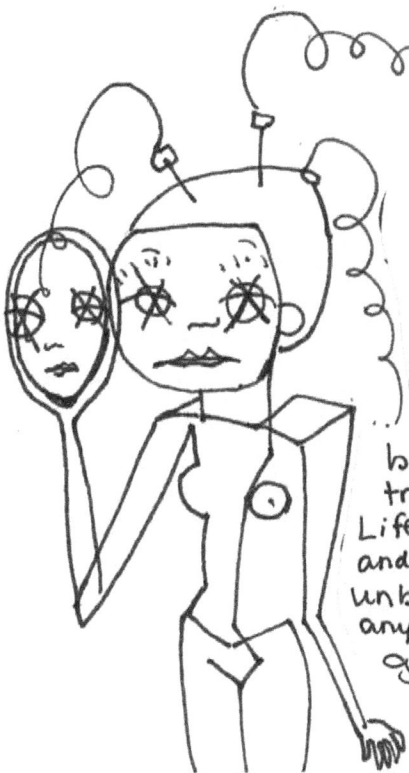

Outta CONTROL

~Birthday~

I hate to sound campy, but it is true. Real Life is scary and can be unbelievable anything, good or bad.

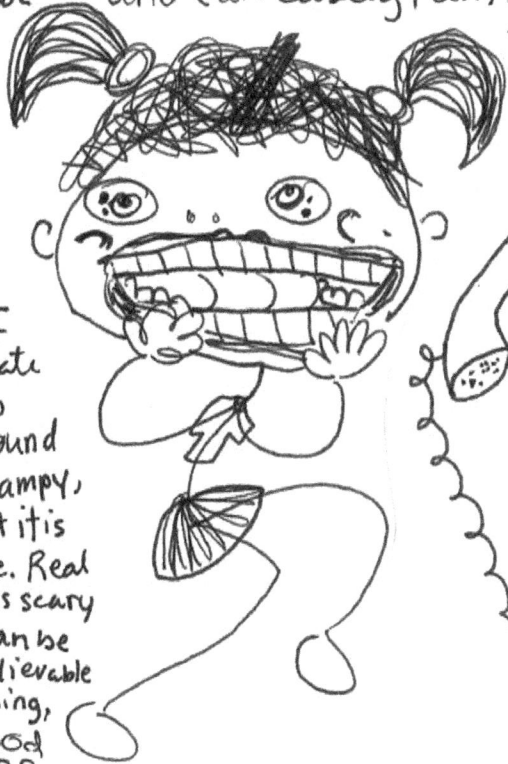

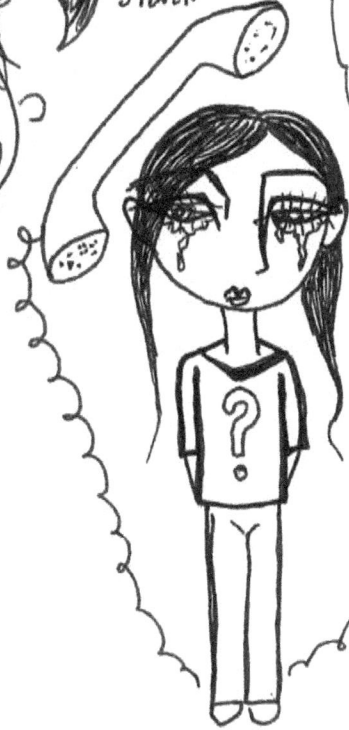

What did I do?!?!?!

DUI → Driving Under the Influence
Drunk Driving

Who is the least drunk to drive?
Who is the best drunk driver?

fly fly fly fly fly fly fly fly fly fly fly fly fly fly fly fly fly

Vehicle accidents are the #1 killer of young adults. Young adults do not have enough experience to have a "gut reaction" as a result. Drunk drivers are over-confident, too slow, driving aggressively or being obviously IMPAIRED.

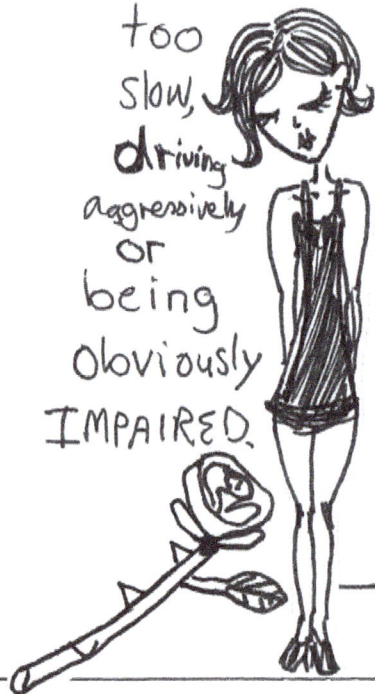

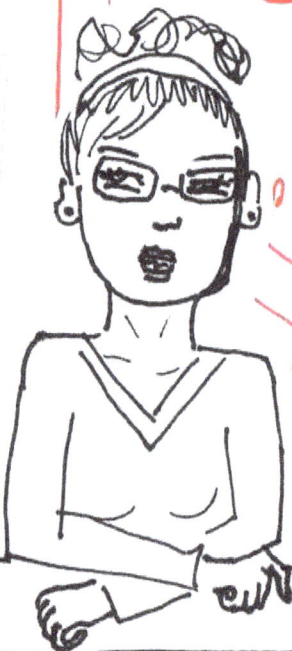

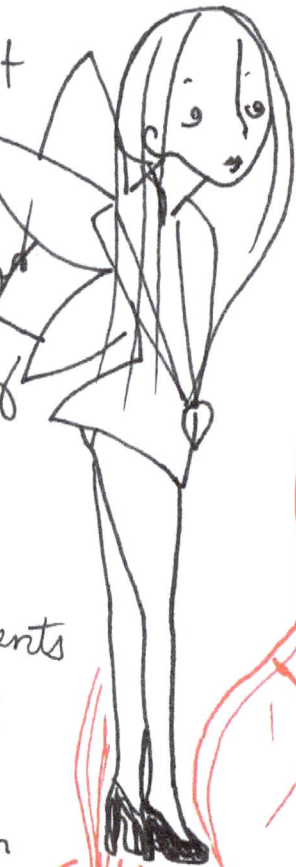

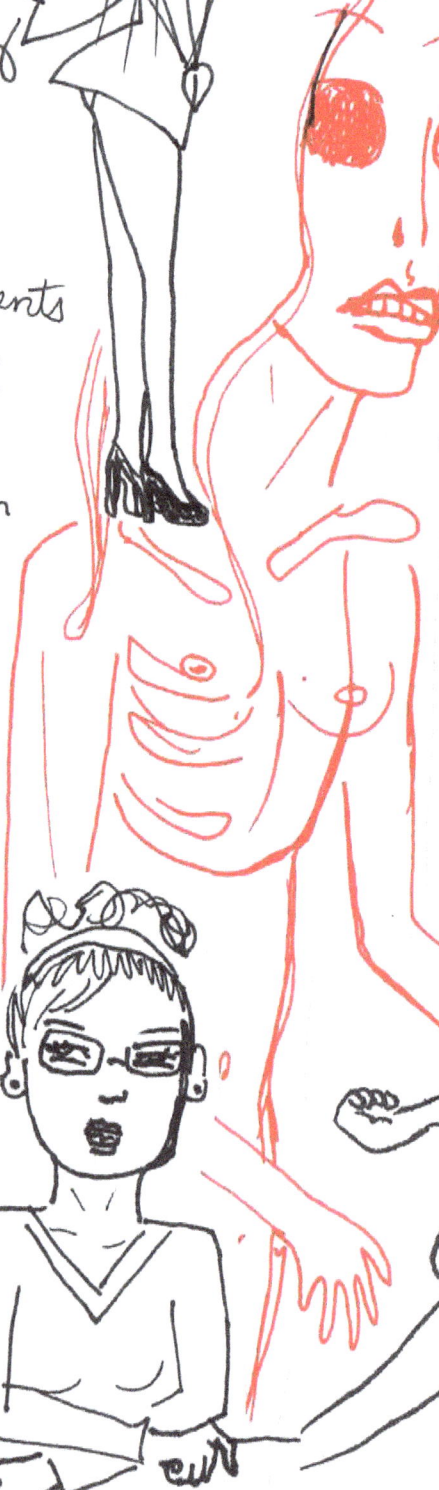

When you live in a small town, everybody you know finds out. They will tell you they saw you pulled over or saw you in the paper. People get bored and that is what they do, they look for people they know, or know of.

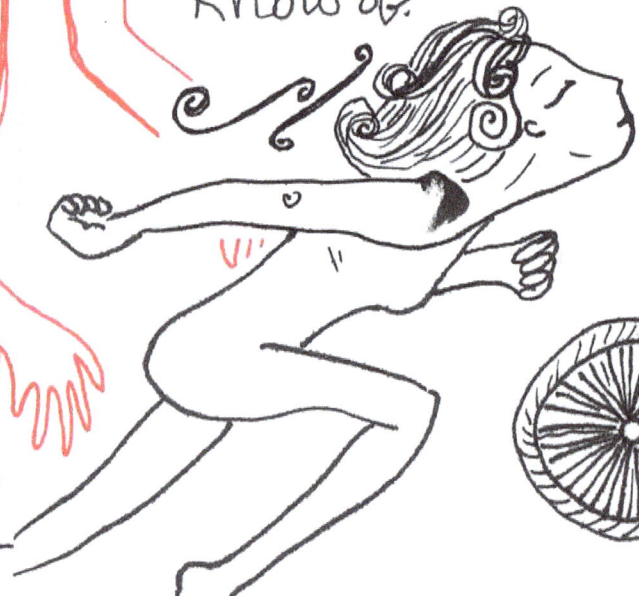

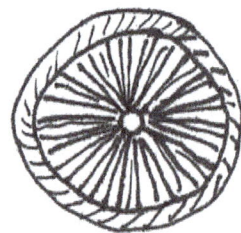

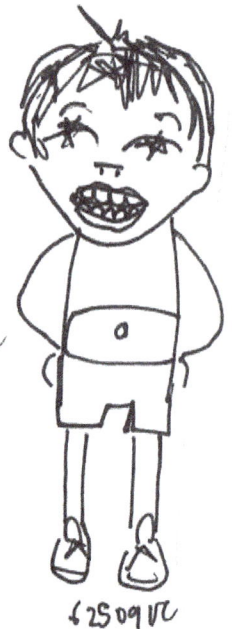

6 25 09 VC

People drive drunk all the time. They think they are actually pretty good at it. They always get caught (or caught again) eventually. By then, they have already caused damage. Drunk drivers ruin property, total vehicles, and they ruin peoples lives by killing or seriously maiming them "on accident." They often get charges for manslaughter, 2nd Degree. This is a lighter sentence than murder or premeditated murder. Justice is not served in our law system. Any person who ingests alcohol is willingly giving up control of their judgement. That means they can commit any crime and get off on a light sentence of a couple of months and a couple years of → PROBATION

Uh. Im trying.

62409 VL

Because the perpertrator was drunk

And "didn't know what they were Doing."

Why is it never "their fault"?

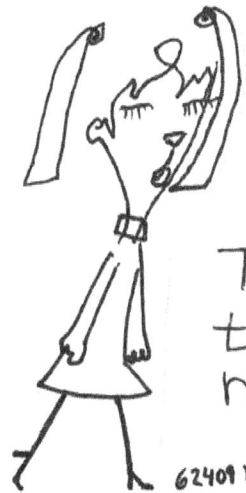

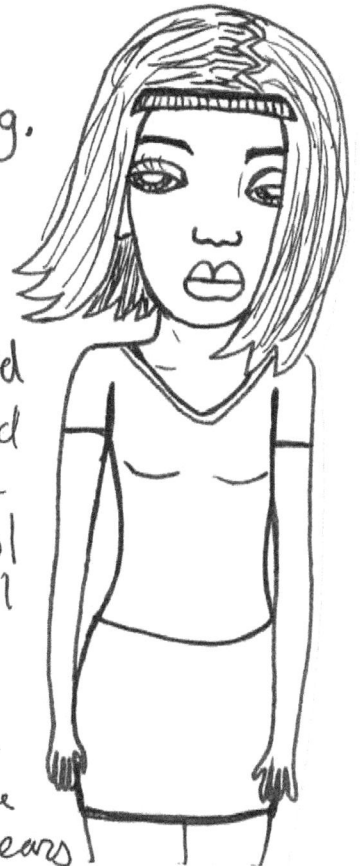

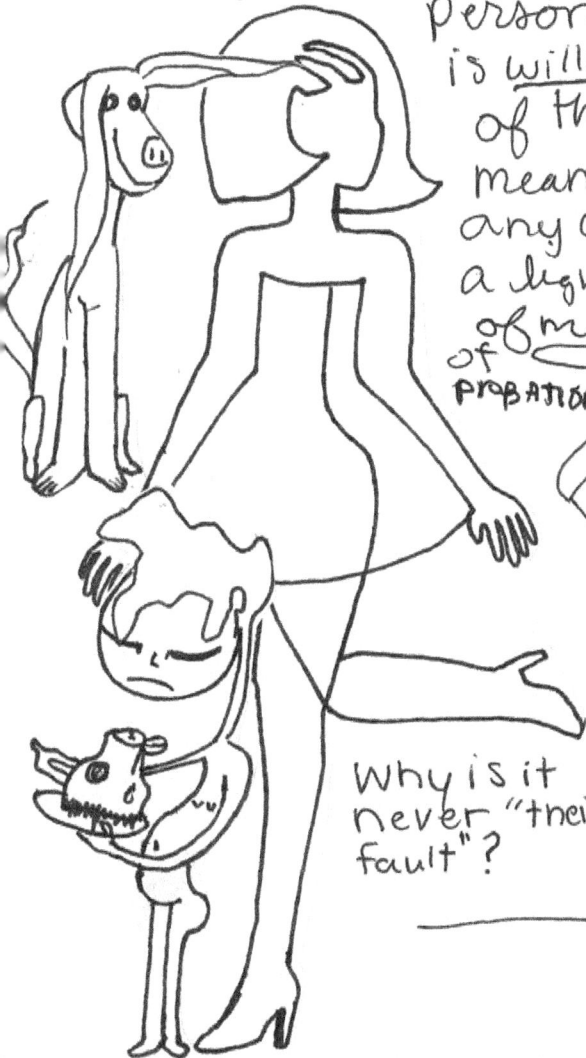

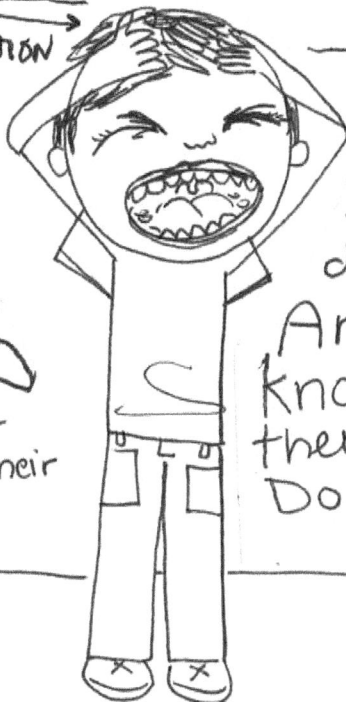

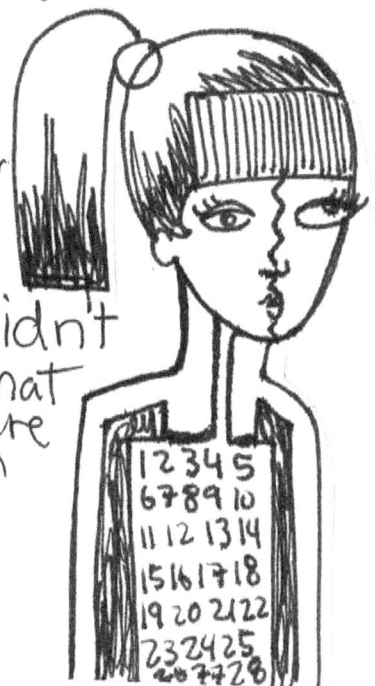

12345
678910
11 12 13 14
15 16 17 18
19 20 21 22
23 24 25
26 27 28

They go free,
someone you
love is dead;
Then they get
Caught again or kill a
couple more people, because
THEY CONTINUE TO DRINK ALCOHOL,
The same fucking thing that got
them where they are in the first place.

ACK YOU GOT ME!!!!

Driving
Drunk is
like this:
- Think of being
so tired you can't focus.
- Then, shut your brain
OFF.
- Put on a pair of goggles
and fill them with
water. Your world is
a watery vertigo.
- Shut down your
nerves, so you are
numb and
painfree.
- Throw out your judgement
and respect for human
life.
- Drive way too fast and
over-correct until you
seriously injure or kill
yourself or someone else.

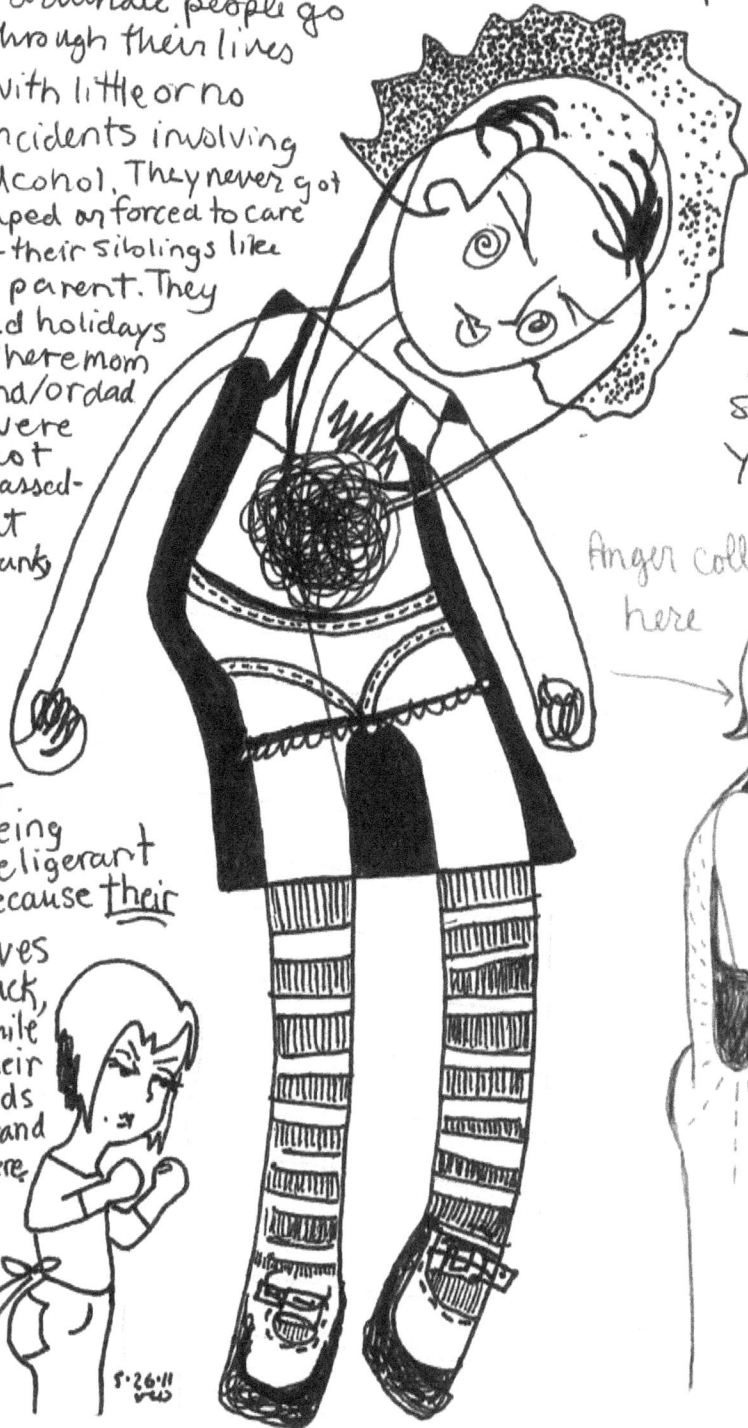

Fortunate people go
through their lives
with little or no
incidents involving
alcohol. They never got
raped or forced to care
for their siblings like
a parent. They
had holidays
where mom
and/or dad
were
not
passed-
out
drunks

Or.
being
beligerant
because their
lives
suck,
while
their
kids
stand
there.

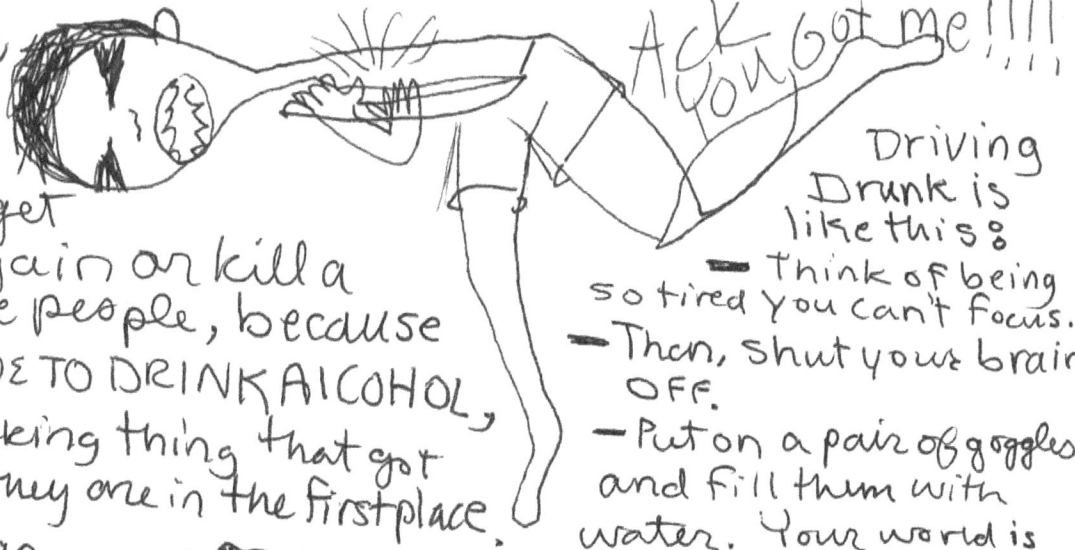

5-26-11 VCB

Anger collects
here

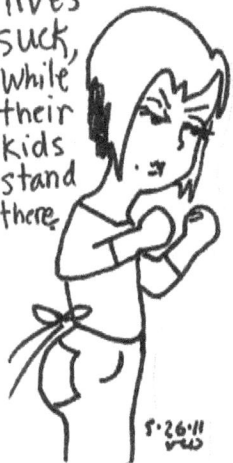

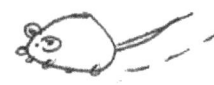

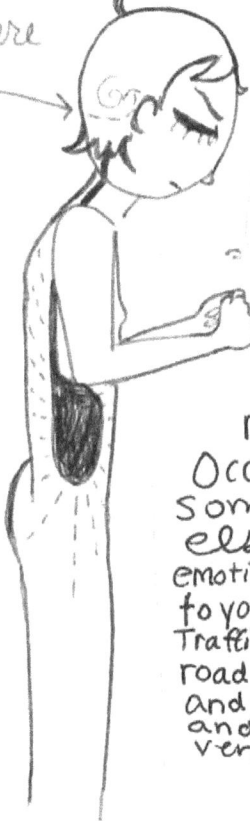

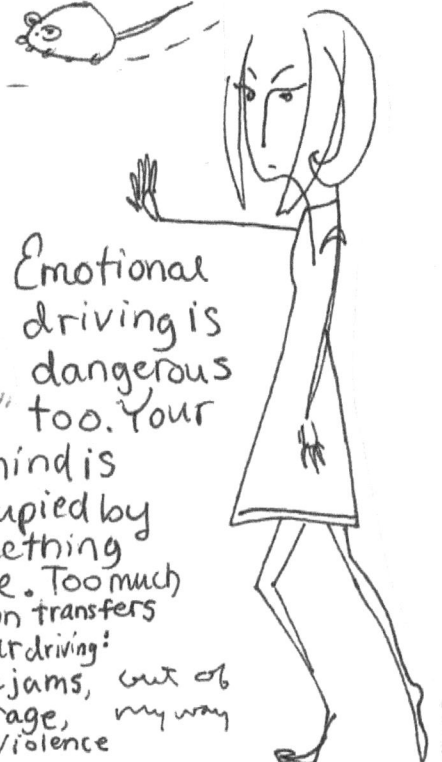

Emotional
driving is
dangerous
too. Your
mind is
occupied by
something
else. Too much
emotion transfers
to your driving:
Traffic jams,   out of
road rage,   my way
and violence
and
vengence.

8/18/09 VCB

5-5-07 VC

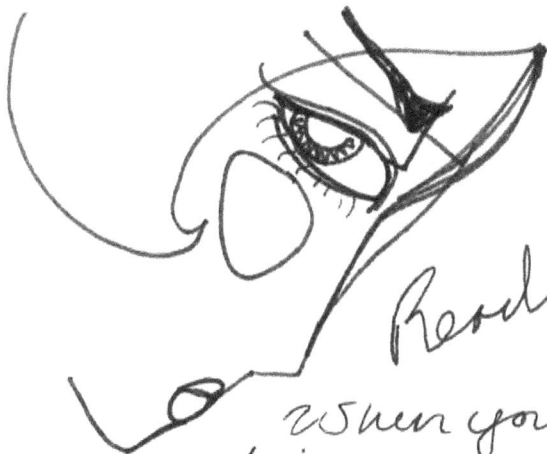

Ready set GO!!! hahahaha

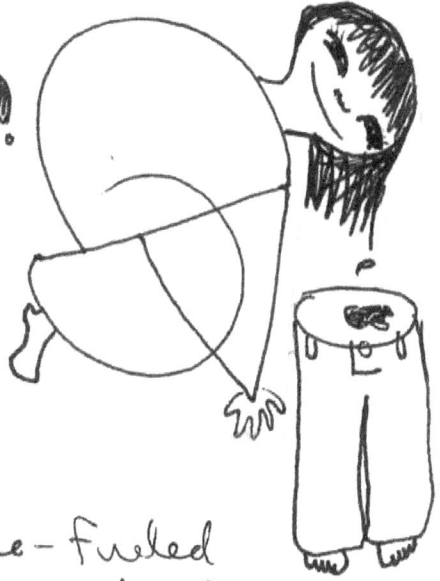

When you drive a vehicle, You are the operator of a gasoline-fueled internal combustion engine in over two tons of structure. You control off and on, stop and go, speed, direction, and destination. When you are on a substance that alters any of these, thats when the shit hits the fan. 3 days in jail and money money money. No more PFD Required classes, probation officers, and making money to pay enormous fines and penalties.

Drunk drivers are in a system that makes it easy to get busted. Alcohol establishments are usually in places you have to transport yourself to. You can take a taxi or drive most people drive. You never want to leave your truck or car there overnight Soo...

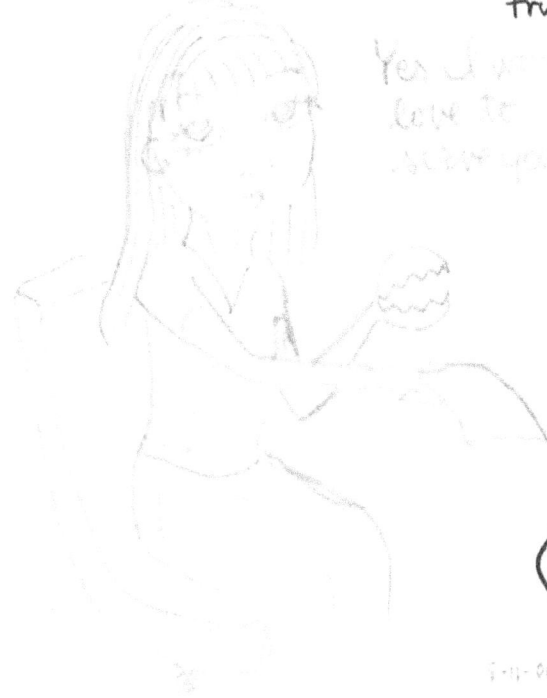

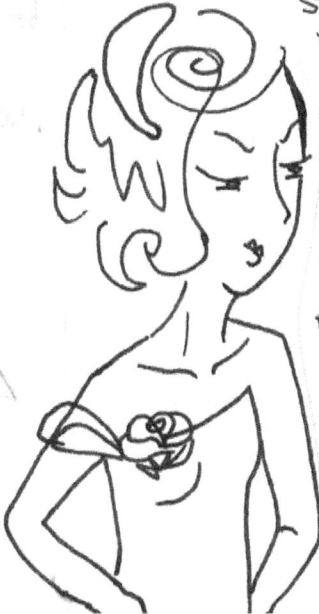

you risk it. "IT" means everything. Job, jail license Freedom.

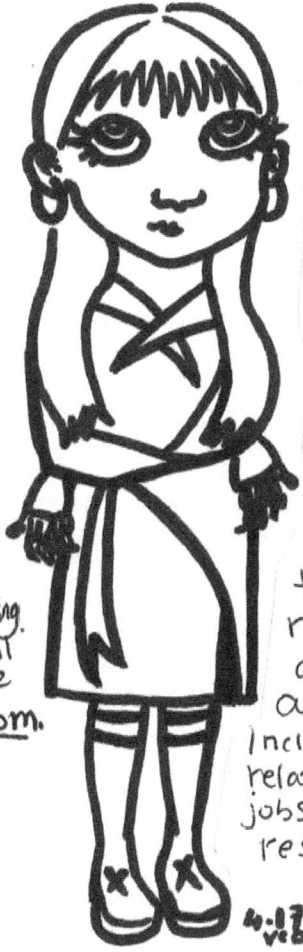

People can't deal with their lives, So they drink. That way, they do not care about anything. Including kids, relationships, jobs, and responsibilities.

Our government ♡Loves♡ it when people drink and smoke. They pretend to care about the wrong things, like drugs. Alcohol and tobacco products are taxed because they are legal and can be taxed. Government also loves the social control aspect. Alcohol consumers are easy prey for law. They break laws and cause mahem, but law inforcement officers are good at what they do. They use tricks to get people to convict themselves. People who drink alcohol get in trouble easily, they get caught easily. Grouse get wasted off of rotten cranberries and lose their survival instincts. You can kill them with a rock.

Drunk dumbasses get in trouble and get a good old criminal record and probation. They keep drinking and screw up again until the drunk trouble-maker goes to prison. Being a felon is not easy. You are kept track of and nobody will hire you. So, the governments gets rich off of addicts; drugs, you screw up again and persecute your freedoms away. Poverty social class control, cheap, available and accepted.

yes sir. yes ma'am.

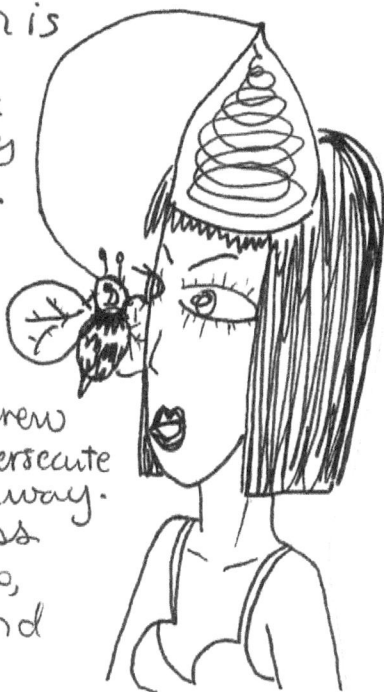

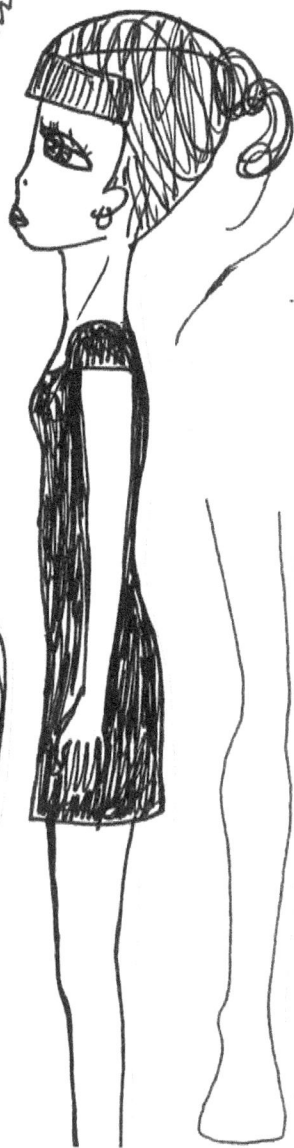

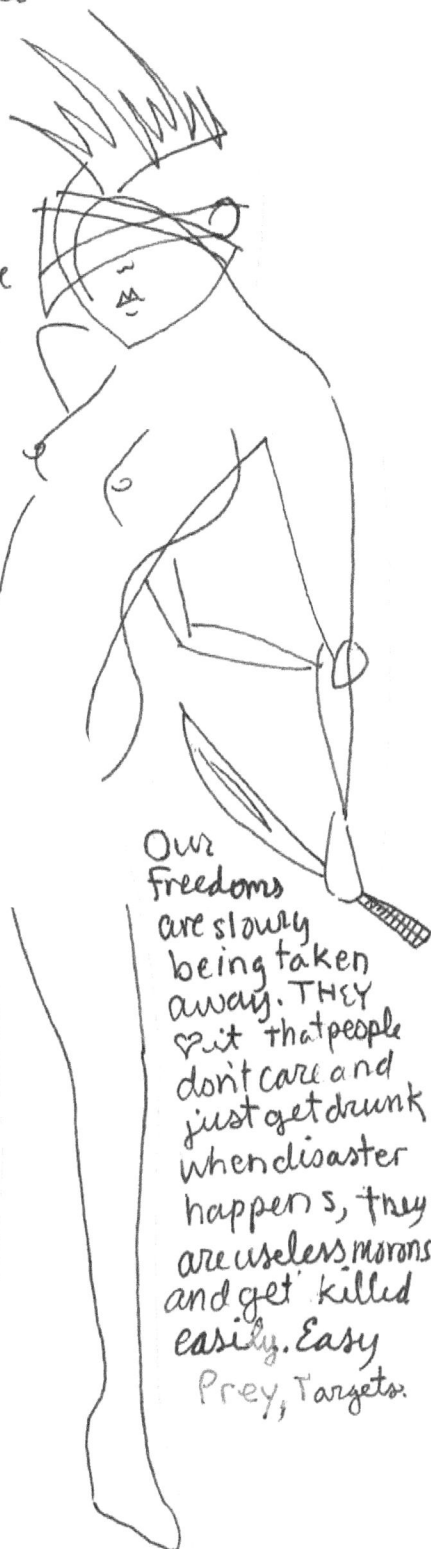

Our Freedoms are slowly being taken away. THEY ♡it that people don't care and just get drunk. When disaster happens, they are useless morons and get killed easily. Easy Prey, Targets.

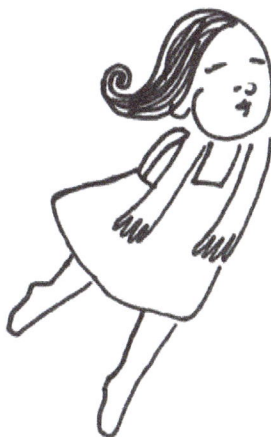

122808 Vc

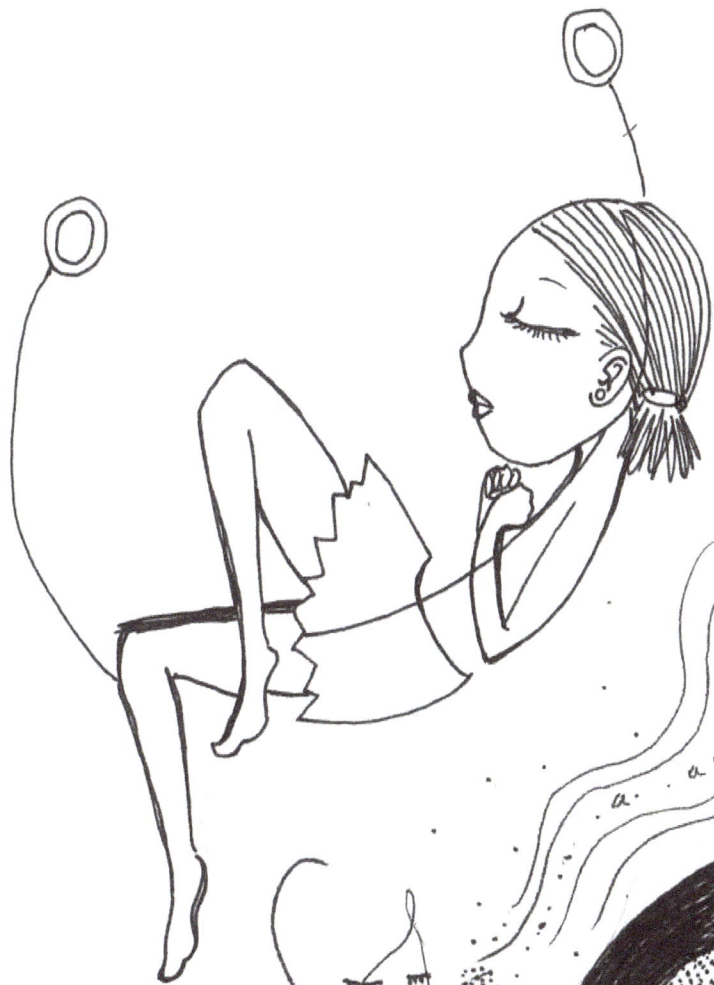

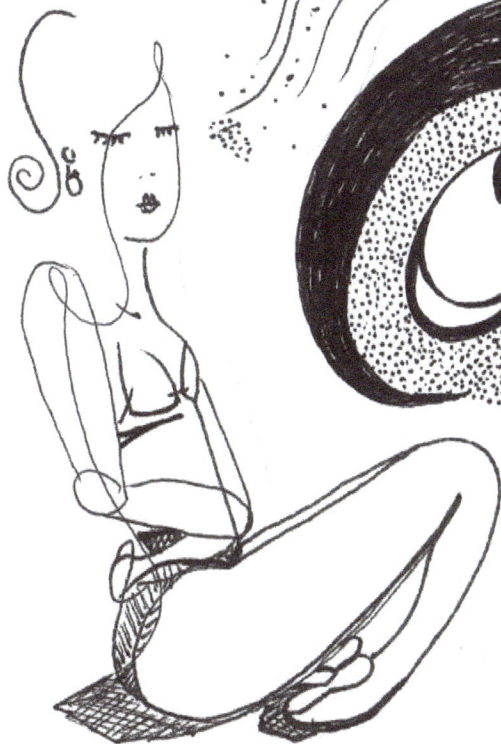

2.7.09 Vc

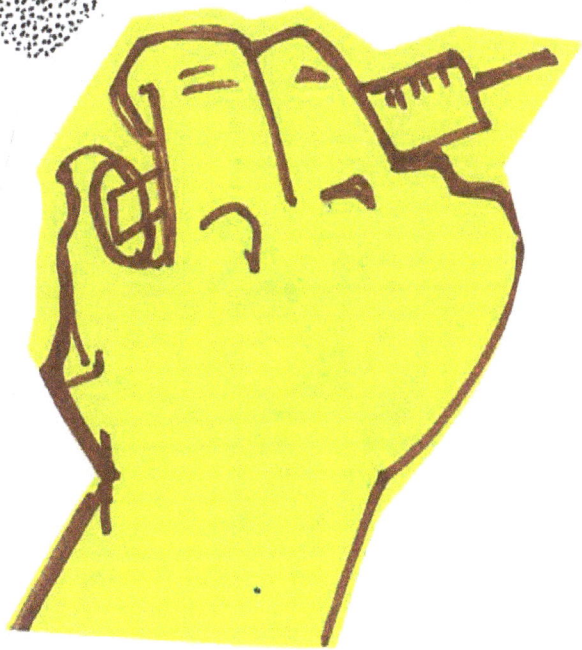

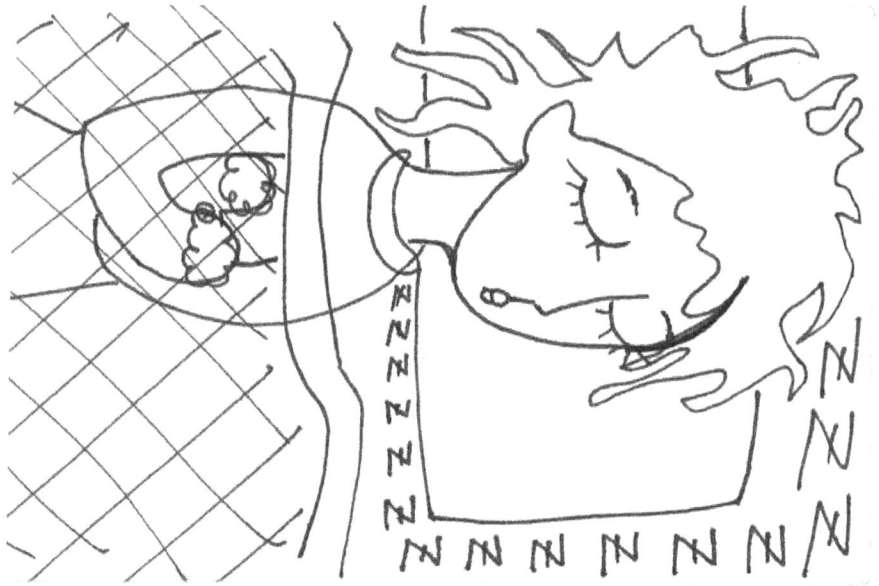

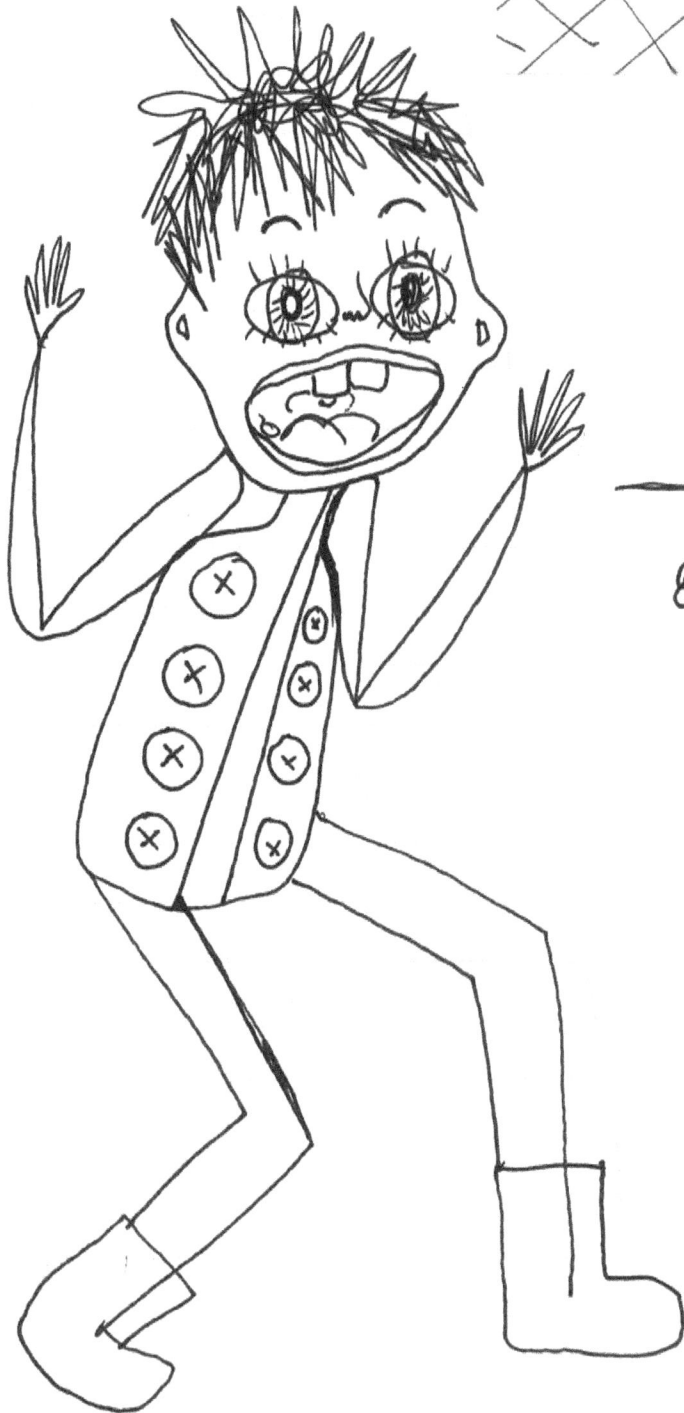

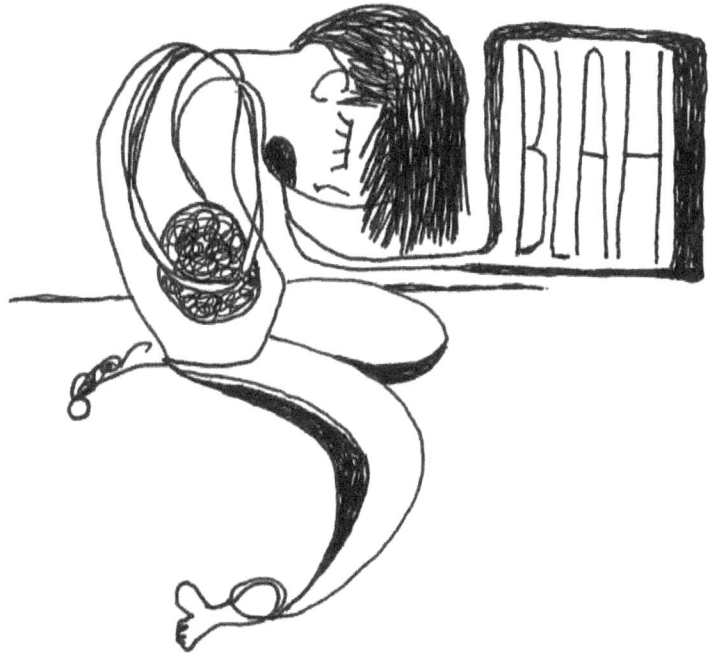

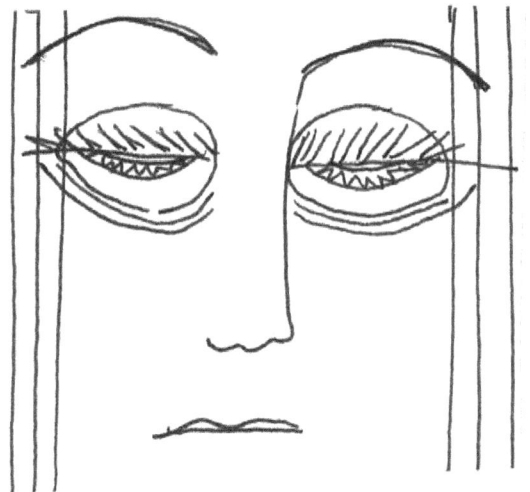

Opiates

Hello, my name is Mike. I am Val (the author)'s husband. I am writing the section on opiates because unfortunately I am the expert on this subject. I'm not saying that I know everything about them but, I do know alot. I will do my best to educate you and pass on what I've learned. I'm a recovering opiate addict and will be for the rest of my life. I was in my teens when I started to do opiates. I'll get back to my story in a minute. First I would like to explain what opiates are for those of you who may not know. An opiate is any drug that is derived from the opium poppy. These include: Heroin, morphine, oxycontin, oxycodone (percoset, vicodin, percodan), dilaudid, + fentanyl to name a few. Opiates have become so widespread due to their ability to relieve pain very well. I know many people who became addicts because of a surgery they had or cancer. The doctors give them large quantities of strong opiate pain-killers then just cut them off after a long period of time. This causes them to have withdrawals. The withdrawals from opiates are horrific! Its very difficult to explain how bad they are to someone who has never experienced them. Symptoms include: Extreme body aches + pain, fever, chills, cold-sweats, shakes, nausea, vomiting, diarhea, fatigue, insomnia, "creepy crawly" feeling in your skin, as well as several other bad things. This feeling is so bad that you will do absolutely anything to get more opiates so it goes away, BAM! .... addiction. I myself started to do them with my friends. We had already been heavy "partiers" and drinkers for years. We would do coke, meth, and whatever when we drank. When they would hand me a straw and say "do this line", I didn't think twice about it. After a while I started noticing that I felt really shitty during school. I didn't figure it out until one day I came home and they gave me a line of this stuff and then I felt all better. Oh crap! I'm addicted. What they had been giving me was oxycontin, usually just called oxy. After I had that realization I tried to get out. My father had passed away several months before that and I had some money from his life insurance. I used some of it to move out of town into my own little cabin. I still had the same friends though so it didn't work as well as I hoped. I even went so far as to go out to West Virginia and live with my aunt. However, I couldn't get away from myself. My addict brain devised a system to have my friends up here in Alaska send me pills. An addict can justify anything. Anyway, after about a year I got really homesick and came back to Alaska. As soon as I got back my friends had a big fat line of oxy waiting for me. Such good friends, yeah right. Things went from bad to worse. I lied, cheated, and stole all the time to feed my addiction. Anything to keep from being (In withdrawals) sick. I rarely ever got high, I would just get well. Every single day was the same. I would get up

WTF?!

french back dog.

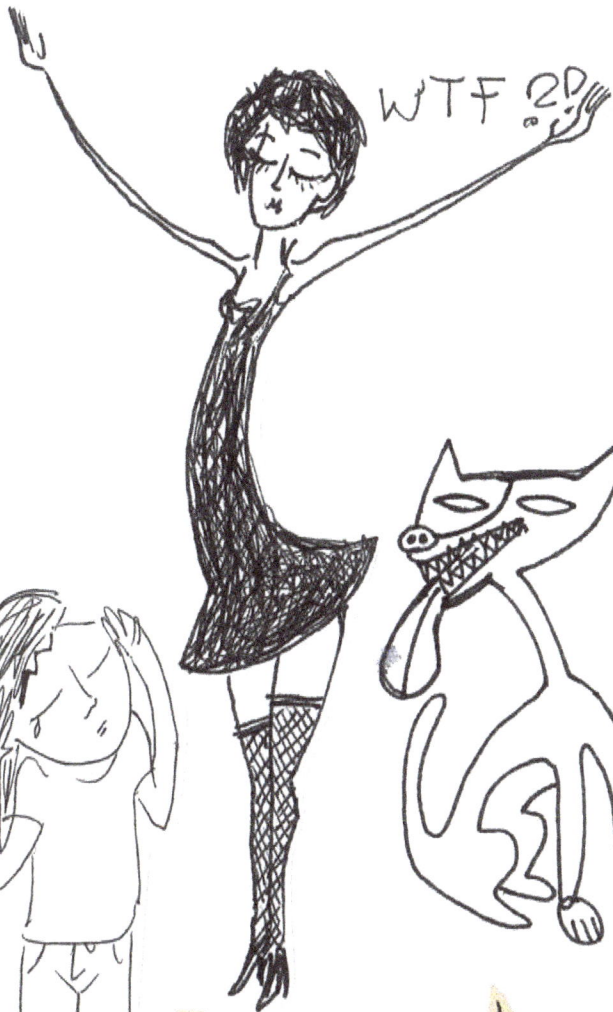

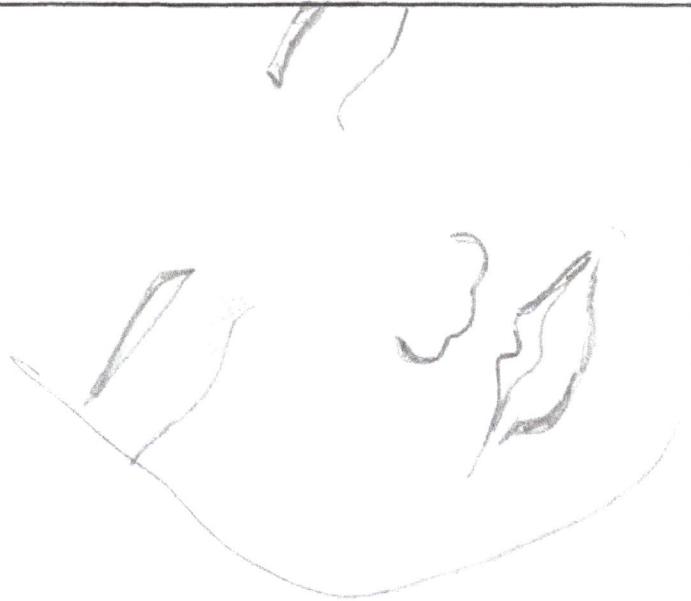

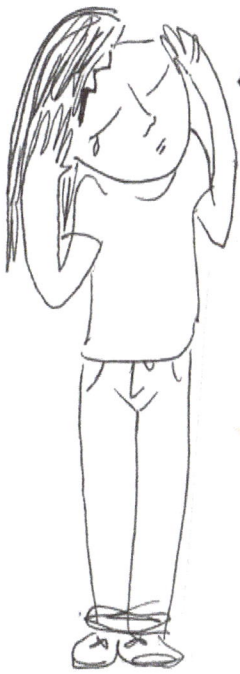

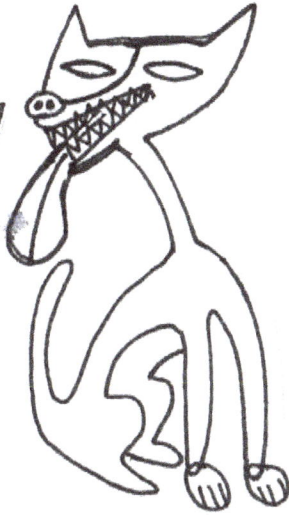

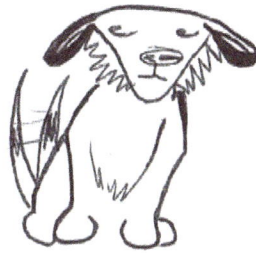

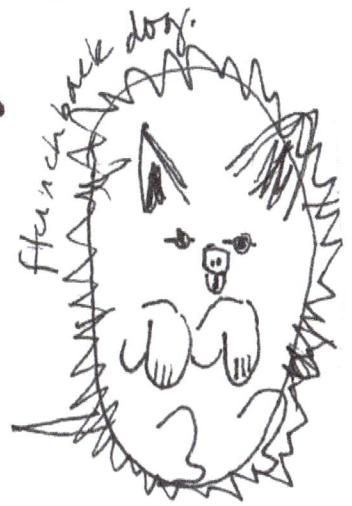

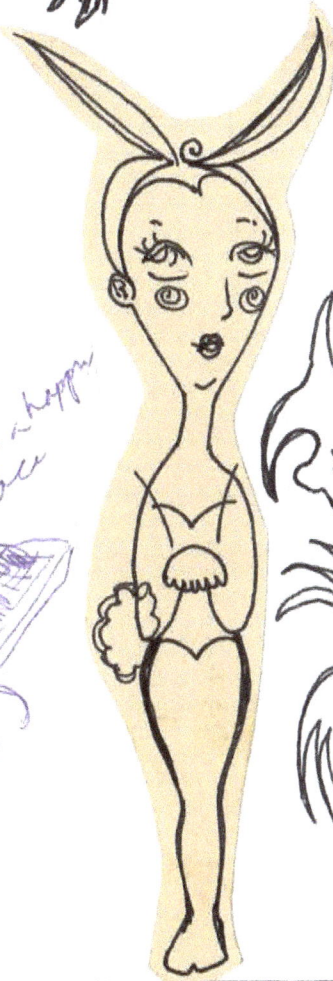

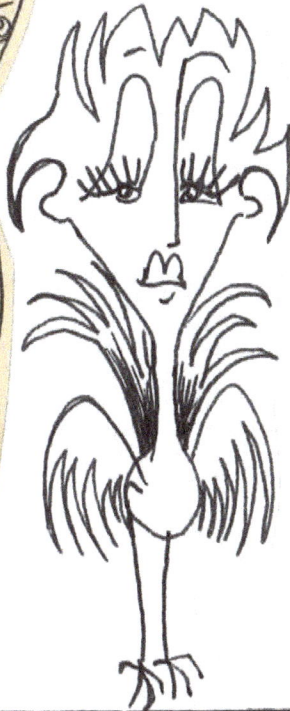

Always planning someones demise.

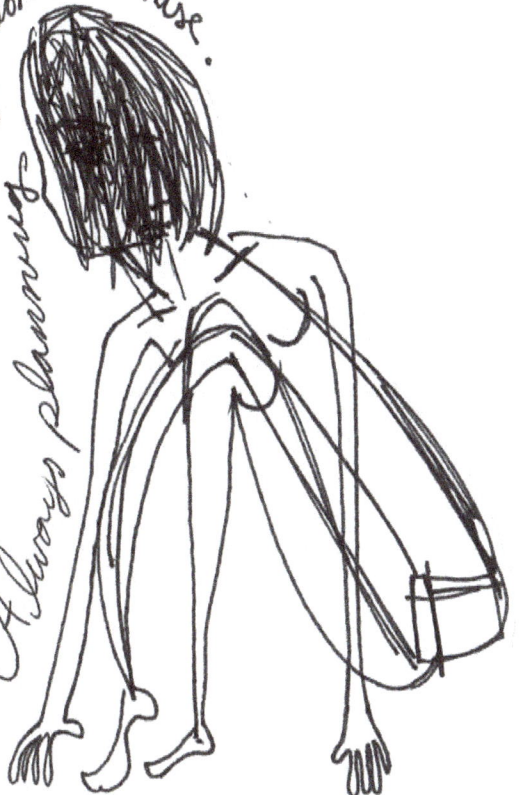

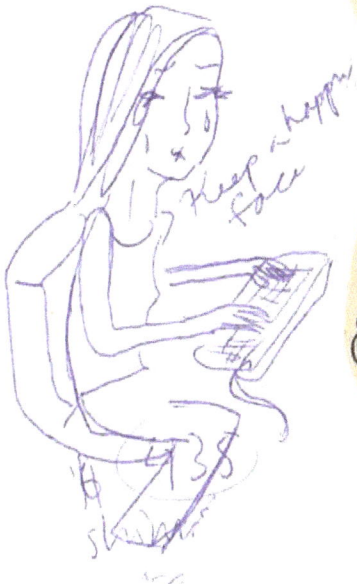

Keep a happy face

stay away from my babybe

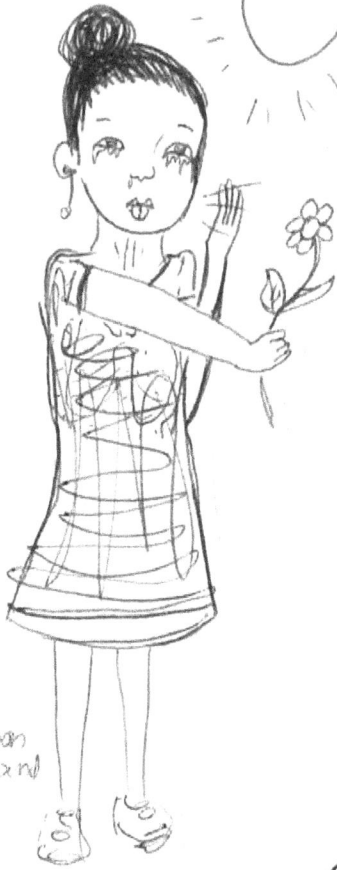

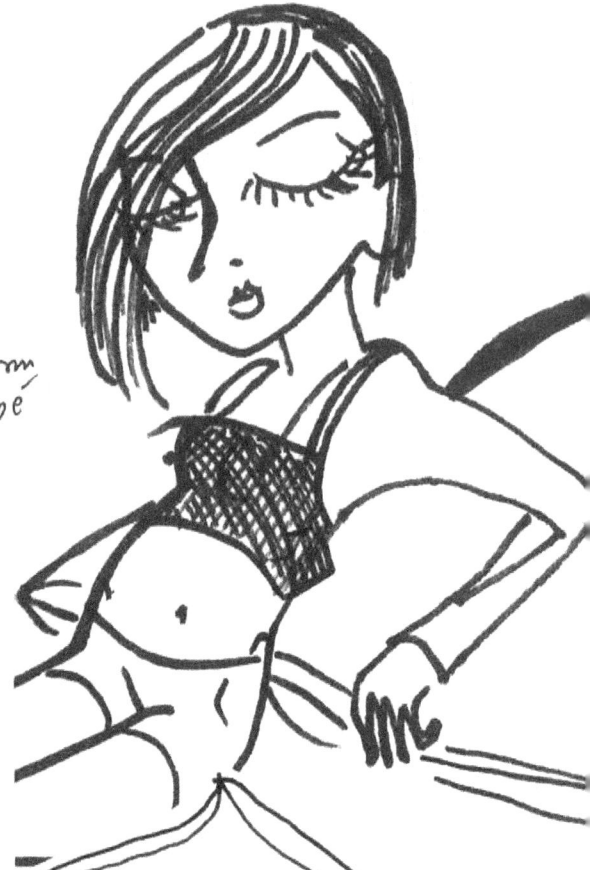

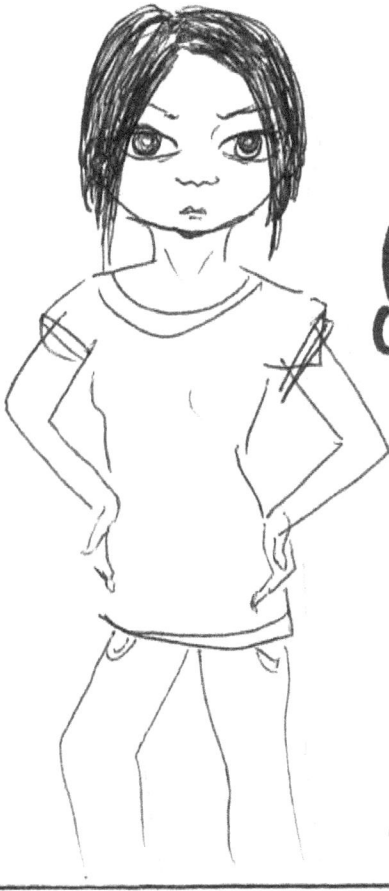

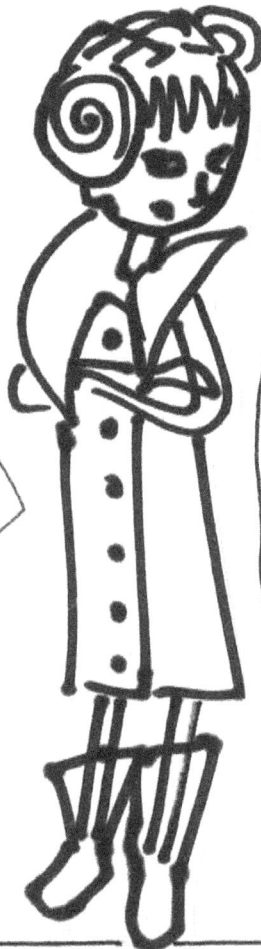

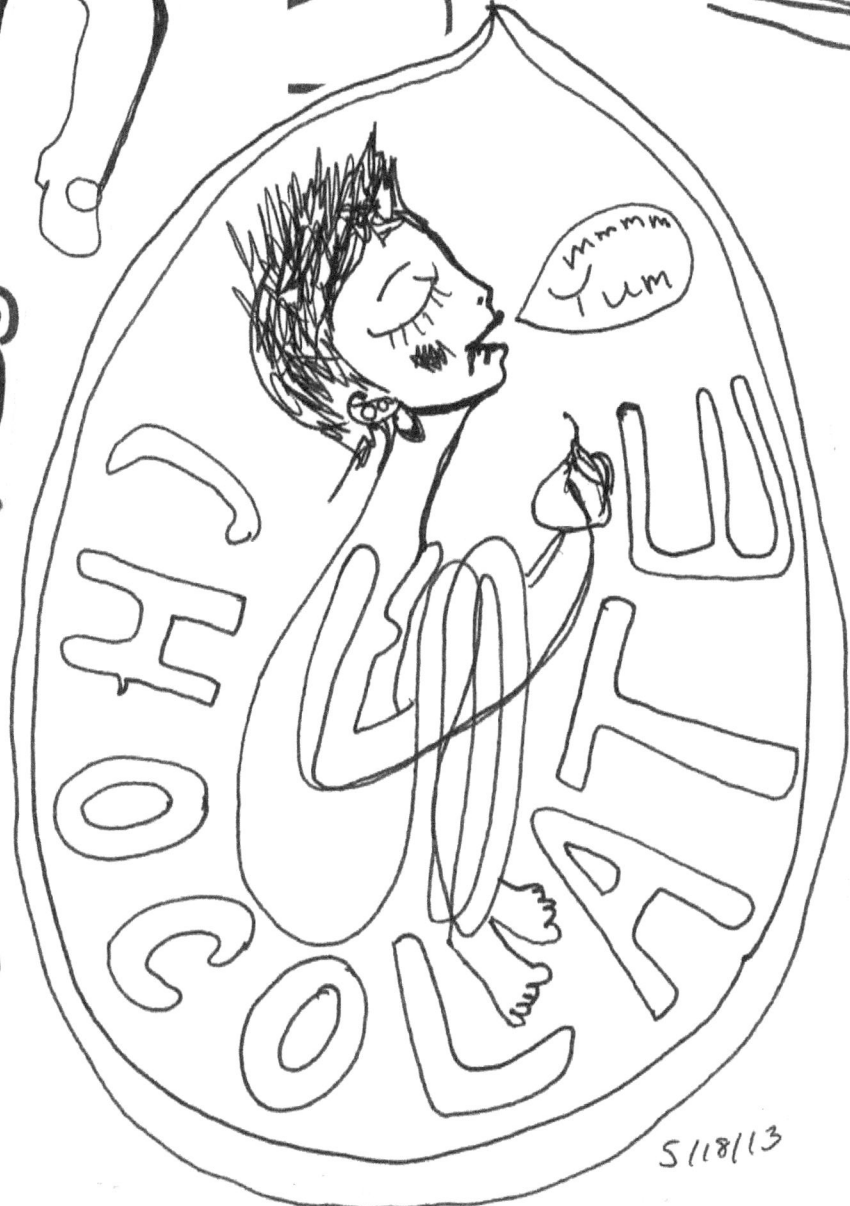

Allergic to certain plants and Sun

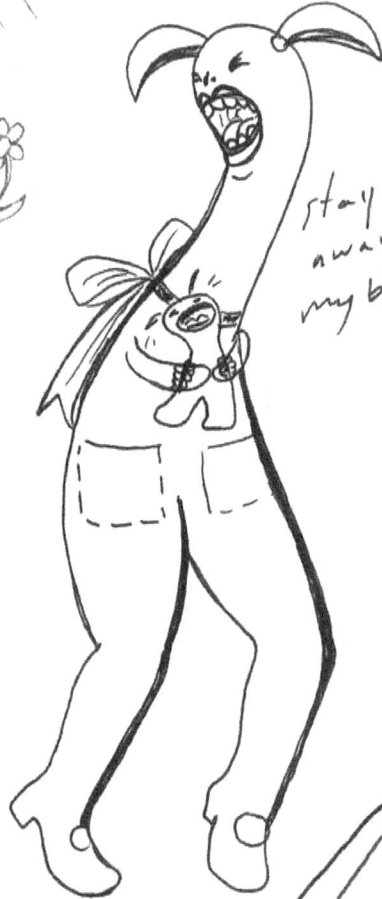

mmmm Yum

CHOCOLATE

5/18/13

feeling like shit and have to come up with some scam to get money, Then I'd have to find the drugs, go get them, and finally use. By this time it was usually late in the day. I would maybe try to get something done or take care of business but, most of the time I wouldn't get anything done, That was my life, Day after day, every day, for seven years. When your an addict your priorities are screwed up. You spend your rent money, or whatever money you get on opiates, (pills or heroin), It's actually the same for most drugs but, I'm focusing on opiates because that's my area of expertise and that's what this chapter is about, You don't pay your bills or buy food or anything that you . should spend your money on. All money is for drugs. This life, the opiate addict's life, is a very sad and harsh reality. Basically a living hell from which there seems to be no escape. The withdrawals that you go through when you don't have any drugs is so bad that you'll do anything to feel better, That's why people lie and steal from the people they love the most. You will do ANYTHING. I have seen some really messed up stuff. It's basically impossible to put the feeling into words to explain it to someone that has never experienced it. It feels like your dying and sometimes you pray for the sweet relief only death can bring. I personally have always thought of suicide as the "bitch way out". Like your giving up because you can't handle life. That's why I never killed myself. My own personal relationship with God and my faith also helped me get through alot. I'm not trying to force religion on you at all. I'm just saying that my beliefs helped me quite a bit. Anyway, it's easy to think that you are doomed for life when your an opiate addict. However, this isn't the case. There usually comes a point in every addict's life when you decide you want help, enough is enough, or your sick and tired of being sick and tired. You can't force someone to change. They have to want it. If you try changing for someone or something else it won't work either. Ultimately you have to be doing it for yourself. You might think you can't change but, you can. If ya want it then you can do it! I was an opiate addict for seven years which was a third of my life by the time I got into treatment. I had heard that there was a methadone clinic in the town where I live. It took me a while to finally decide to apply because I'd heard there was a waiting list + it took months to get in. A friend of mine said to me "the time will go by either way. It's better to be on the list than not.". I finally applied. I had to wait eleven months but, I would meet with one of their counselors every week and knock out some paper work. They even let me go to all the required groups. When I finally got in I had all my stuff done. I will never forget that date! April 7th 2006. Let me back up a bit. You might be asking, "What is methadone. It's a synthetic opiate medication with an opiate blocker in it. Therefore it keeps you well and keeps you from being in withdrawals. Also it blocks the

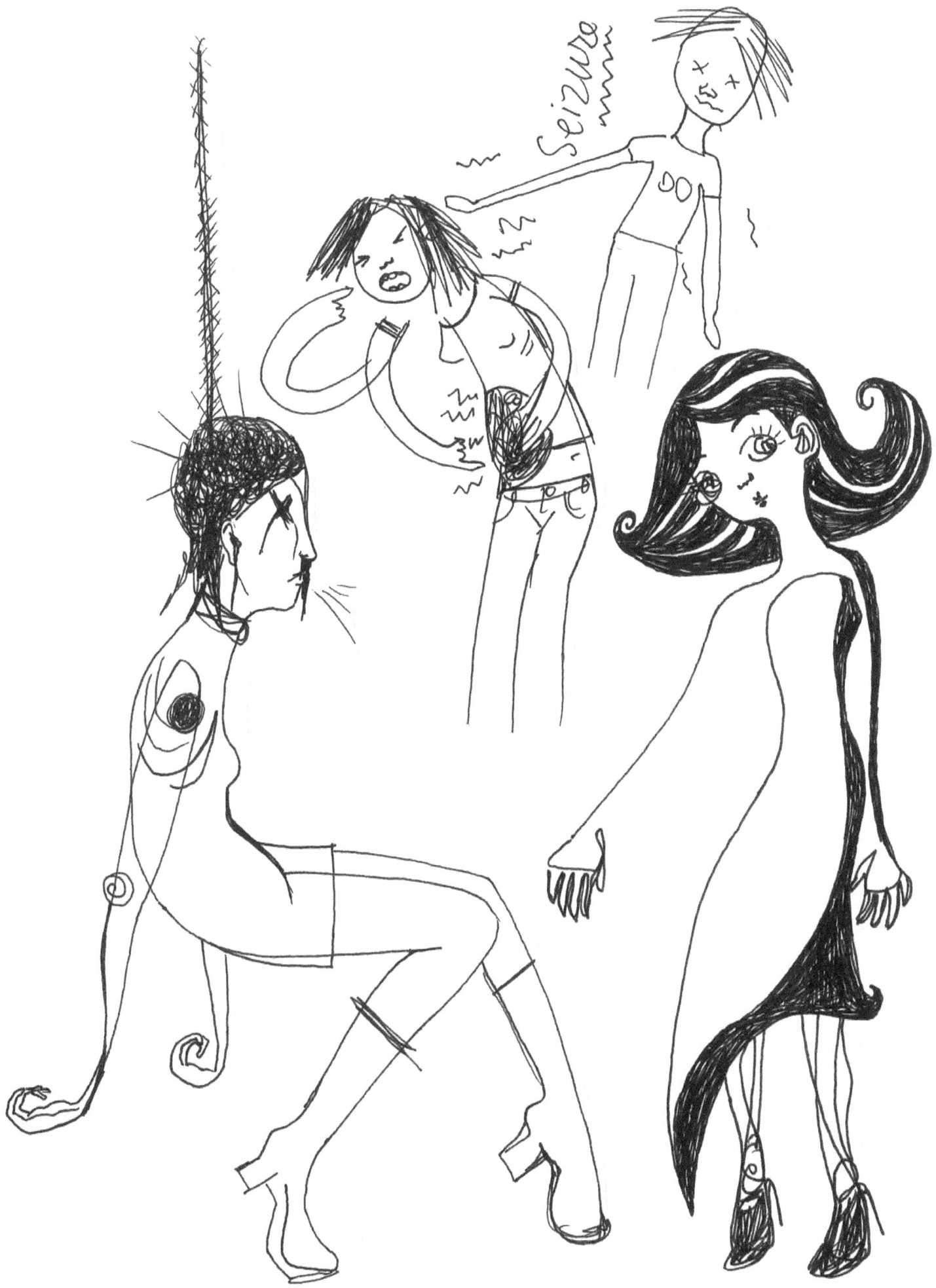

Seizure

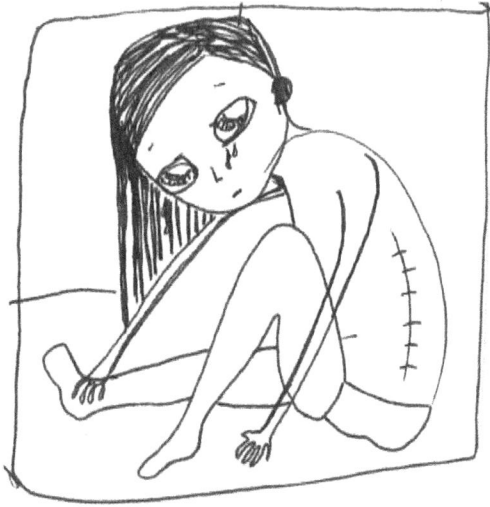

Yeah..

I'm trouble.

And I love

YOU.

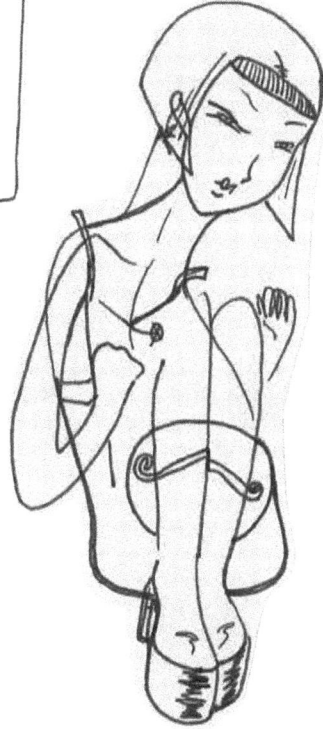

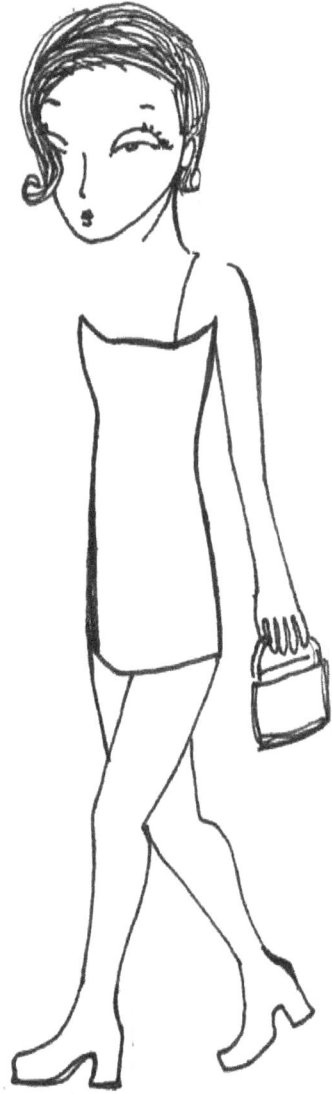

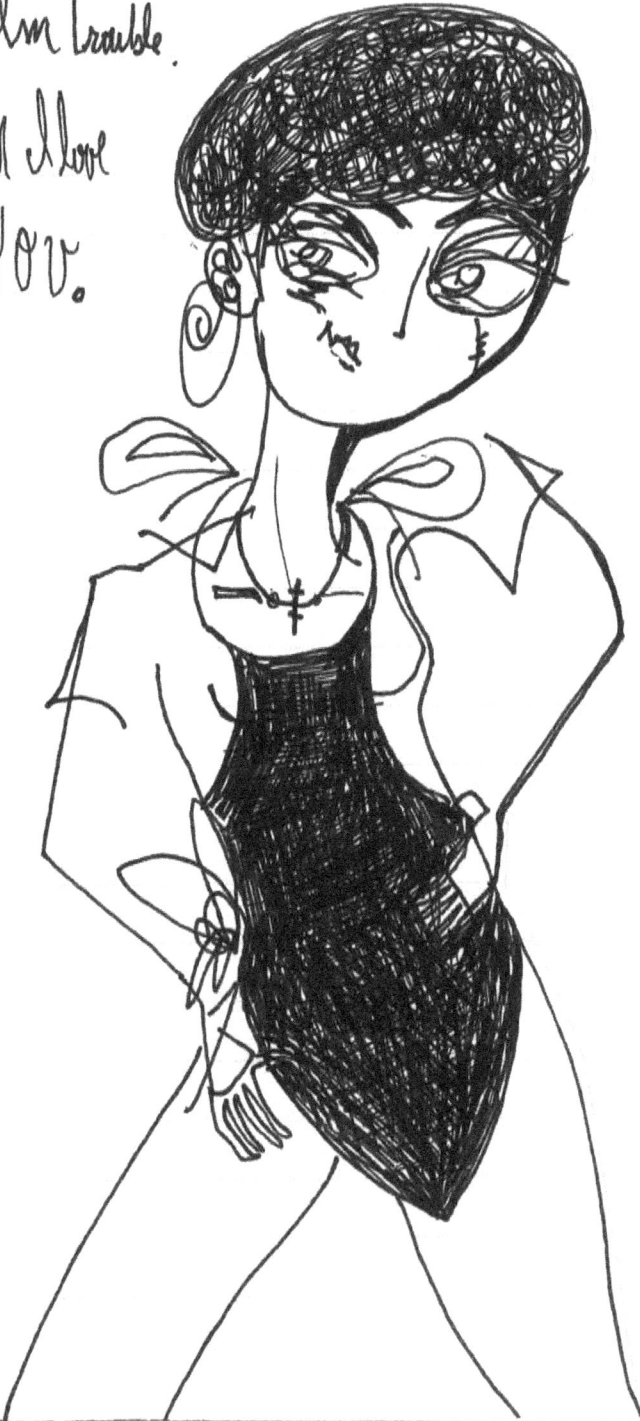

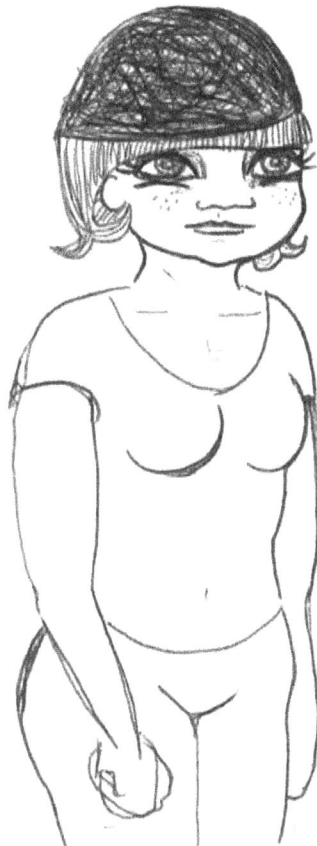

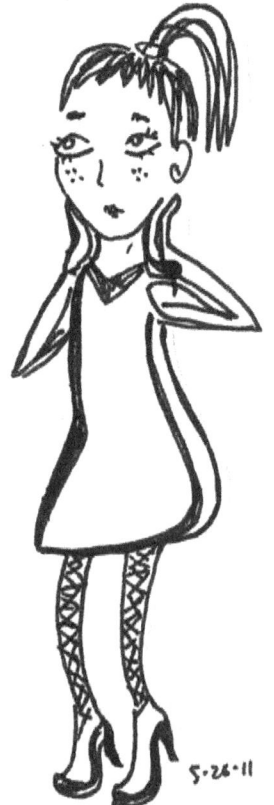

5-26-11

effect of other opiates so if you take anything else you won't get high. It allows you to feel good all day long and be stable so you can live your life. Actually have a job + take care of business and put your life back together. I owe my life to methadone treatment. Since I got in I have gone to school and got my degree in automotive technology. I also met my wife at the clinic. She started working there as the receptionist. I got laid-off from the job I had at the time. I then started hanging out at the clinic more. I didn't have any friends because as soon as I got clean they stopped calling + didn't want to hang out with me anymore. Some friends huh. Fuck 'em! That's how I felt about it. Anyway, we started talking and after a while I found out that she liked me. Shortly after that I got up the balls to ask for her number. Actually, I think I gave her mine and she called the same day. We met up when she got off of work. We immediately hit it off and knew we were meant to be together. One month later we got married. It's been awesome + we have a really cool son together. My life is way more awesome than I ever thought it could be. When I was using I never thought I'd live to be 21. I've almost died several times. I have overdosed on several kinds of drugs, I've stared down gun barrels and had an AK-47 pressed against the back of my head. I've been in many car wrecks too. Obviously I'm supposed to be here. Maybe so I can pass my knowledge on to you, who knows? The addict life is not one I would recommend or even wish upon my worst enemy. There are many ways to get the pills or heroin into your system. Intraveinously or "shooting up" is probably the most effective but, is also the most detramental to your body. I have known people that were addicted to the feeling of the needle prick itself. It doesn't matter whether you shoot, snort, smoke, or just swallow pills. Once your addicted your addicted. People who have never experienced addiction don't understand it. They often say things like; "Why don't you just quit?" or "Suck it up!", They are full of shit! It's not possible to "just quit". What happens is when you flood your brain with opiates + dopamine it stops making it's own natural opiates. Therefore when your not putting the drugs in and your not making it on your own, your brain freaks out and this causes withdrawals. This is why when you do some opiates again you feel normal and good again. This is also why replacement therapy works so well such as methadone treatment like I'm on. Now there are other options too like suboxone (buperorphine) and vivitrol which is a shot that lasts for 30 days, You just have to find what works for you, Some people go to meetings also for support outside of whatever type of treatment they're doing. Unfortunately NA or narcotics anonymous is against methadone and anything like it. They believe in total abstinence and think your trading one drug for another. However there are groups like MARS (medication assisted recovery services) groups. I think I got that right. I'm just not sure about the last letter. My point is that there are alot of different options for you to get

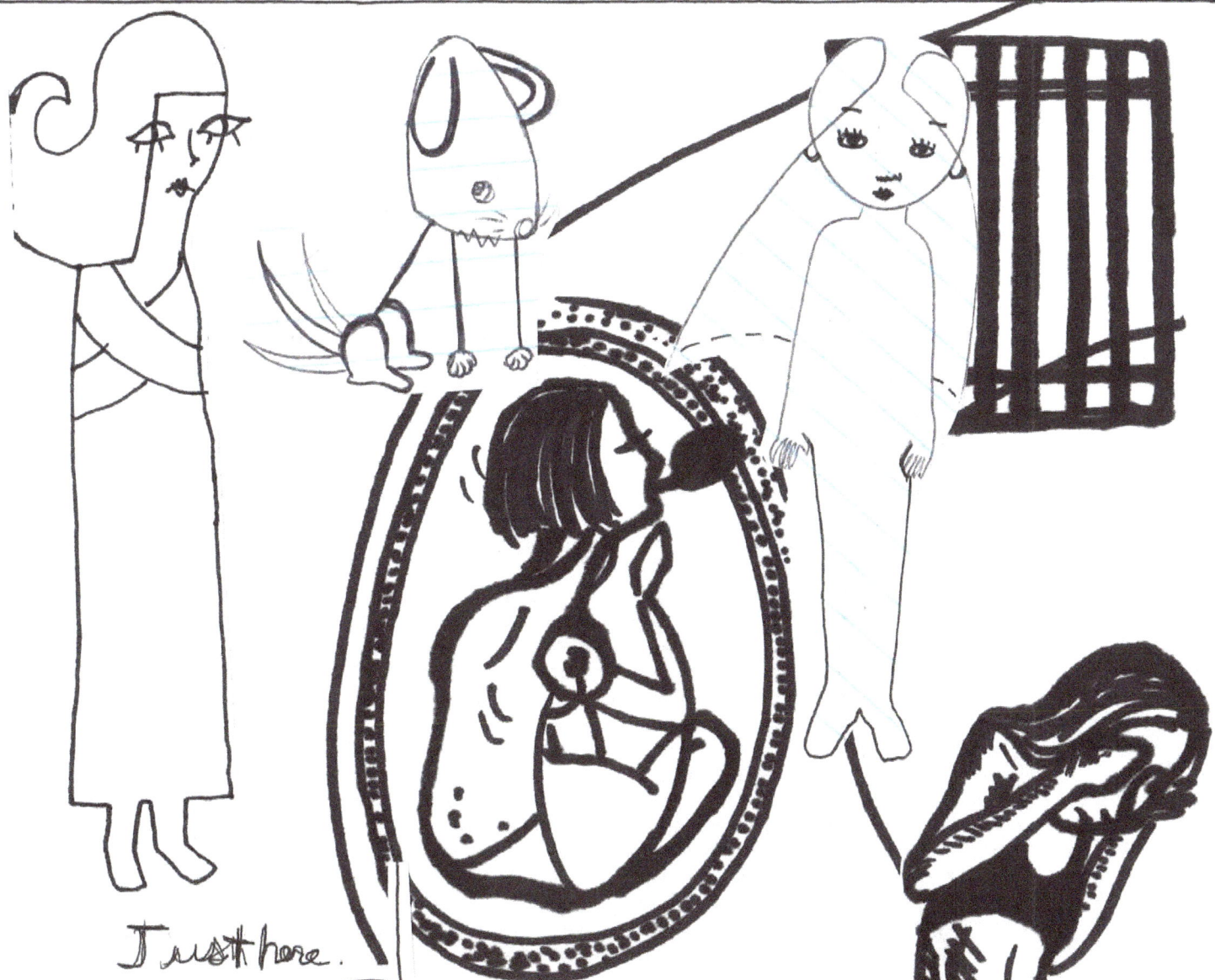

Just here.

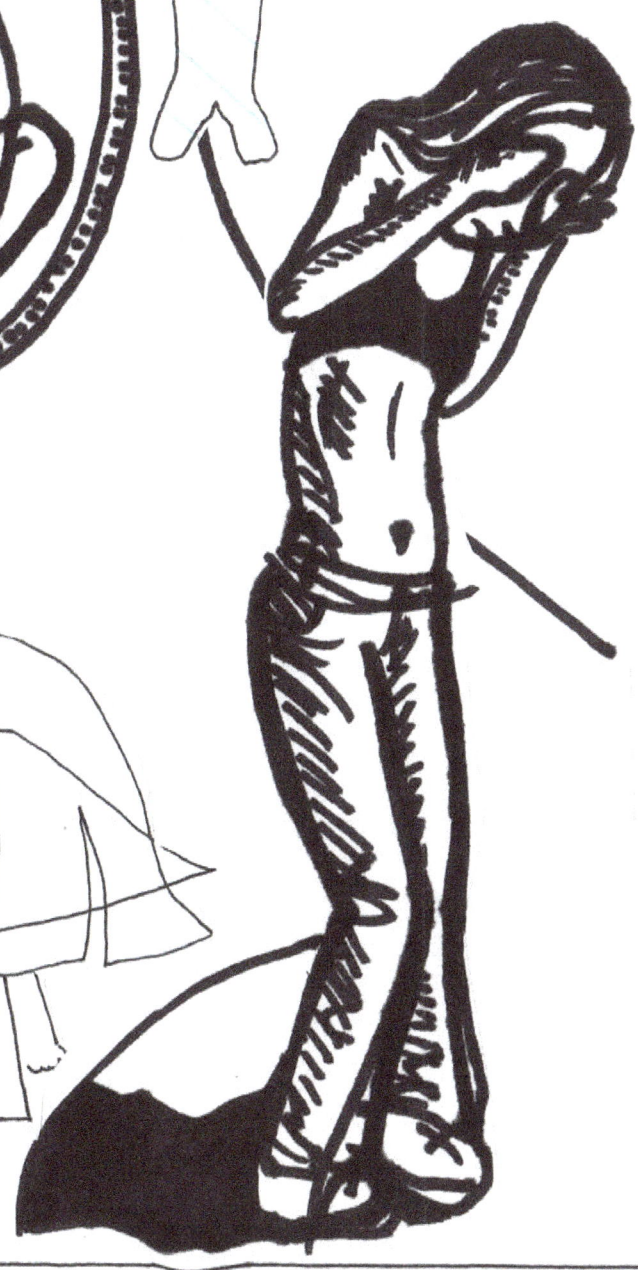

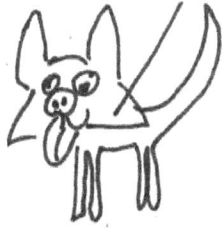

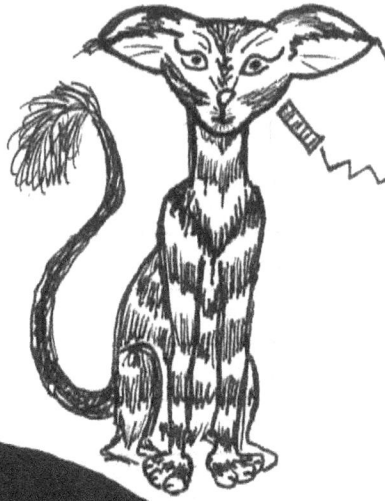

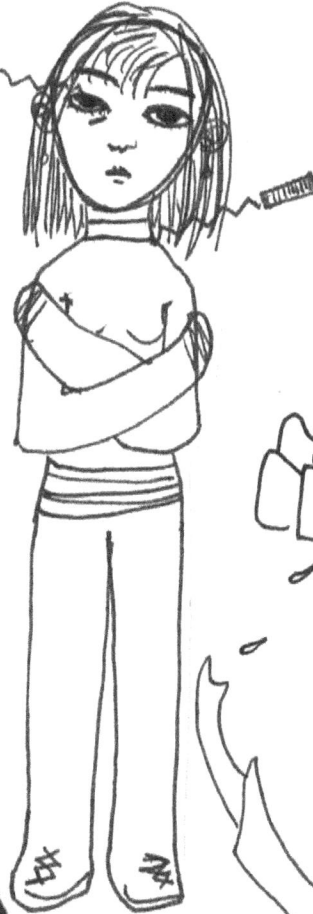

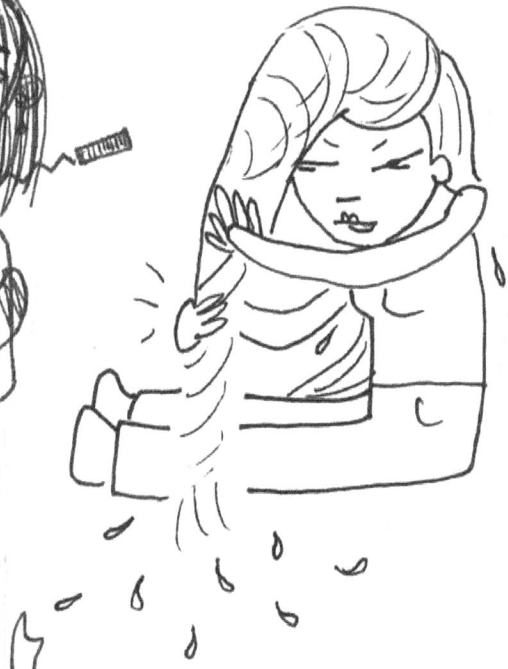

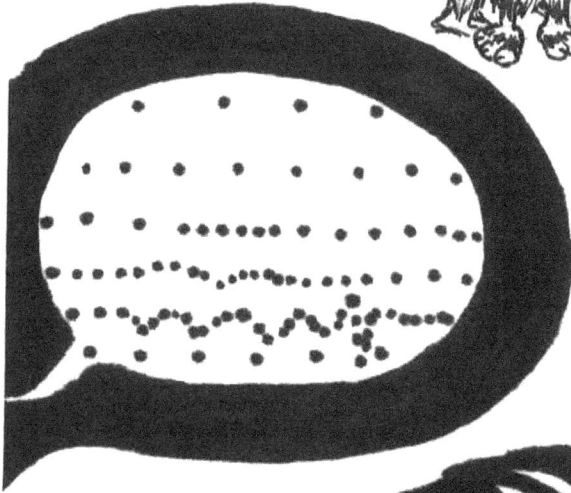

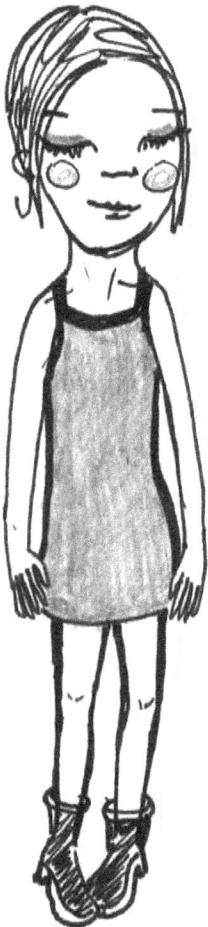

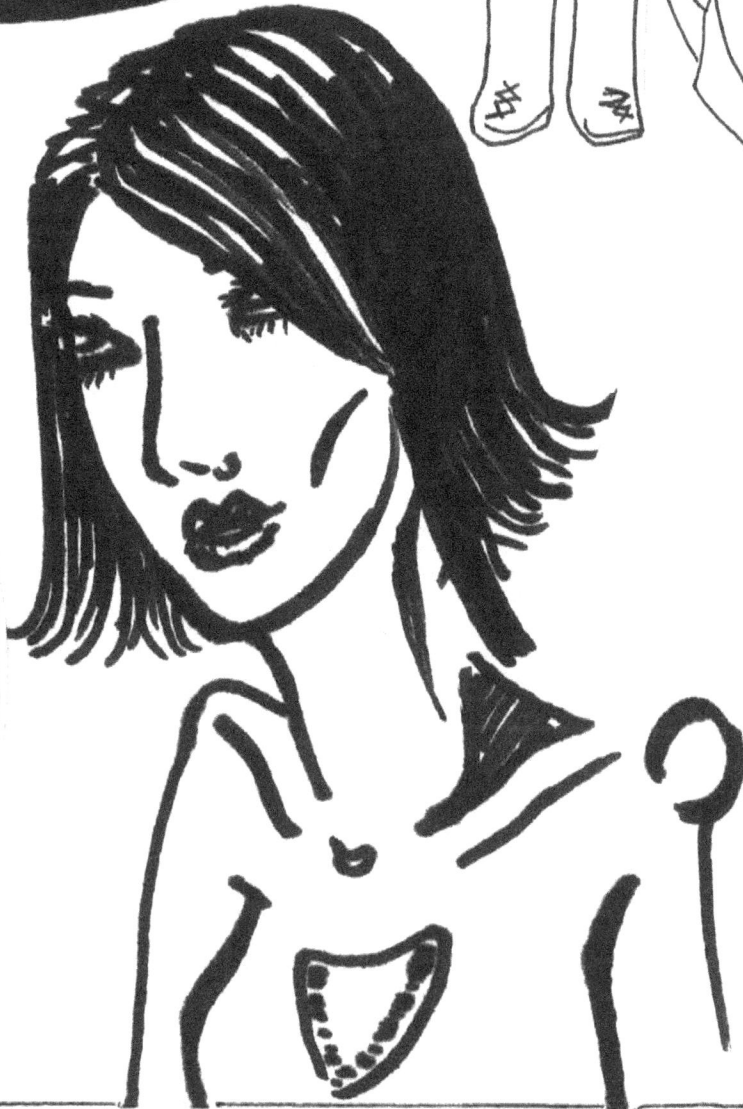

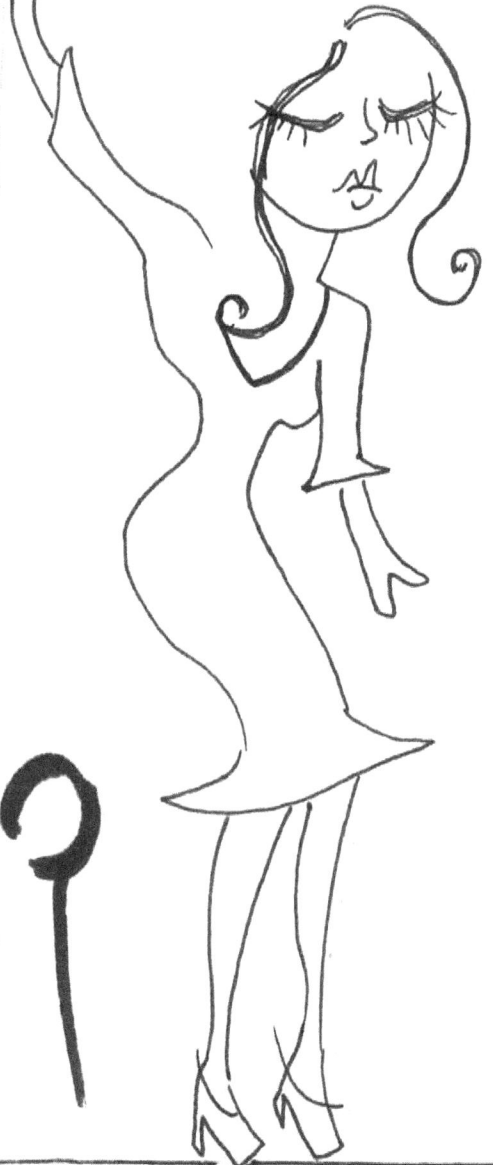

back to normal and move on with your life. It doesn't matter how long your addiction to opiates lasts. No matter if its several months or several years you do quite a bit of damage to your life. After you get clean you will actually have to deal with your problems and pick up the pieces left from your path of destruction. This can take a while and be overwhelming at times. People often get discouraged during the period of time right after getting clean. Its probably the most difficult time and many people will relapse at least once. Relapse means you use your "d.o.c." or drug of choice and get high again. For an alcoholic relapsing would be having a drink. For an opiate addict it means getting high on opiates, shooting some heroin, whatever. This can be very discouraging because you feel like all your hard work of getting clean has been undone. You can't beat yourself up too much though. Recovery from any addiction is a process. It takes time. Also it is like quitting smoking. It takes practice to quit. You have to keep trying. You have to want it. Life after addiction is possible and it is awesome. It's not always easy as triggers can be anywhere and not always avoidable. However, you will get stronger and learn more and more coping skills. I hope that I've given you some good information as well as a bit of advice. Perhaps my experience with opiates that I've shared with you can help to keep you from having to go through such a horrible thing that would destroy your life and hurt many others close to you. If you or someone you know is addicted to opiates or even just doing them recreationally I encourage you to get help for you or whoever it may be. If they aren't ready to change or don't want help right now that's okay. Don't beat them down or lecture them because that doesn't help at all. Just be supportive and be a good friend to them. Trust me, sooner or later they will be ready to get help. There are many resources out there for addicts. A really good organization is one called; SAMHSA. Substance Abuse and Mental Health Services Alliance. Just go to SAMHSA.com on the web or google it. You can also find out where your nearest methadone clinic, suboxone provider, or NA meetings would be. Find what works for you. Treatment isn't one size fits all. Don't let someone else force you to do what "worked for them". Also, you can't compare yourself, your experience, or your addiction to anyone else's. In conclusion; when your ready seize the opportunity to live and have an awesome life. Remember how easy it can be to become addicted so Please, be careful. You are smart and special so don't let anyone make you feel like crap. Even if you are already or become addicted in the future, your not worthless. Know in your heart who you are & who you want to be. You CAN do anything so Fucking DO IT!

Law — Know your Rights

You are a United States citizen, that means you have rights, Freedoms, and protection.

Law enforcement can be helpful, sometimes they can be tools. Many abuse their power and act like they have more power than they actually do. They are not always correct. Law Enforcement officers often offer deals for less penalty on you, they try to turn you and your passengers against the other to stumble out the truth. They bypass your freedom of unlawful search an seizure. That means that they need a warrant to search your person, personal belongings, and private vehicle. They may tell you to empty your pockets and take your bag, turn it upside down and shake it.

Do not be afraid of their word against yours. You do not have to answer unreasonable questions, specially accusatory judgemental questions. 6·8·07 vz

Unless they have Reasonable Cause, they have NO right to search anything. People give up their rights, skip the whole process, and usually convict themselves by admitting information, BECAUSE they think they have to. Research your rights as an Alaskan and U.S citizen.

- Reasonable Cause is when they "feel threatened", smell something, see something, "THINK they see something suspicious", "suspicious" behavior, a past record, and looking Dead-Giveaway.

★ If you don't know your Rights, they are NOT going to tell you. They want you to volunteer information. ★

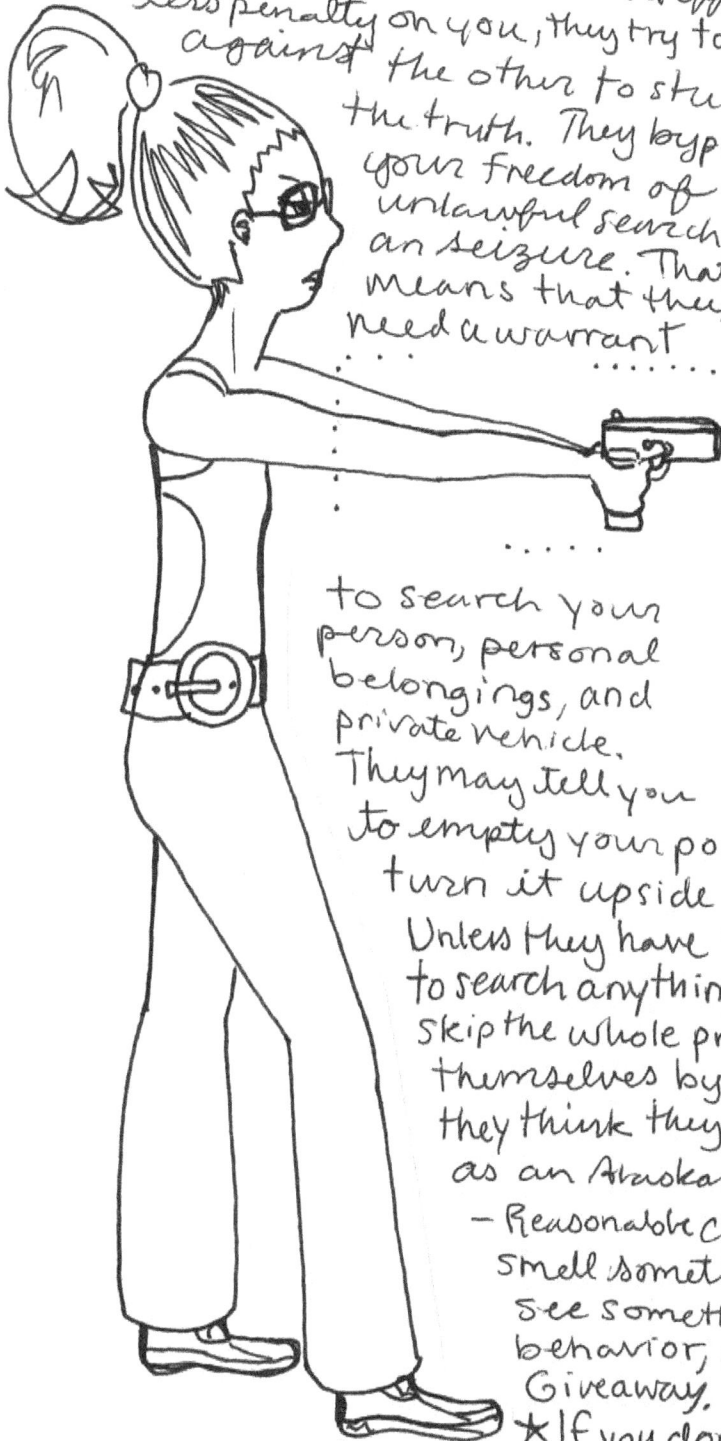

I was a victim of unreasonable search and seizure. I was with my friends and we got pulled over on the expressway. We were surrounded by officers who held us at gunpoint and told four girls to lie face down on the pavement, hands up. They thoroughly searched the car and our personal belongings that were in there.

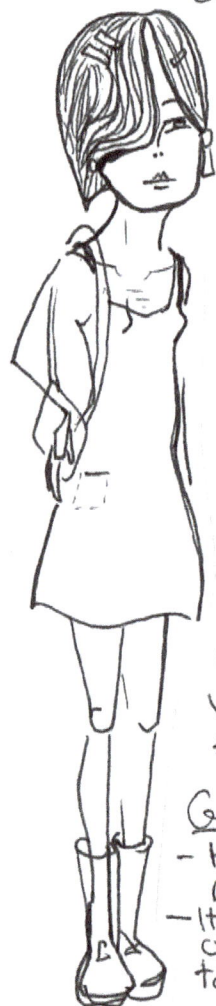

Then they took whatever they wanted and sent us on our way. They told us after the constitutional violation. That they got a report of someone waving a handgun around in a "car that looked like ours". We were terrified and didn't tell anyone. I guess I CAN say I have been held at gunpoint.

Know your rights, stay calm, and don't panic. Police officers KNOW when you are scared. I don't know much about law, but I will tell you what I know.

＊ You are Innocent Until Proven Guilty ＊

Getting Pulled Over

- Have your paperwork ready and extra lights in a visible place. Don't panic, they always take forever.
- It helps to have a cleanish vehicle. If you have bags or purses, close them. Tell your passengers to have their ID's ready → When they ask if you know why they pulled you over, say no. An answer to that question is admission.

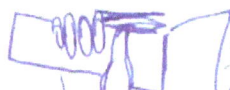

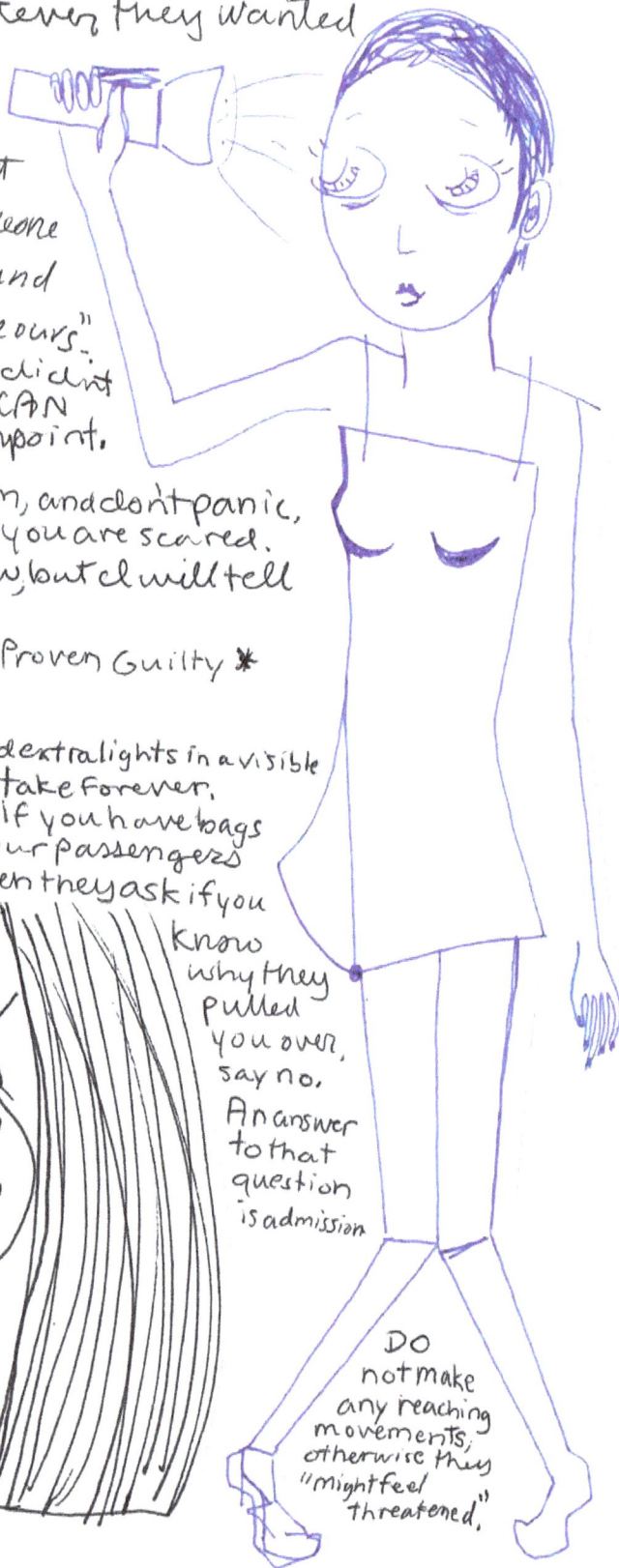

CH—EEK!

Do not reach in your pocket or bag. They are searching every visible surface for reasonable cause.

DO not make any reaching movements; otherwise they "might feel threatened."

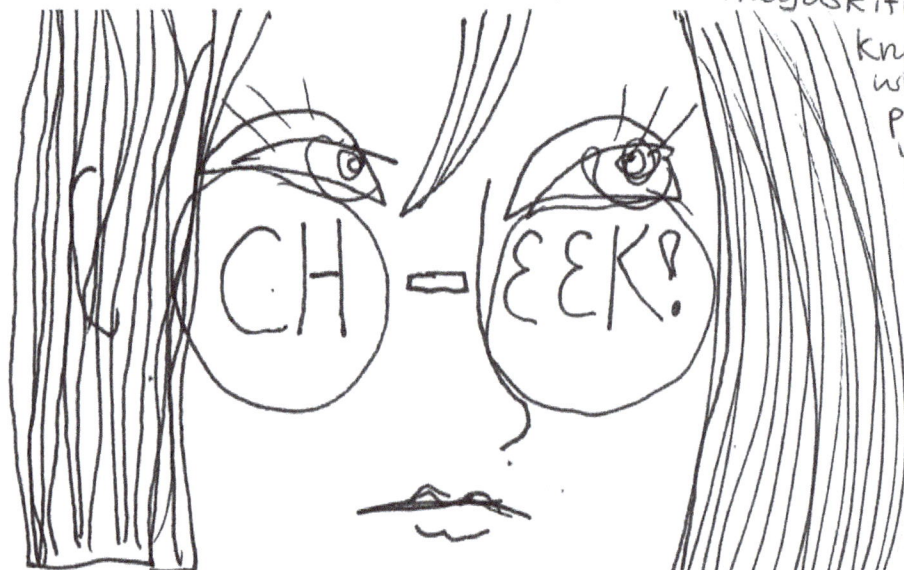

You are a U.S. citizen, that means you have freedoms, or Rights, that are protected by <u>our</u> U.S. Constitution.

Among these protected freedoms, the important ones to know are the Fourth, Fifth, and Sixth Amendments.

invoke = to put into action
revoke = to suspend (ex: Revoked drivers license.)
seizure =
waive = to give up something. (ex: waived fees.)

FREEDOM CARD - Carry 2 copies of this card, in case the officer takes a copy.

★ I hereby <u>revoke</u> and <u>refuse</u> to waive all of the following Rights and Privilages afforded to me by the U.S. Constitution.

★★ I <u>invoke</u> and refuse to waive my Fifth Amendment
5th → Right to Remain Silent. <u>DO NOT</u> ask me any questions.

I <u>invoke</u> and refuse to waive ~~any~~ Sixth Amendment
6th → Right to an Attorney of My Choice. Do NOT ask me any questions without my attorney present.

I <u>invoke</u> and refuse to waive all privileges and rights pursuant to the case <u>Miranda vs. Arizona</u>. <u>DO NOT</u> ask me any questions or make any comment to me about this decision.

4th → I <u>invoke</u> and refuse to waive my Fourth Amendment Right to be free from unreasonable searches and seizures.

I <u>DO NOT</u> consent to any search or seizure of myself, my home, or of any property. Do not ask me about my ownership interest in any property. I <u>DO NOT</u> consent to this contact with you. If I am not presently under arrest or under investigatory detention, please allow me to leave.

ANY statement I make, or alleged consent I give, in response to your questions is hereby made under protest and under duress and in submission to your claim of lawful authority to force me to provide you with information.

Law Enforcement may not like that you will not make their job easy. If the officer fails to honor your rights, remain calm and polite, ask for the officers' identifying information and ask them (him/her) to note your objection in their report. DO NOT attempt to physically resist an unlawful arrest, search, or seizure. If necessary, you may point out the violations to a judge at a later date!

Law Enforcement and Your Home

If you are home, always talk to them or they can enter by force. ① Talk to them through the door OR ② Go outside, lock and close the door behind you.

Do not invite them in. Do not hold the door open a crack and talk to them.

Every surface is pored over. Nobody ever invites a vampire in. If you do, that's it. If they see any reasonable cause, that's it. Be calm and explain what is going on and you will fix it. Again, do not volunteer information.

Law enforcement officers should be addressed as OFEICER, not SIR. Don't let them threaten or intimidate you, they are supposed to be the good guys. Don't fall for their tricks, don't make it easy for them to violate your rights.

So many people make police officers' jobs easy. People are cowo when it comes to authority, it is scientifically proven as a social science experiment. If you are going to "waste their time", they should be out catching drunk drivers instead of hasseling young adults who take their rights for granted Justice is not fair. Non-violent criminals fill prisons, taking up the room that should be for rapists and murderers. Prison is college for criminals.

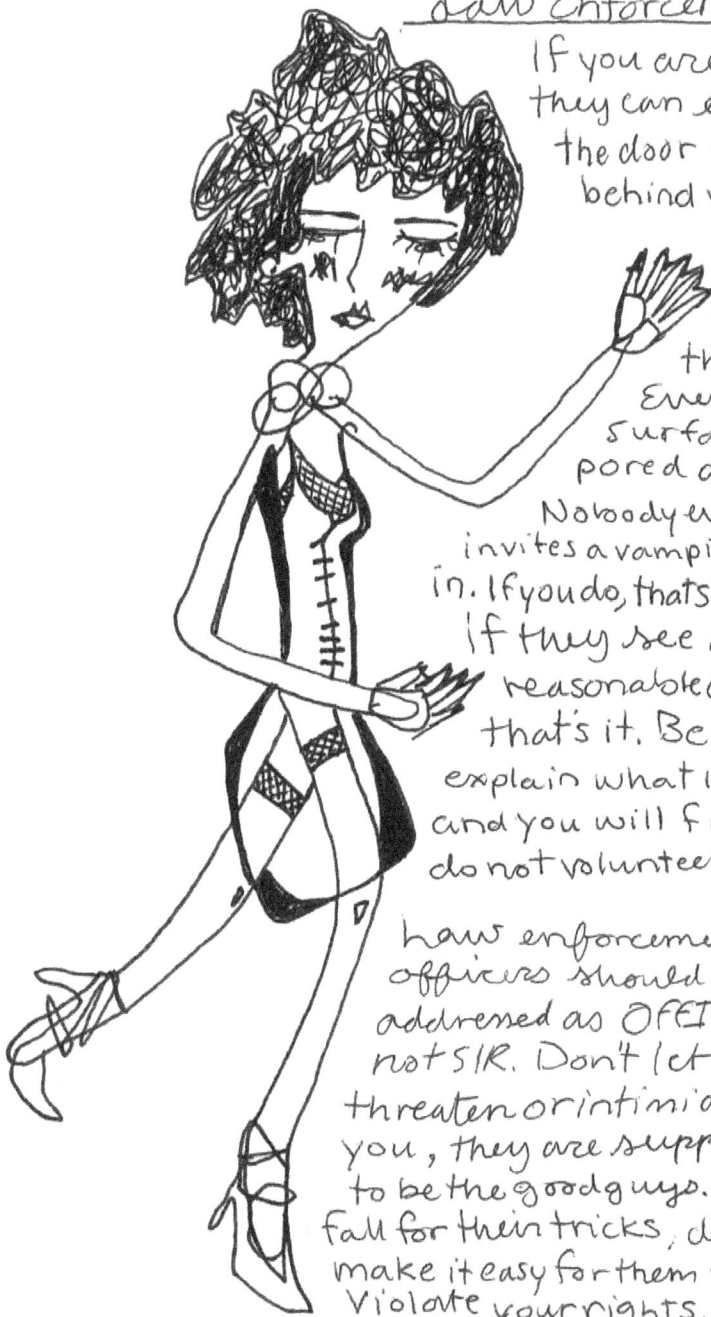

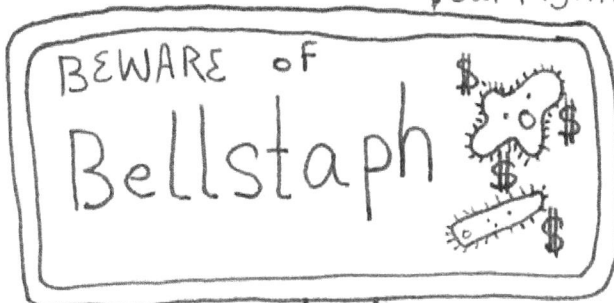

BEWARE of Bellstaph

If they do, report them. Get their car number and badge number.

3/1/02

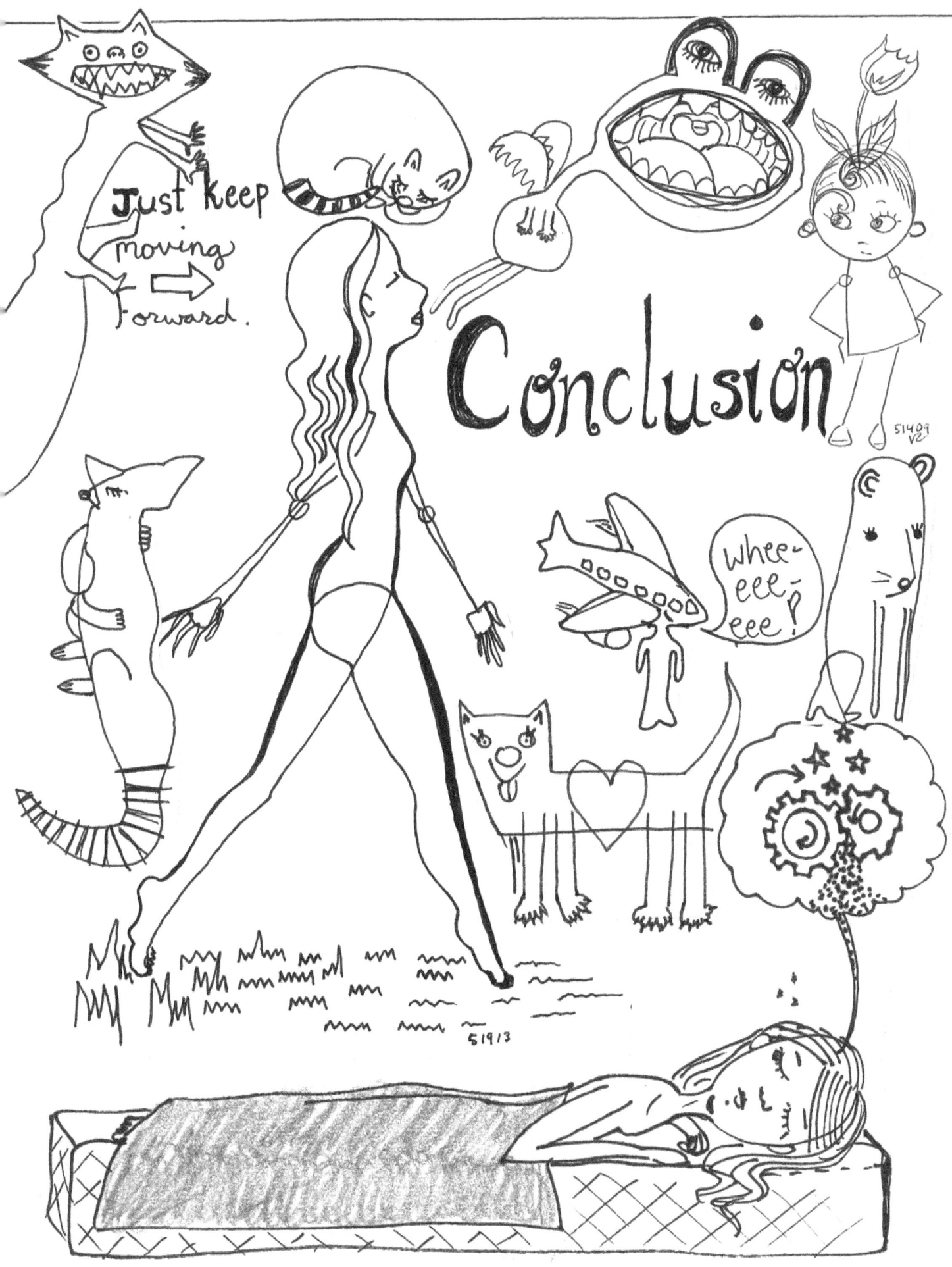

Just keep moving Forward.

Conclusion

whee-eee-eee!?

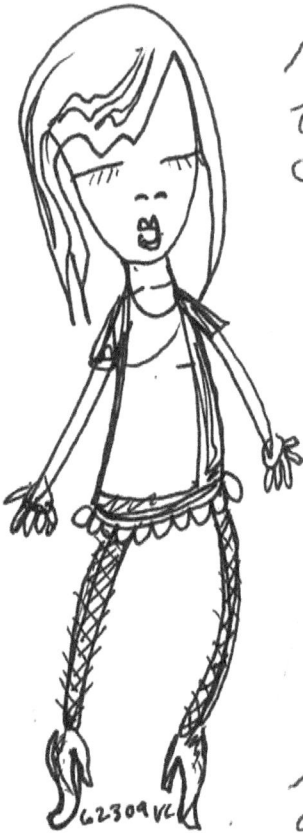

Nobody lives forever or stays young, we are all going to die. There are no magic cures for addiction, depression, and anxiety. These can and do happen to anyone. When it feels like everyone and everything are against you, and your mind is spiraling down uncontrolably that is not real. WHEN YOU HAVE THESE FEELINGS AND DRINK ALCOHOl, YOU WILL PROBABLY COMMIT SUICIDE. If I got into hard drugs or alcohol, I would not be alive today, happy and loved. I would have died, or became a crackwhore, both bad outcomes for me. Sometimes I feel like I missed out, but the truth over powers the fantasy every time. I know myself, both good qualities and Flaws.

Nobody is perfect, except for God.

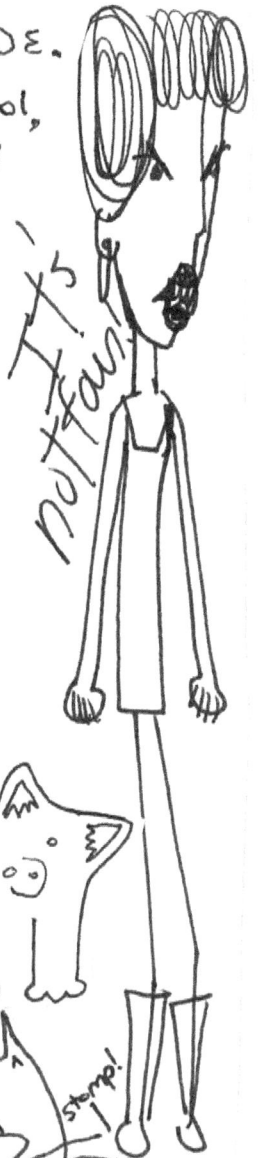

It's not fair.

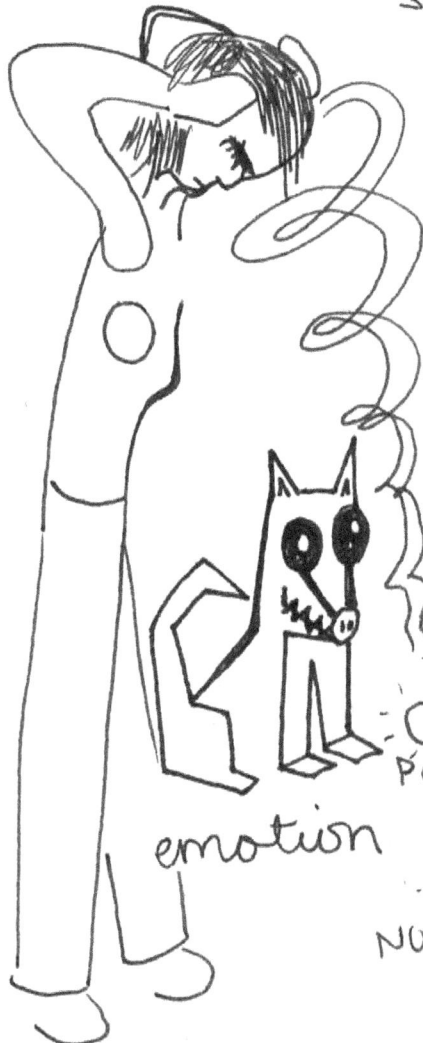

emotion

POP

NOTHING

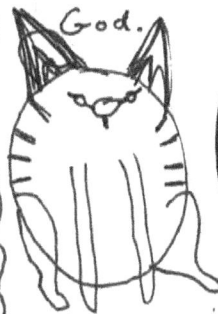

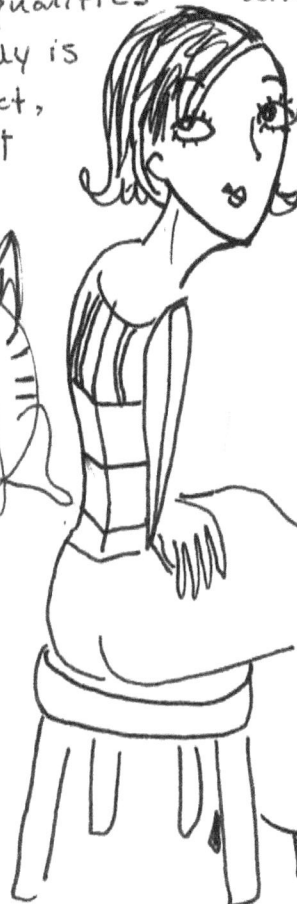

. . . . . .
_____
. . . . . .

They said to just wait patiently

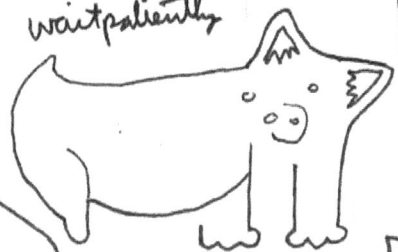

stomp!

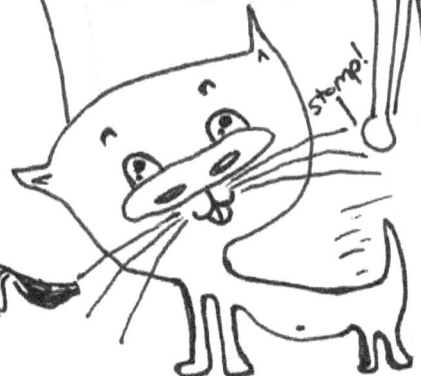

So, you will probably get in trouble, screw up, and do crazy things. It is such a short amount of time, being a young adult. It is also the easiest time to get lost, killed, addicted, and commit suicide. When you become an addict, years can pass. if you get into recovery, you a' recovering addict, but still an addict.

— You should be treated like a person.

- Your body should not be an object for people to use. Your body belongs to you. Some girls and guys will use either giving or withholding sex as a power, to get what they want.

When you have to do things for people to love you, that is

CONDITIONAL Love. For example: If you have sex with someone, then they will love you.

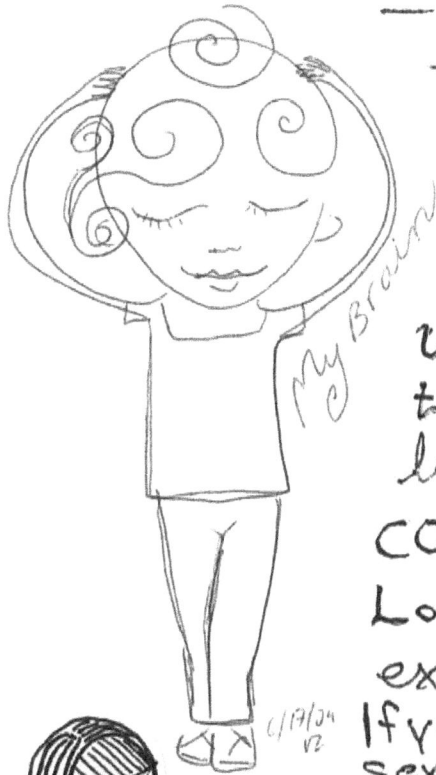

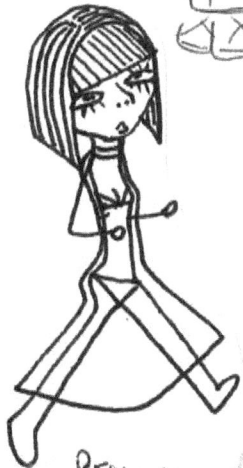

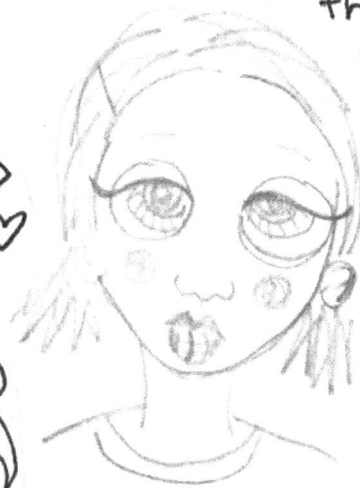

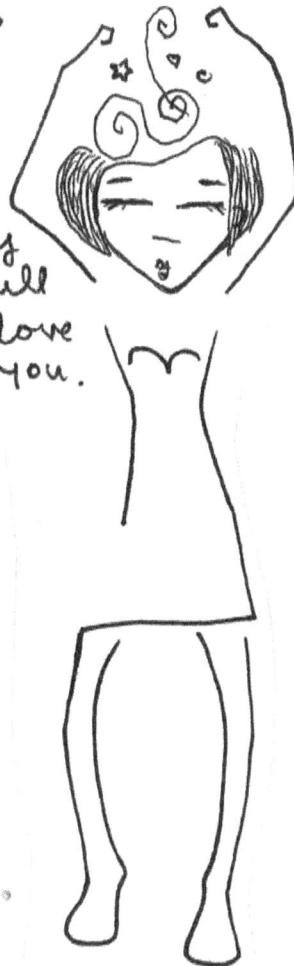

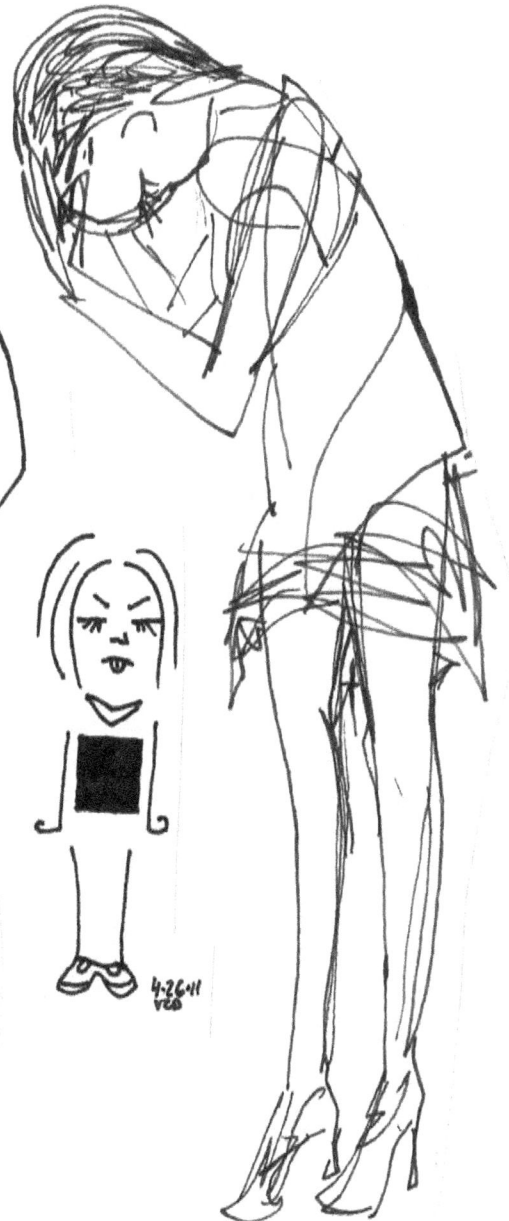

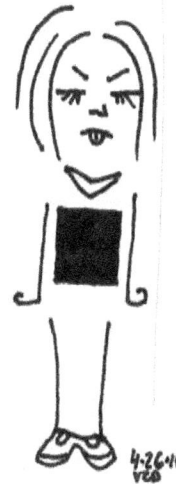

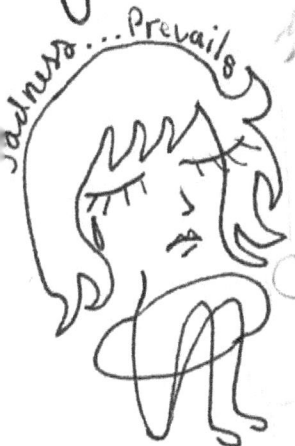

My Brain

Sadness... Prevails

I feel like crap.

4-26-11
VCO

I didn't know unconditional love until I was 27.
UNCONDITIONAL Love is when a person loves
another person for who they are.
Unconditional love is the kind that God has
for each and every person. Everyone
has dark and light in them.
Sometimes the dark overpowers
the light, but the Love
and Light in a persons
heart never dies.
We all want to be perfect
and for things to be fixed.
Heres the thing:
No one person
can be perfect,
Only human.
Sometimes
things can be
Fixed; other
times it
Just keep   may take
going...   a long time
            or may never happen.
It is good to treat
other people with
the compassion and
respect like you would
like to be treated.

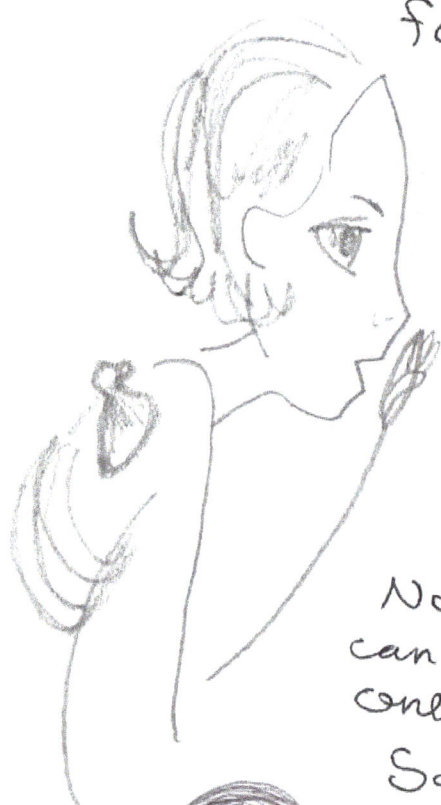
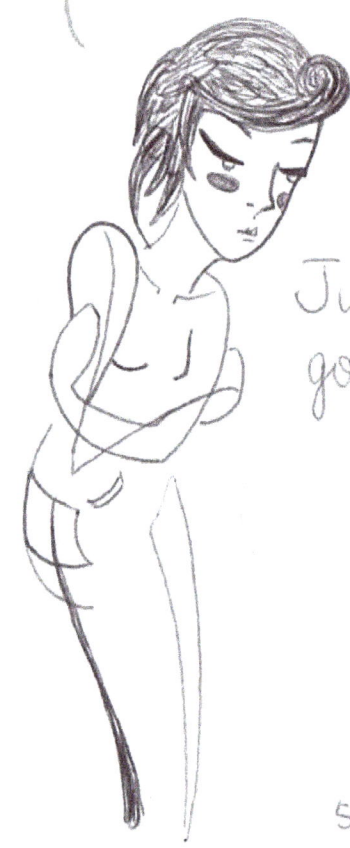
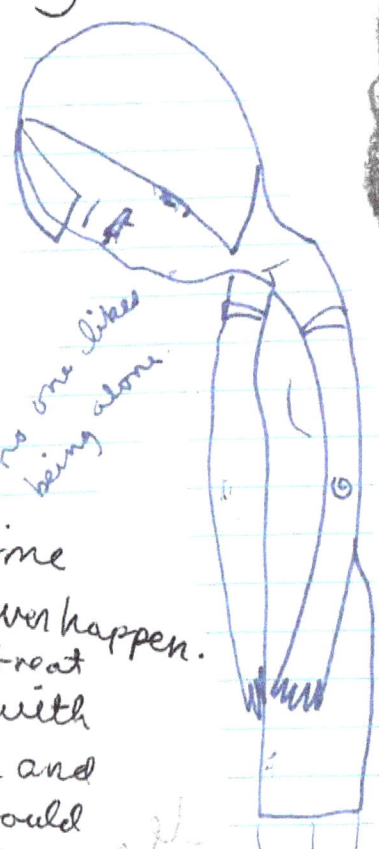
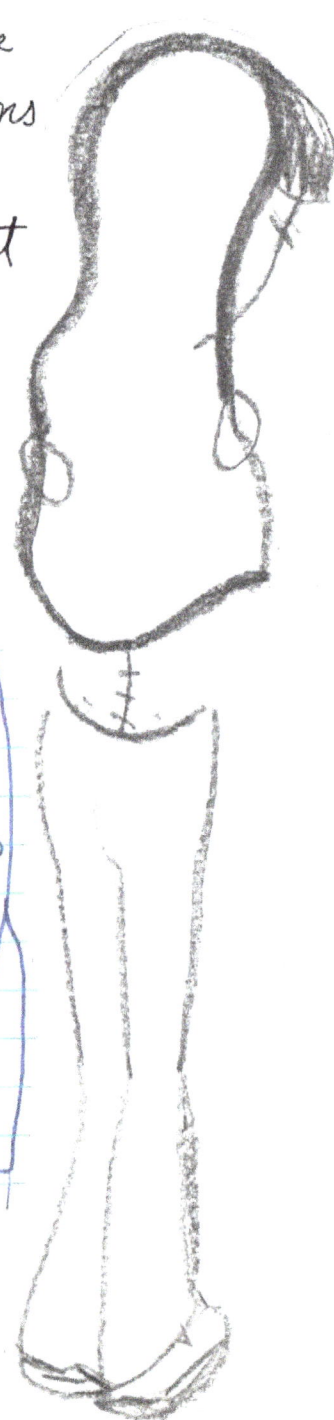

hey!

no one likes being alone

5-5-07

HOT FRY SIZZLE

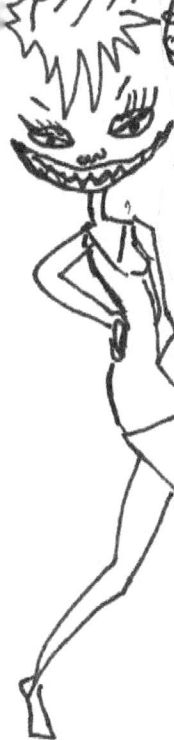

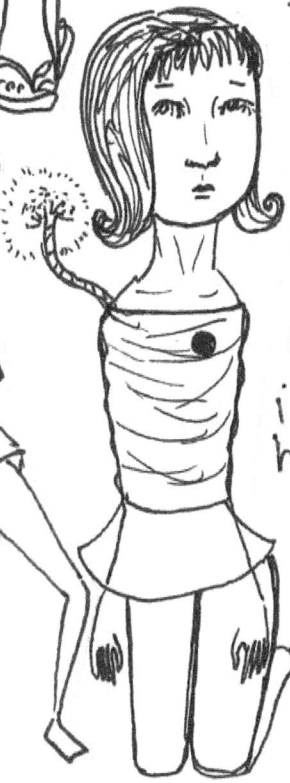

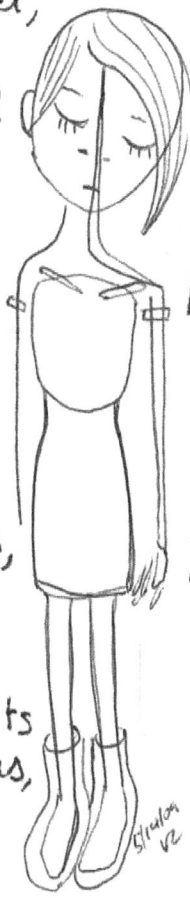

Each person gets one chance to be alive in their body. When god you die in reality, you become only a memory in someones head. You are somewhere else, but not here with all the living. People die naturally with the passing of time, either by accident or body breakdown. If you are worried about suicidal people in your life, Tell Someone. Don't weigh down the problem with alcohol. Your problems just get pushed deeper down, if you are suicidal. When you don't deal with your hurt, Sadness, and a worthless feeling existence, harmful thoughts and memories can stay with you and potentially ruin your life. I was suicidal for 17 years. You have the power as individuals or groups to help stop molestors, rapists, and anyone who treats another person with disrespect or indignity. Children and young adults should be sacred, precious, and loved.

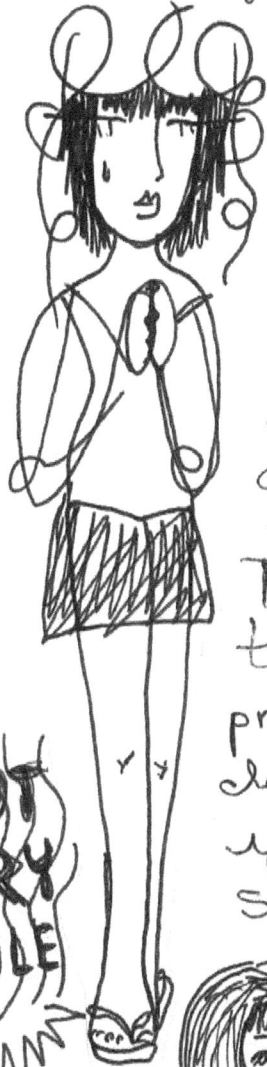

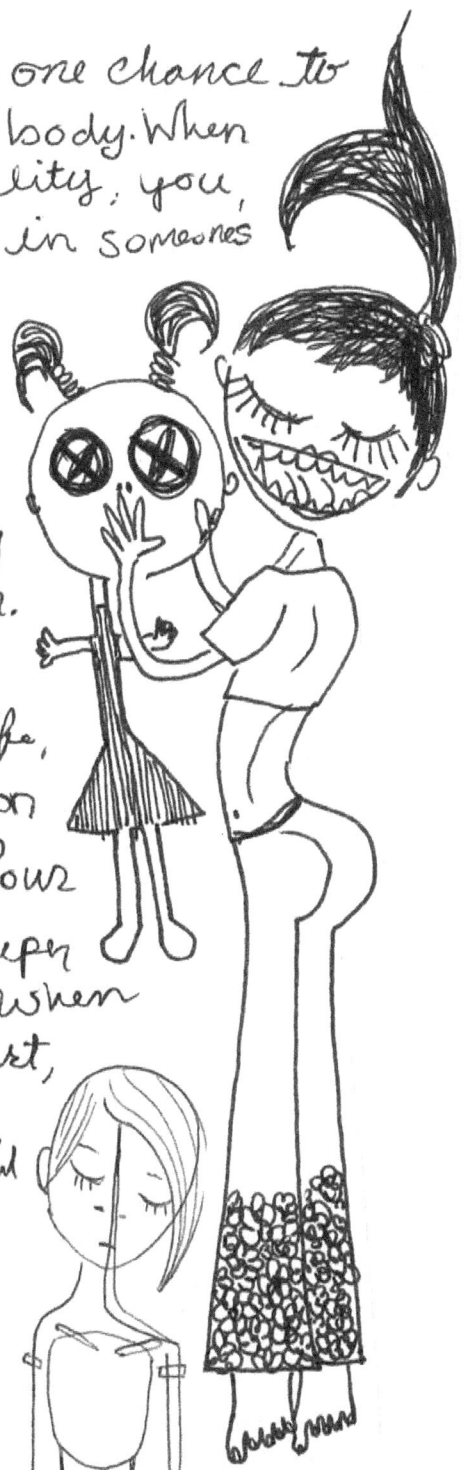

When children and young adults are not loved, they die by suicide or Fail to Thrive.

If you are, or have been a victim of emotional and physical abuse or neglect, know that you are not alone and people can help you.

Whatever atrocity was done to you, has been done to more people than you think. You are not the only one whose dad or grandpops is abusing them. You might feel powerless, shamed, worthless and dirty. Abusers do not want their victims to feel control or to feel good about themselves. All it takes is one, it could be you. When 1 person comes forward with the horrible and unacceptable Truth, it makes other victims confident to come forward as well. It will probably be a huge effing deal, but none of "them" are on your side and they were never going to rescue You.

I'm Fucking SUPER.

Why don't you just tell me You Don't Know Shit. Fuck!

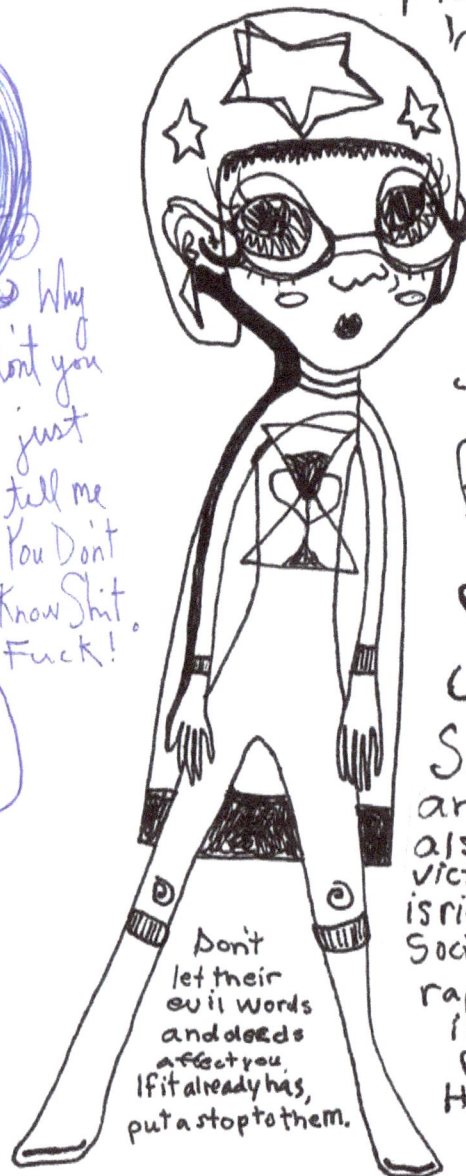

Abusers threaten homicide or suicide. Do not believe them, they are too important in their delusional sickass world. Whatever happens to THEM, is never ever your fault.

Don't let their evil words and deeds affect you. If it already has, put a stop to them.

Saving yourself and fighting back also saves potential victims. You KNOW what is right and what is WRONG. Sociopaths, pedofiles, and rapists might know it is wrong and feel proud of it. Help put them behind bars.

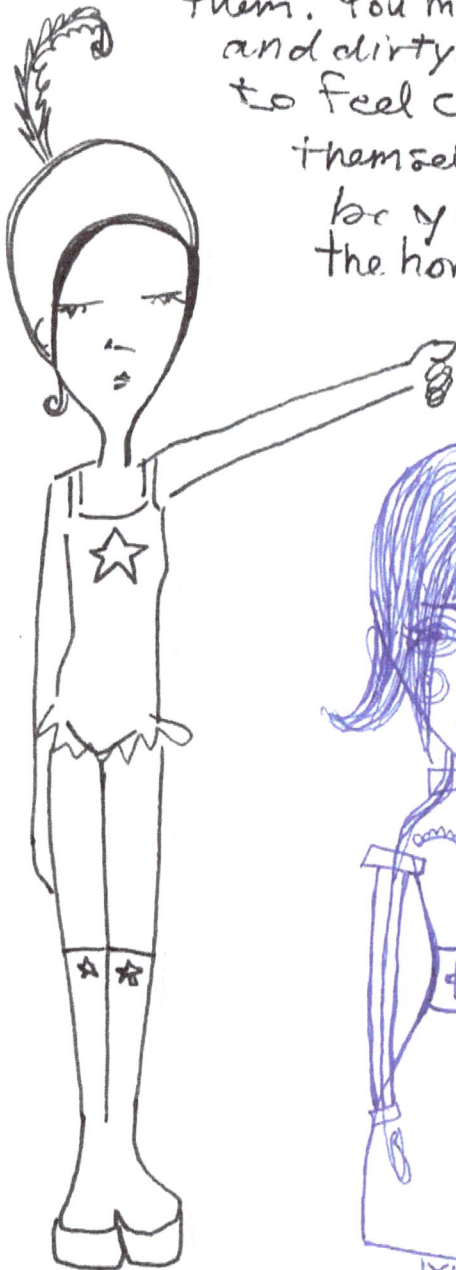

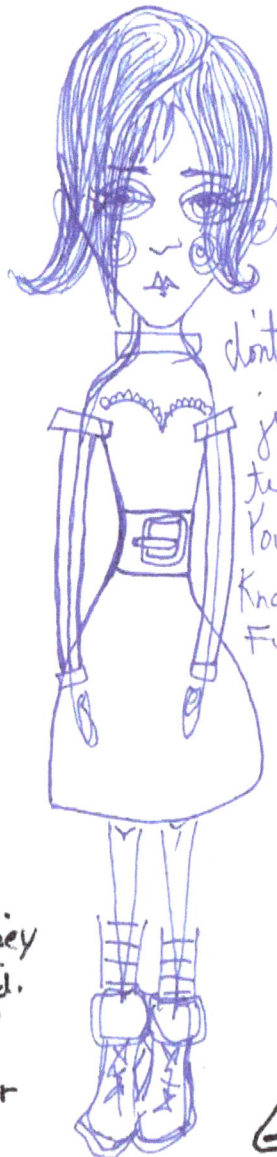

I have known many young adults who grew into adults. A lot of them suffered badly and are wise beyond their years. I was one of those that suffered. It is sad to see young adults who raise themselves and their siblings as a mother or father figure. It is not easy being a SCAPEGOAT, a person who takes the blame for everyones problems. It is sad when young adults, even children, are more functional. Big Sisters and Big Brothers, you are your siblings' role models, their safety. Children are waiting to be rescued ** and comfort; YOU are their HERO. If you had your personal boundaries violated by your father, brother, grandfather, uncle, family friend, or anyone else, the law is on your side. If they are not doing it to you, they are doing it to someone else. Innocence Reapers are sick sick sick. They are social deviants who feel good about themselves when they don't get caught. People do horrifying things to children every day. These children grow up to be promiscuous, addicts, suicidal, suspicious, and anxious or depressed. My childhood was in a village. I was shy, scared, distrustful, and withdrawn. I was violated many times, each time I told my mother. She didn't do anything about it. The most help I got was "Stay away from THEM." There were no confrontations, no criminal charges, and another molester goes on to others, whose mothers say the same.

The headline on No Shit News today is this: THINGS ARE STILL THE SAME WAY 25 YEARS LATER.

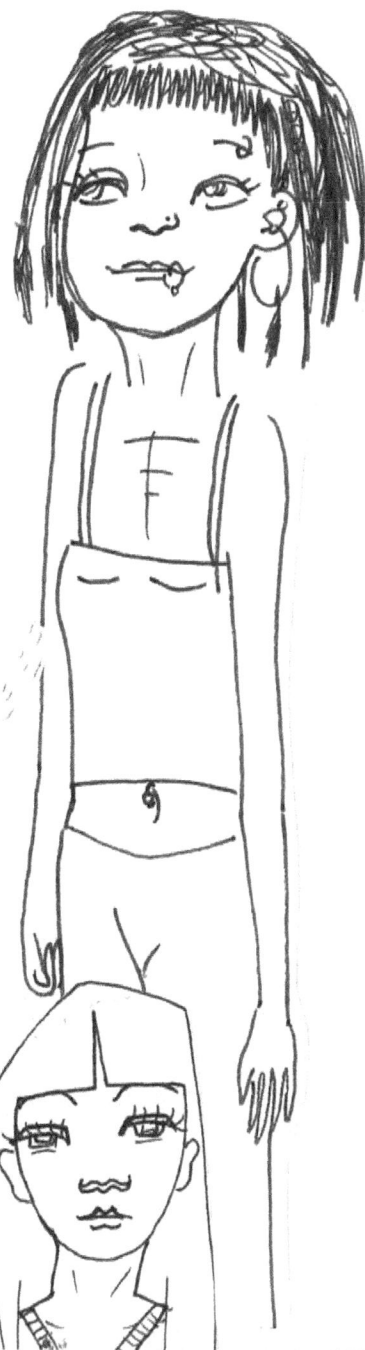

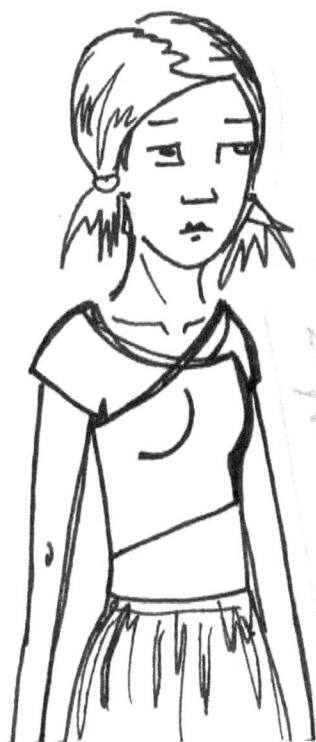
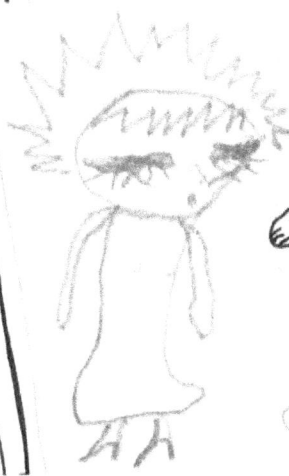
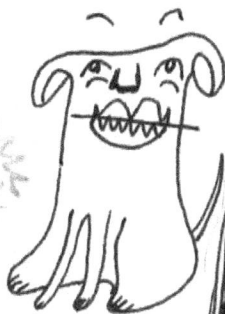
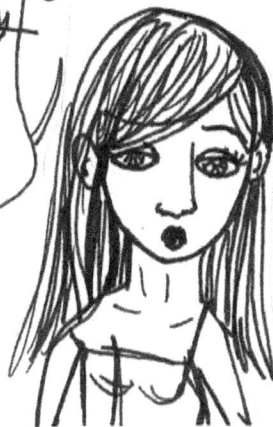
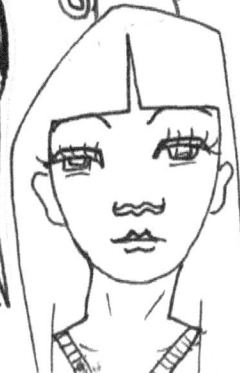

Adults need to...

stop stop

stop STOP **STOP** STOP

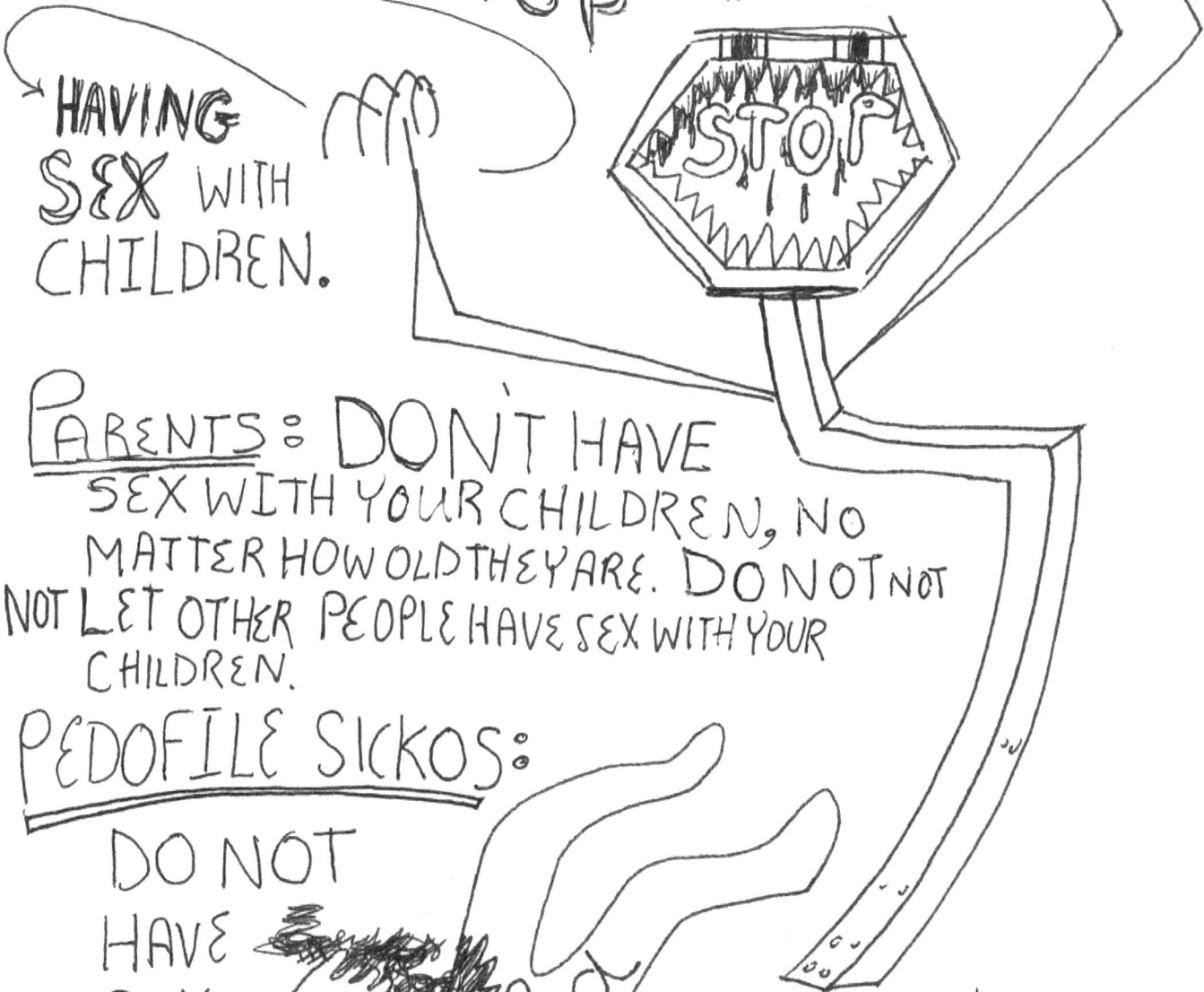

HAVING SEX WITH CHILDREN.

PARENTS: DON'T HAVE SEX WITH YOUR CHILDREN, NO MATTER HOW OLD THEY ARE. DO NOT NOT NOT LET OTHER PEOPLE HAVE SEX WITH YOUR CHILDREN.

PEDOFILE SICKOS:

DO NOT HAVE SEX WITH ANY CHILD.

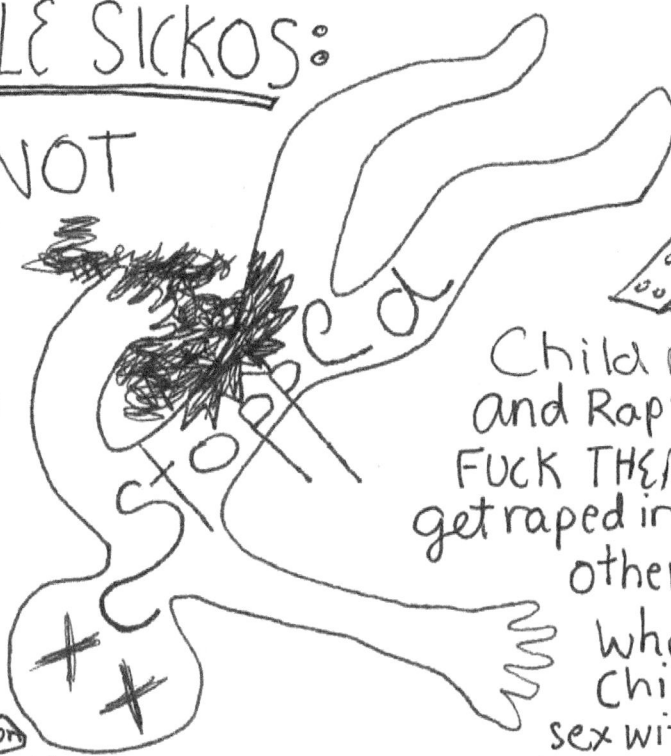

Child molestors and Rapists can go FUCK THEMSELVES and get raped in prison by other prisoners who have children. Having sex with a child is an UNFORGIVABLE CRIME. Many have not been caught, But they will.

Child Rape Equation
Loss of Innocence as a child
= WORTHLESS-FEELING existence
+ alcohol = SUICIDE.

The End of this
Book.

Suffering sucks. No person asks to suffer, life just happens. As humans, we adapt. We have intelligence that we can express with learned language, but we are a young species and far from perfect. Our weakness is our ability to think and have feelings, both things that can consume a life. Our own brains can convince us that dying is better. No other animal does that, only us. We are fragile, but stronger than we give ourselves credit for. Damage and experience make us resiliant to life totally sucking. In 2013, I almost committed suicide and my husband had a relapse. It was tough and horrible,

CAUTION! SADBLOCBH. Do not get too close.

It's MY BIRTHDAY I WILL TRY TO BE Happy ... I promise.

but we saw the true colors of people we thought we knew. People that we thought were family.

Things can be bad, get bad, and feel like they will STAY bad. Remember, change is always happening. We can only move forward. Each Day is Brand Spankin New.

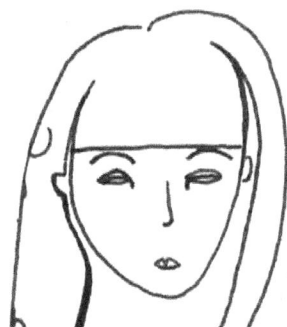

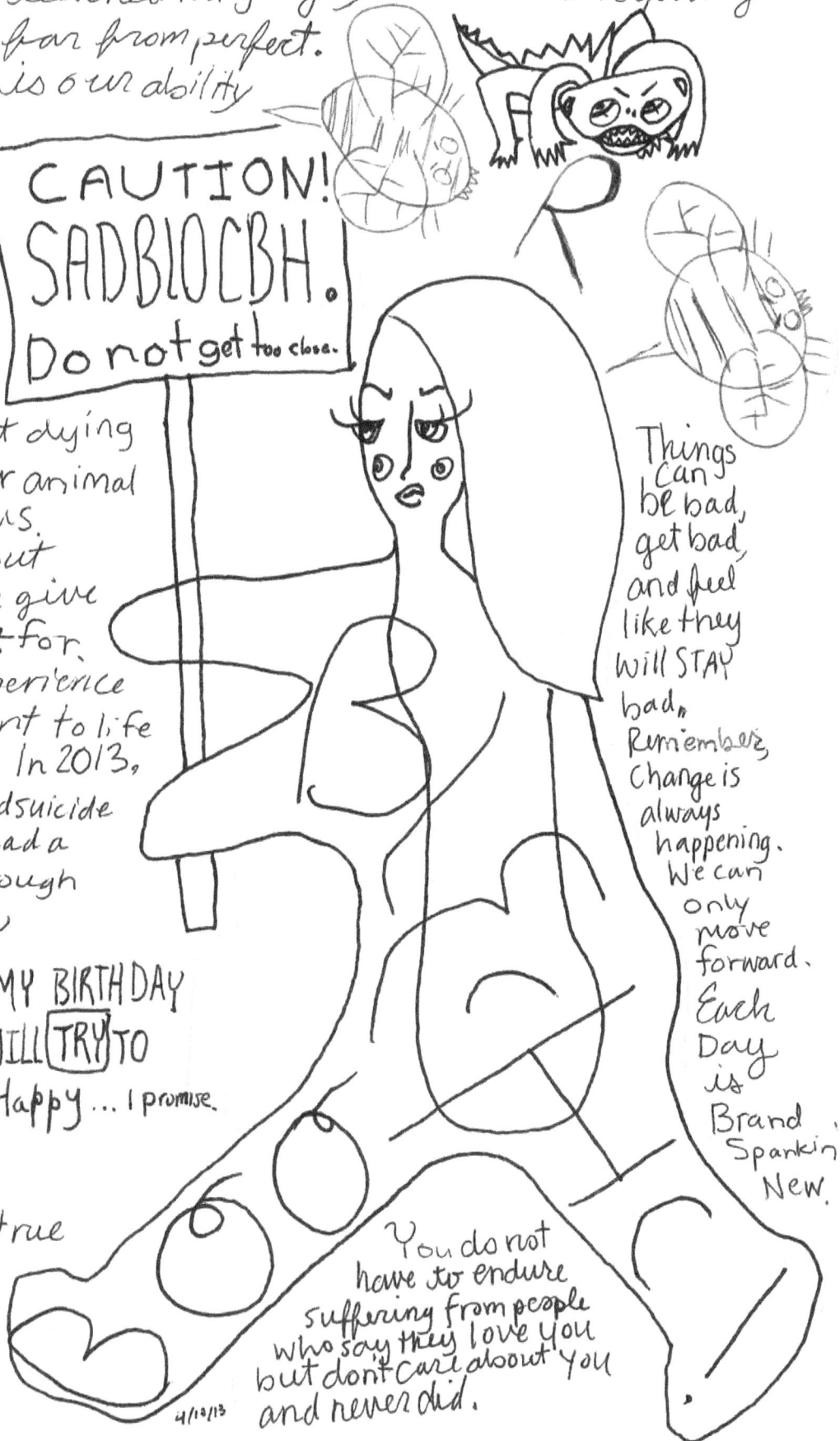

You do not have to endure suffering from people who say they love you but don't care about you and never did.

4/10/13

Being alive is a gift. How we are alive in a body that lets us perceive and experience the outside world. Every person was created by 2 single cells. You might not feel like you have a purpose, but you do. Just because you don't understand why you suffer, that has a purpose. If you have siblings, they need you to protect and save them from the suffering that ruined your life. It is sad to know you are a more responsible adult and better mother or father figure than your own parents, who are disobedient, indignant, drunk, and immature children. If you suffer in society, remember that The First Will be last, and the Last First. I remember that the tallest most beautiful flowers are picked first. They demand to be looked at and worshipped. They lose their beauty first and their slow death makes them unfruitful.

Humble flowers (like me) stay low to the ground, in OUR beautiful reality.

Be someone's miracle Share a Smile and Listen*

Be a Light in the Dark for someone who is lost*

Life and Death are mysteries. So is memory

↓

Consciousness and your Soul.

Any problem can be helped, treated, or put into perspective. Life can be sad and tragic, but it can be happy and fulfilling too. Death never gets any easier. We fear it.

Sometimes you have to fight yourself in order to live your life. Needing help to do that is nothing to be ashamed of.

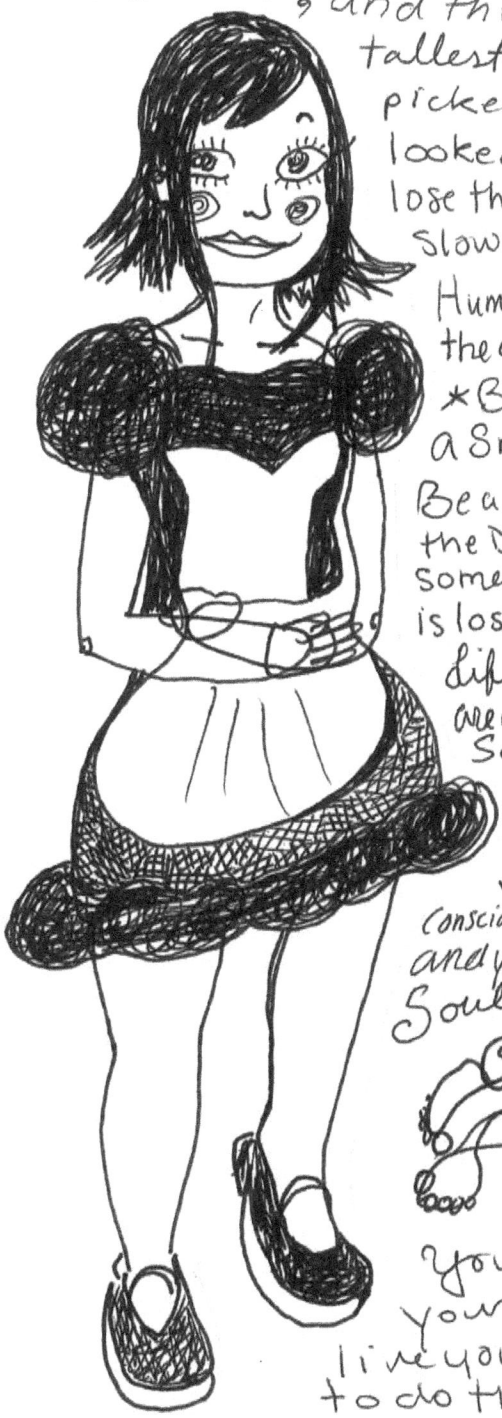

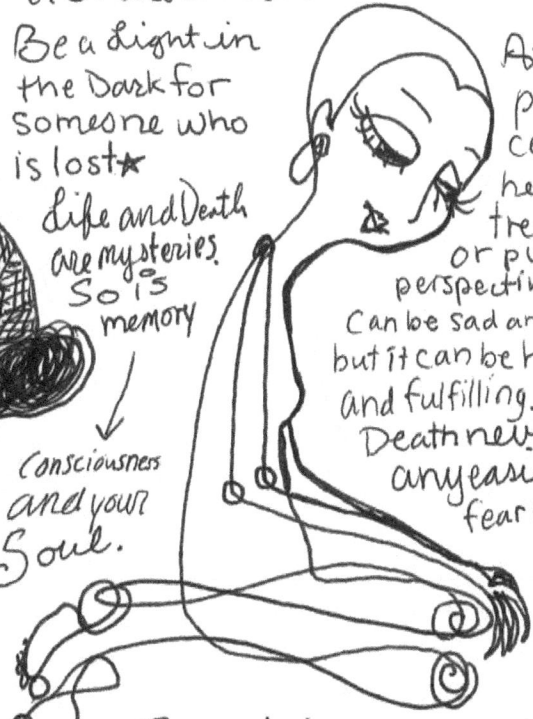

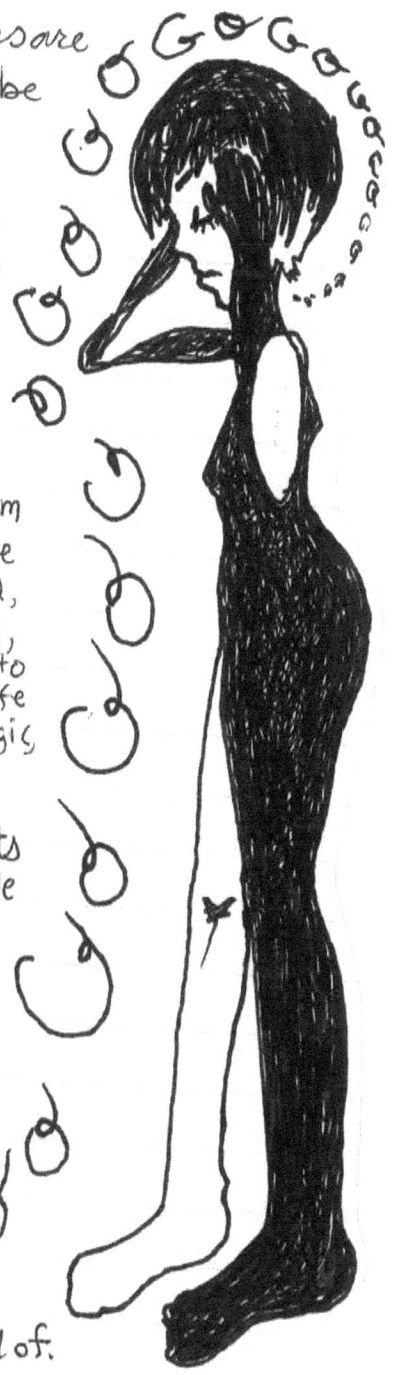

up up and away bye bye?

When nobody expects anything from you, it can make you one of two ways.

1. You can be irresponsible and ruin your own and others lives.

Twinkle

2. You can live for you and achieve good things that will turn into other good things.

Addicts can't "just stop" and a depressive can't "snap out of it" or "man up." They must be treated. When emotions become your reality, it is difficult to know yourself and who you really are. If you get into drugs and alcohol, you don't need to reach the bottom to get treatment. The sooner you get into treatment, the more you will be able to live a life with people you love.

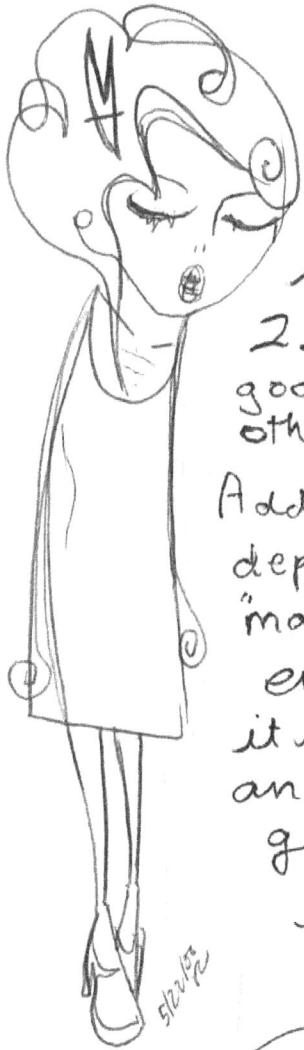

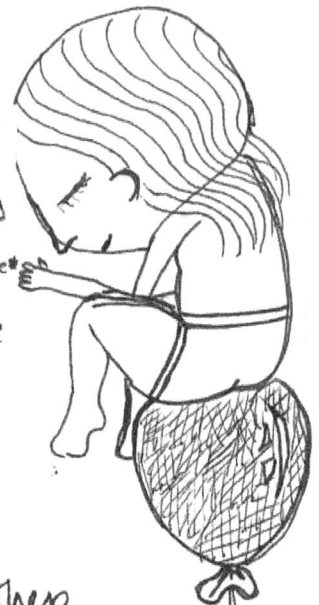

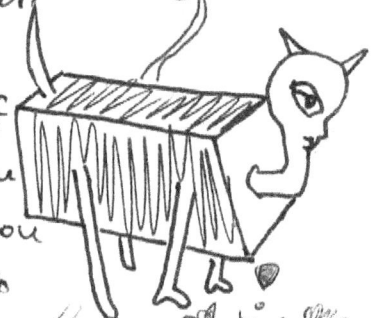

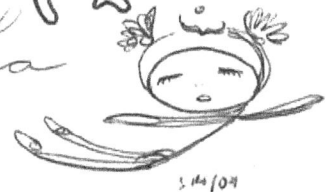

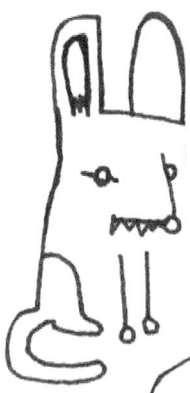

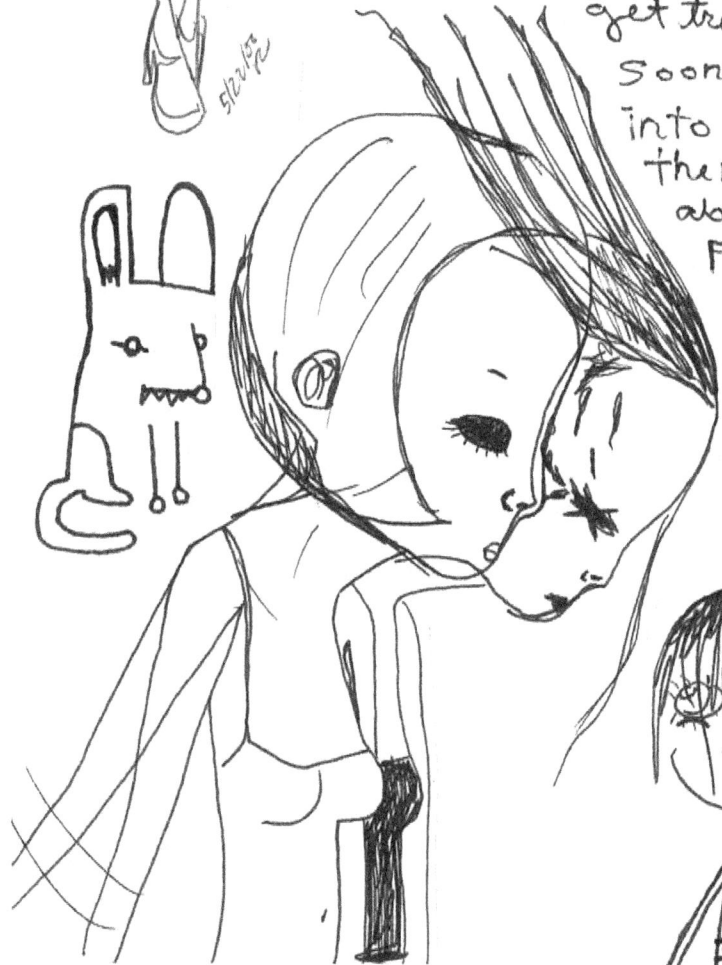

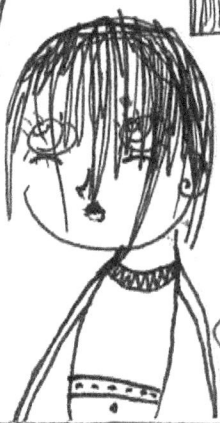

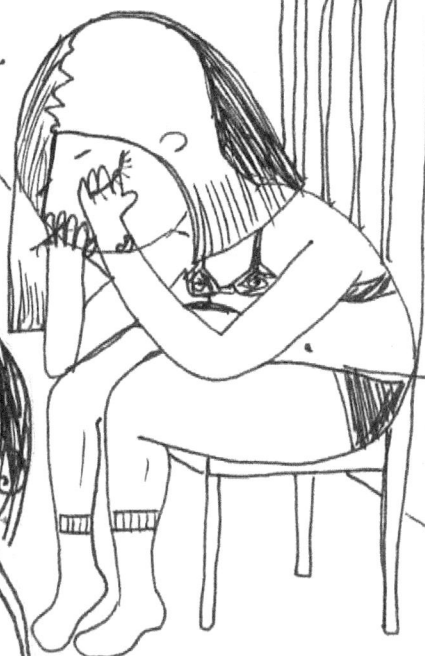

Mental illness and addiction does not make someone a _Bad Person_. They are in anguish, lost and searching for something they can't put their finger on.

If life has not been good for you, it can seem like life will never be good for you. You could feel like you don't deserve love, like I did. I searched for 17 years, feeling alone in the dark and Nobody knew. I have less friends than I can count on my hand, but we have known each other through fun, crazy, and and tough times. Half of us became alcoholics, but we are all still here. There are many times when I could have died, but I didn't want to leave forever and leave only a memory.

5/20/09 DYING IS NOT A BIG PARTY.

You do not get to see your funeral or your siblings grow up.

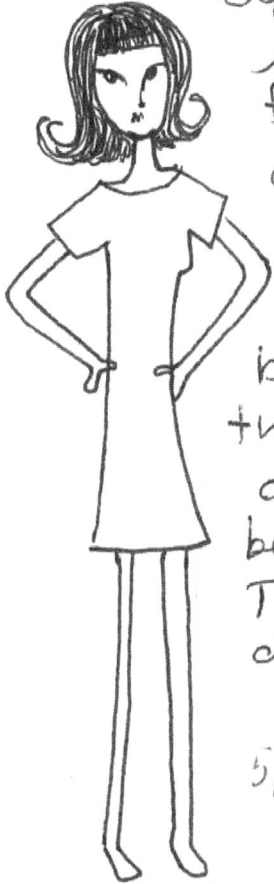

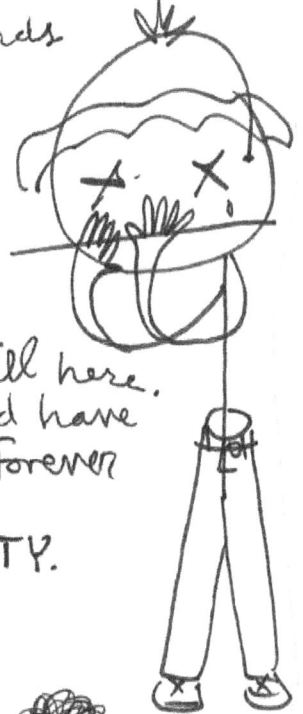

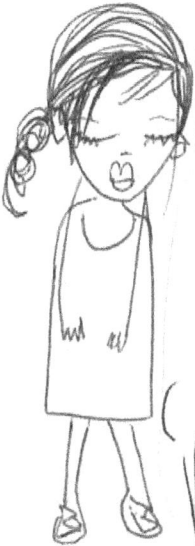

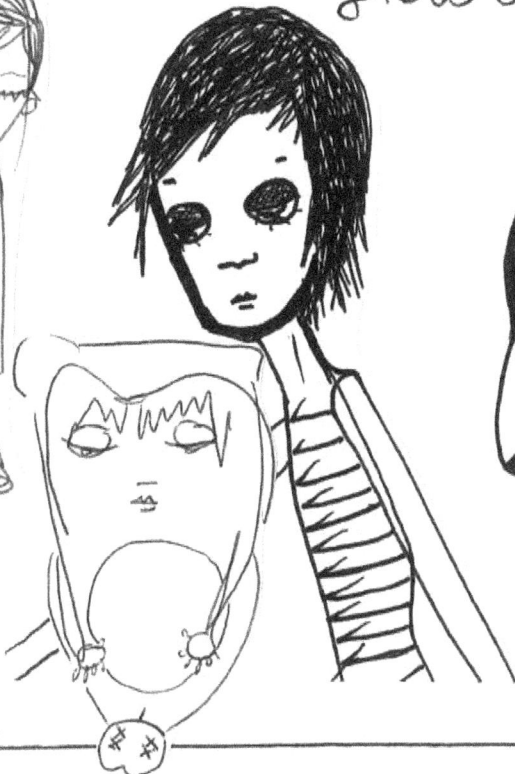

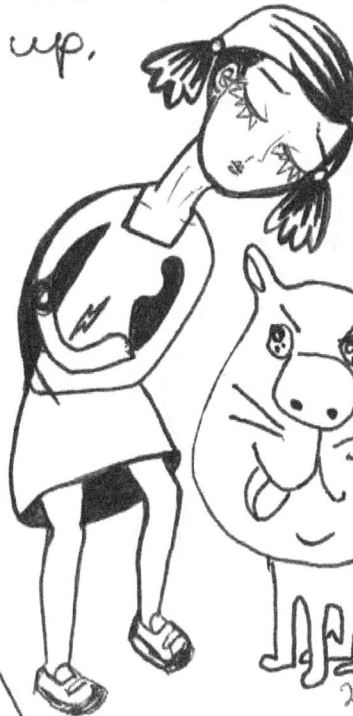

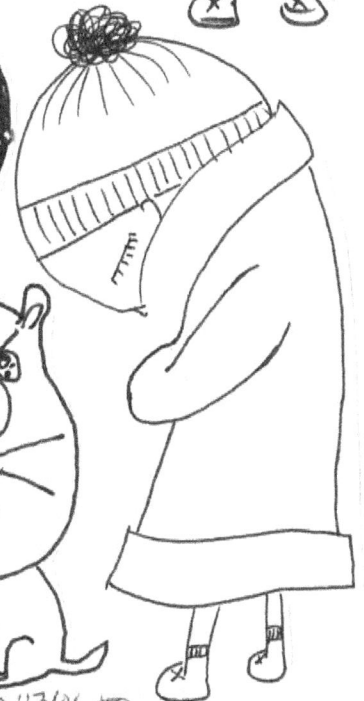

2/17/06

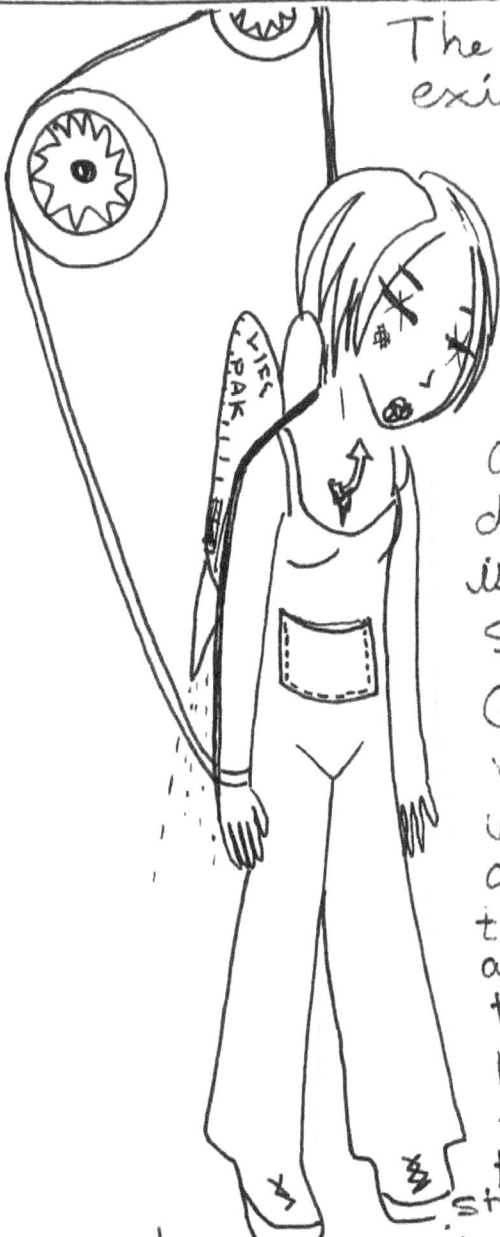

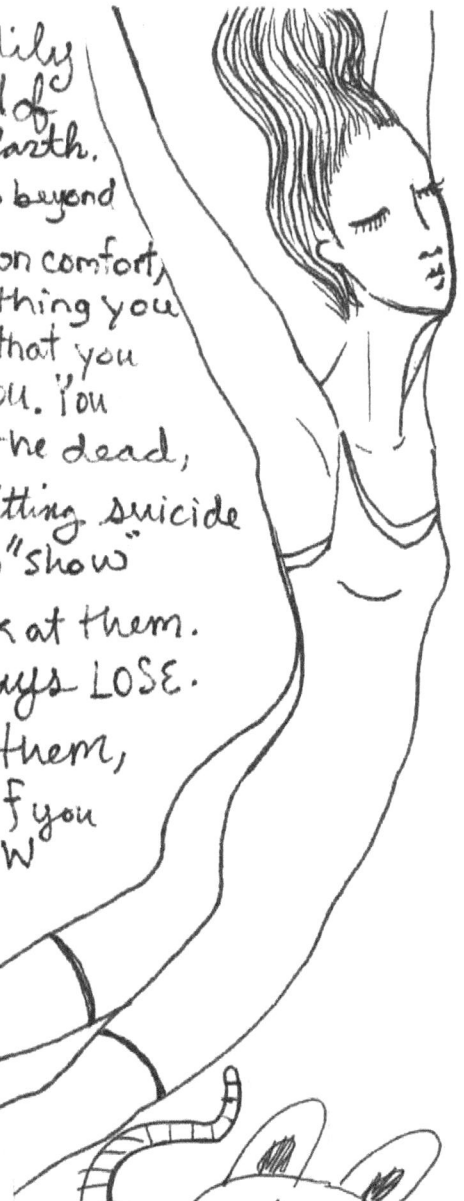

The end of your bodily existence will be the end of you in this reality, on Earth. Whatever you believe is beyond beyond life is your own comfort, you can believe anything you want. All we know is that you won't be HERE. No more you. You can not come back from the dead, dead is DEAD. Committing suicide is never a good way to "show" someone or get back at them. Guess what? YOU always LOSE. When news gets to them, well, problem solved. If you are wanting to die, KNOW that people will miss you and they want you to stick around.

When people die, they come to the end of their story. Life always has a surprise ending and death never gets any easier.

When you are here, you are supposed to be here. If I was not supposed to be here, I would not have a family, future, or be writing writing to you.

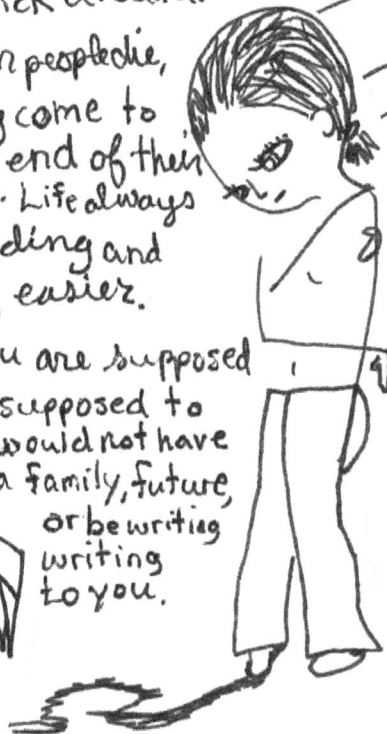

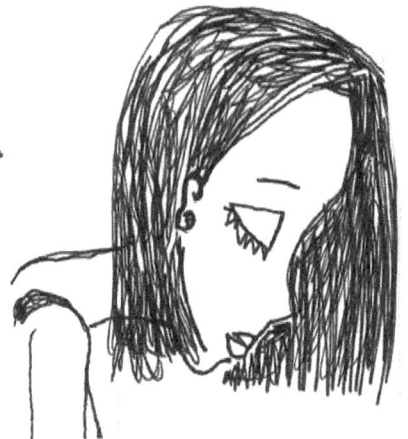

10/22/03

Don't end up THAT GUY. →

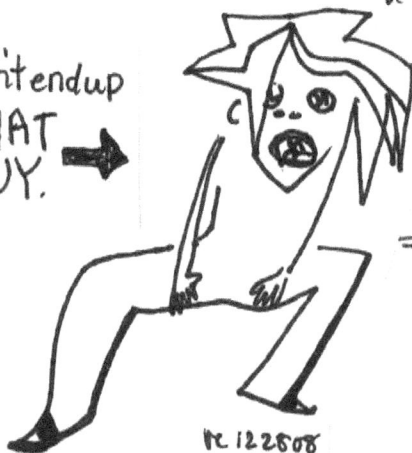

rc 122508

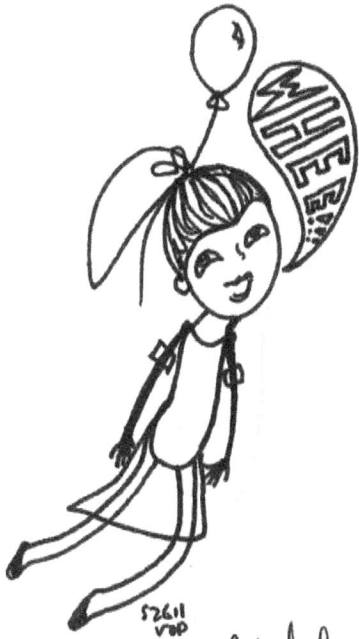

Life is hard for everyone, but we can make the best of it. You can be a recovering suicidal depressive or a recovering addict and make the best of it. When you look for negative bad things, you will find them. Garbage can always be made into something Fruitfull.

WHEE!

BOO HOO

It takes a Very Special Person to Love Me.

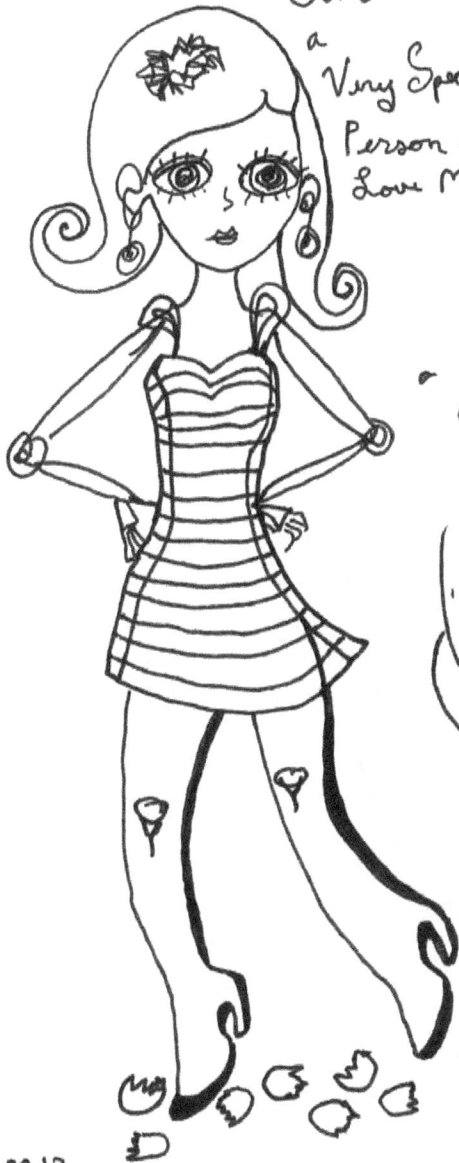

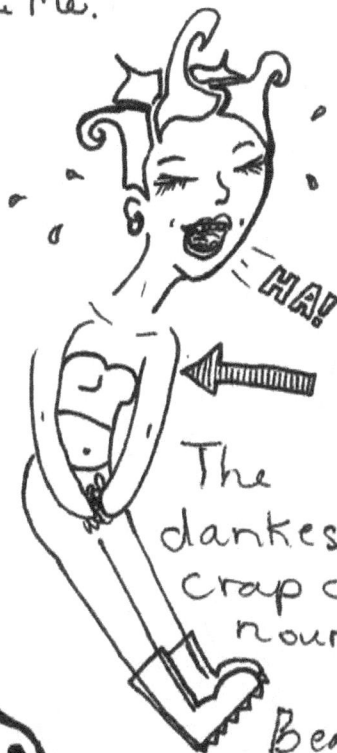

HA!

The dankest crap can nourish Beautiful Flowers. Then, poopy daisys are still daisys.

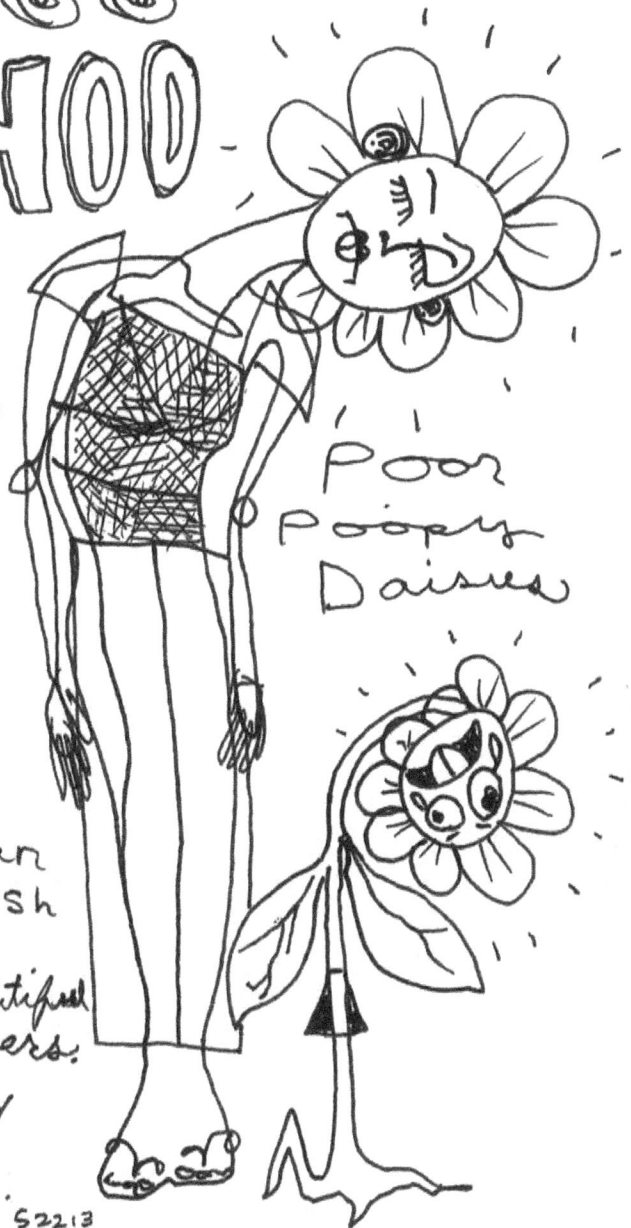

Poor Poopy Daisies

S22 13

S22 13

S2213

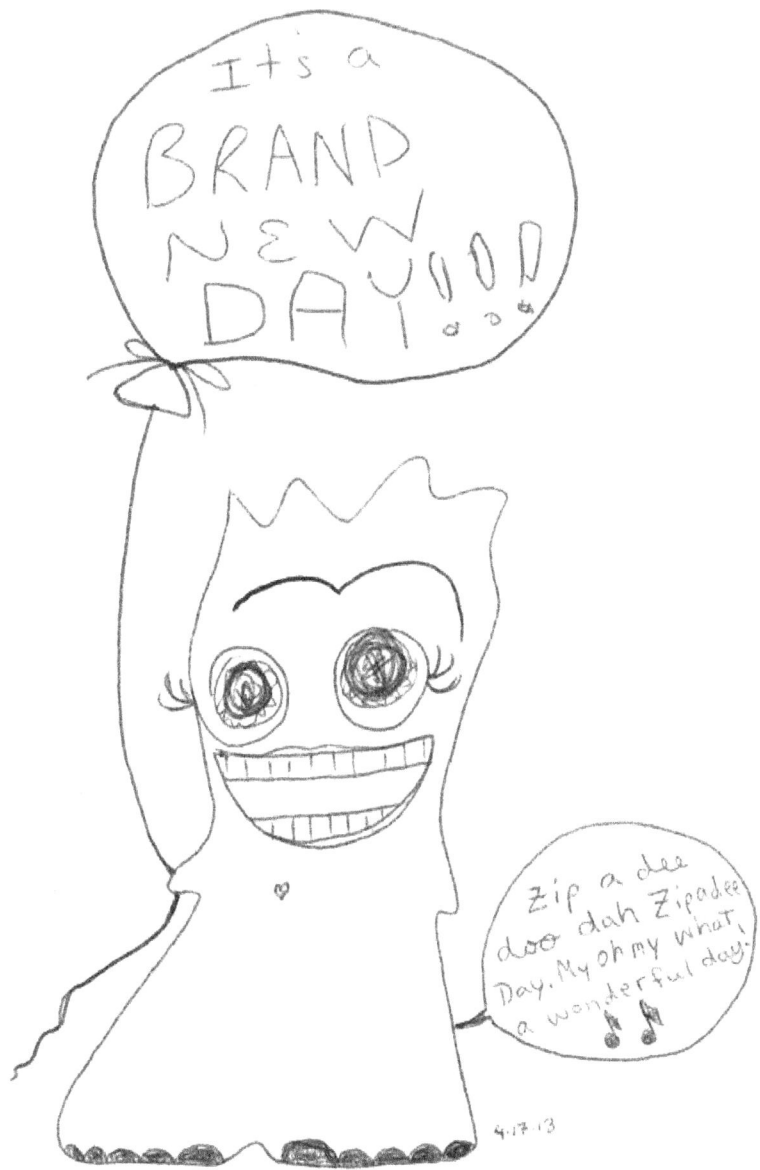

The End.

10 Things I Wish Humans Knew

(Things I teach my humans.)

1. Own your mistakes. Make it right if you can.

2. Be honest, honest with yourself and others.

3. You are in charge of you. You own You.
   Know consequences. When you do bad things, bad things happen.

4. Learn to Let Yourself Be Loved.
   If you don't love yourself, KNOW that you are Loved.

5. Learn about BOUNDARIES. Nope, Just NOPE.
   Learn to say no, enough is enough, this is NOT OK.

6. Sex = pregnant. Sex equals pregnant. Period.

7. Do not touch things that DO NOT belong to you.

8. If you don't know something FOR SURE, don't pass along as a fact. Life is the Telephone Game, but life is not a game.

9. If you don't have anything fair or non-judgemental to contribute, then STFU.
   Keep it to yourself, nobody needs that shit.

10. If something doesn't seem right, you are right.
    If you think there is something you shouldn't be doing, don't do it.
    Wrong is wrong, so simple.

Love, Faith, Compassion, Forgiveness, Kindness, Companionship & Non-Violence

I would like to thank the Lights on My Path. Your direction, guidance, acceptance, patience, and Love made my life possible. Thank you to each one who shared smiles and pain with me. Thank you to each one of you who showed me the kindness of God. Thank you teachers who know your students and give extra attention to children and young adults in need. Thank you to my bosses, strong independent women who gave me a chance. Thank you to everyone who supported my artist dream. Thank you best friends, sisters and brothers. Thank you God for giving me the strength to live and write this book, which was very painful for me. Thank you to everyone who cared to know my good side and accepted that I was going to be a butt sometimes. Thank you to my husband for understanding my pain and being patient with my recovery. Thank you to my son and his best friend Bets who love me no matter what and always make an effort to cheer me up.

Thank you to my psychiatrist and mentor, Mark Andrew Clifford. Thank you to the staff at behavioral health and the staff of FMH who took care of me. Thank you Providence for your outstanding staff and Neonatal Intensive Care Unit. Thank you owners of Alaska House and Well Street for being more family than my own. Thank you to their staff and studio renters for being my friends who make me laugh. Thank you Craig. Thank you Interior AIDS Association for your safety apprenticeship, amazing compassionate staff, and a new perspective on life. Thank you to any addict or person suffering who opened their heart to me. Thank you to all of the dedicated nurses and doctors in my life. Thank you to my friends' parents for being there for me when I had no family to celebrate with. Thank you to my aunts and uncles who made me feel precious, like a princess. Thank you to all of my friends with old souls. Thank you to everyone who comes to visit and cares about me and my familys' well-being. Thank you to everyone who let me get to know them and be their friend. Thank you to all of the misunderstood individuals I have met and known. Thank you to everyone who ever taught me anything valuable. Thank you to each person who let me know I was not alone and existed to them. Thank you to my friends along the way. Guy, Jenny, Mandy, Matt, Chris, Jan, Kell, Rookie, Mrs. Moore, Ms. Dee, Ms. Eddy, Mr. Marshall, Mrs. Husby, Mr. Buckley, Ms. Carlson, D. Mollett, Sam, Colleen, Rachael, Cam, Sara J, Tina, Manny, the late Jean Carlie, Mary, T. Wilson, Diana, Margaret, Tobin, Anthony, Alex, Glenn, Mike D., Dr. Masterson, Dr. Parris, Dr. M.A Clifford, Dr. Brenner, L. Brubaker, R. Brown, and my husbands family. I am sorry if I forgot to mention anyone. Special thanks to you, for reading this book. Thank you Thank you Thank you.
I have the best dad ever ♡

Oh!!! Cupcake

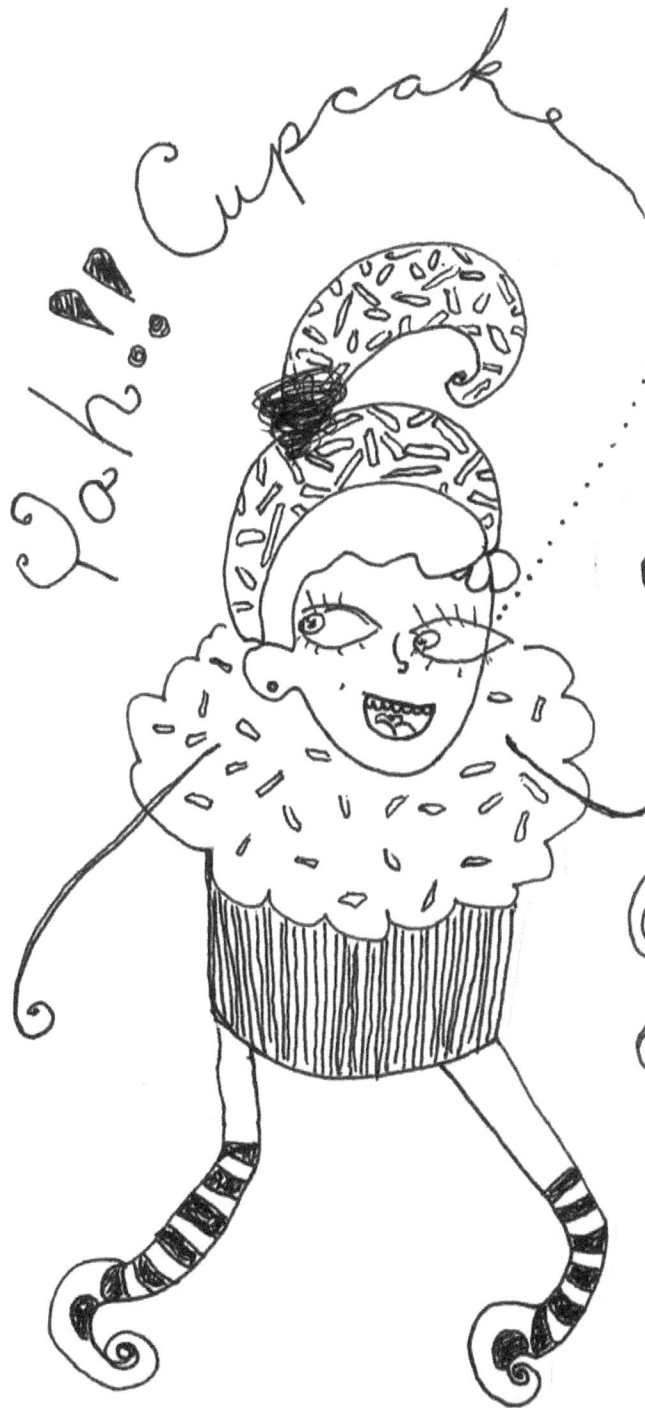

Random Silly Drawings

Notes about me, Valerie (author) of this book) and Madam Awesome DIR.
My name is Valerie. I am a married, Alaska Native, 30th
decade with one child. I have accomplished many things in my
life, but I never did them for me. When I was suicidal, depressed,
and anxious or anything yuck, I drew pictures. My drawings,
my reality. The drawings in this book are from the year 2000 until
2013. None of them were digitally altered or retouched. This entire
book is handmade. I don't have a social network or internet identity.
I don't want the fame, or the fortune. The most I can hope for, is that this
book at least lets a person know they are not alone and they are not
crazy. I am not trying to make alcohol sound bad, Alcohol makes itself
sound bad. Poison in a pretty bottle. The smallest reaction I can hope for
is a smile. Some drawings may look like people you know, but they are imagined.

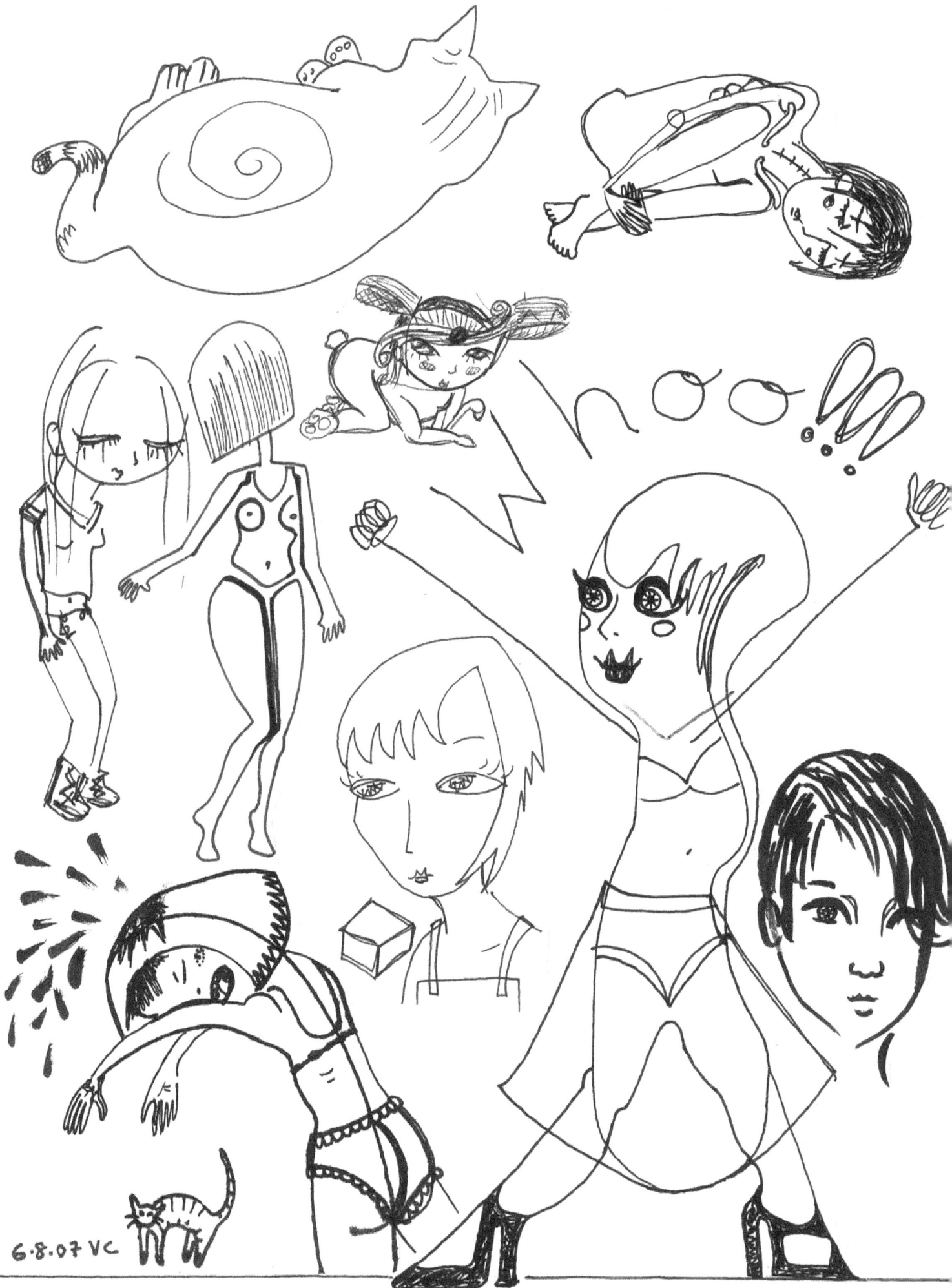

whoo!!!

6.8.07 VC

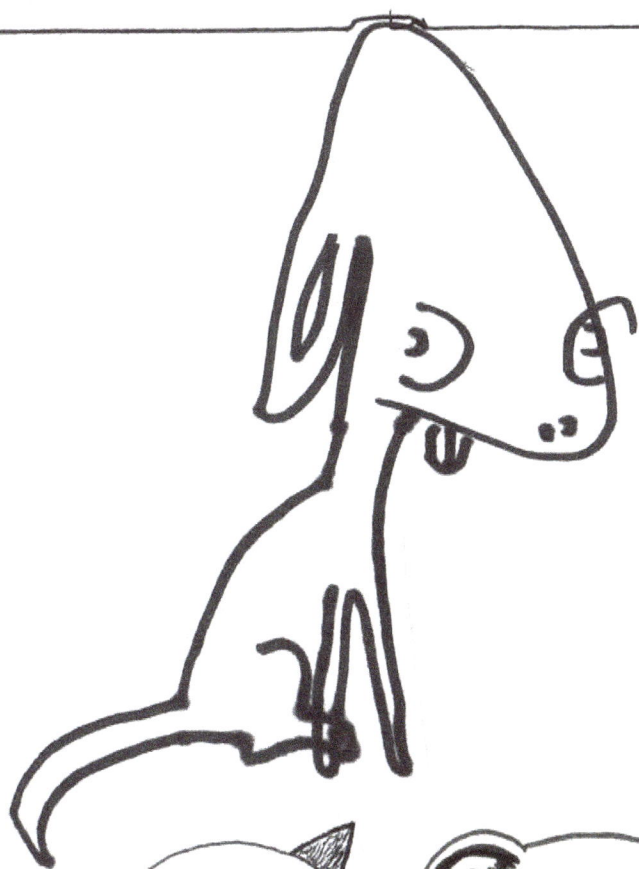

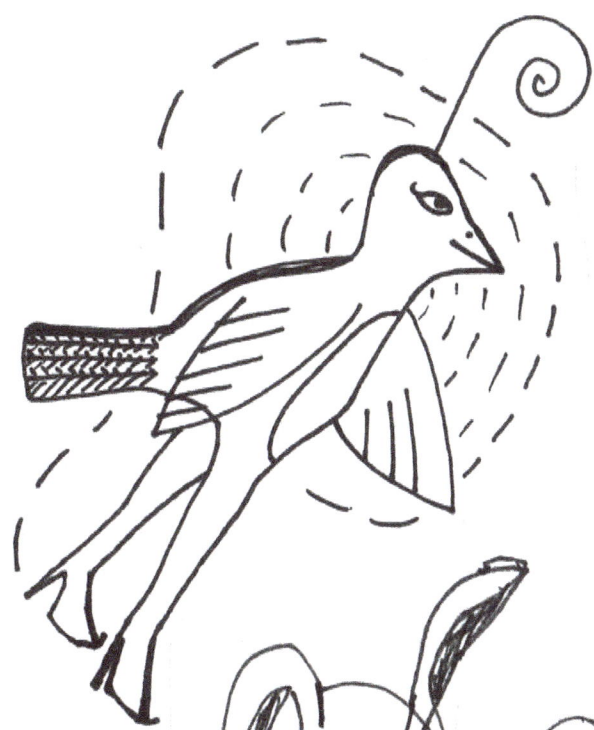

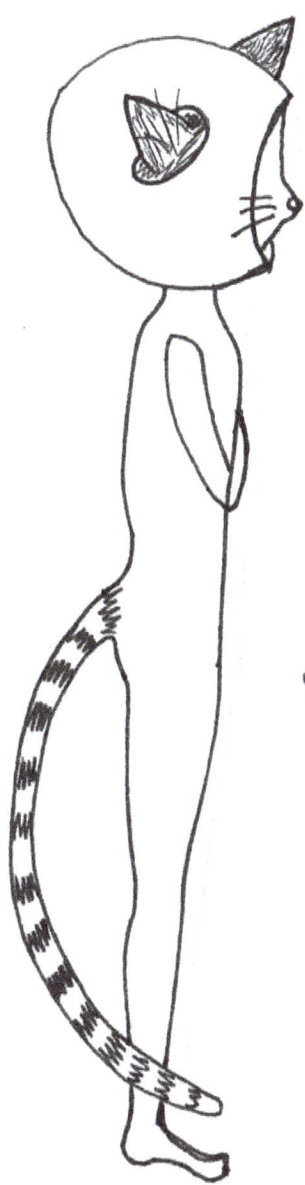

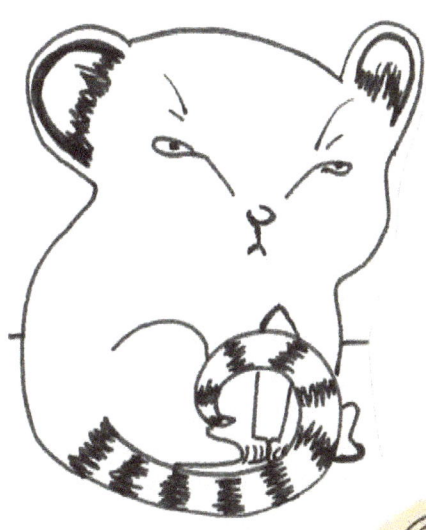

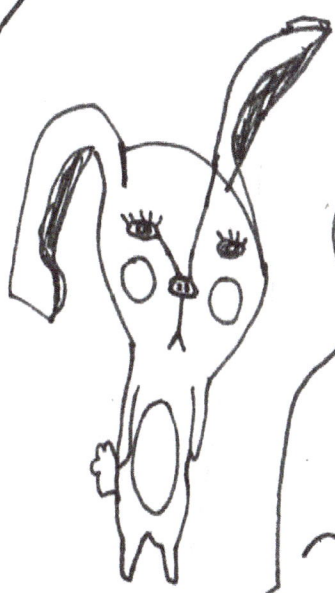

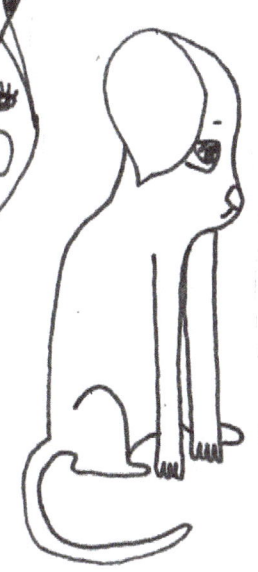

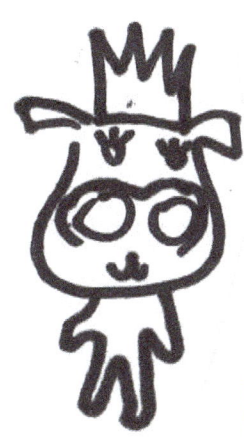

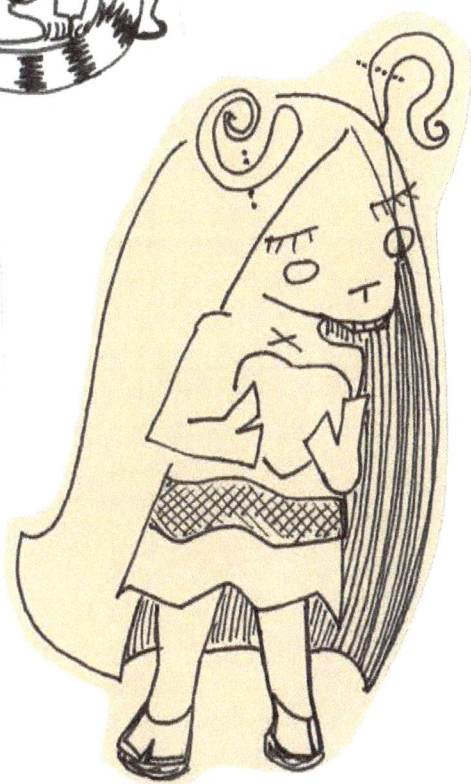

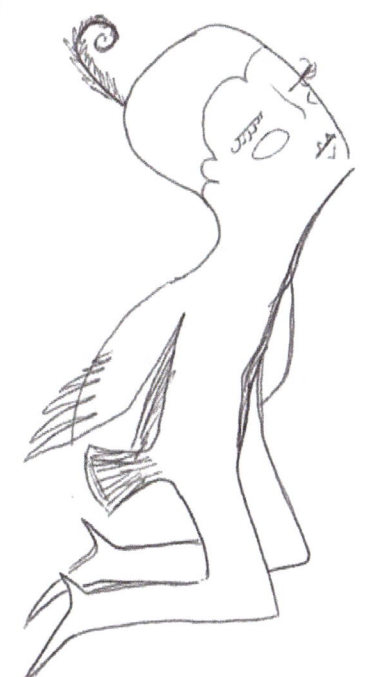

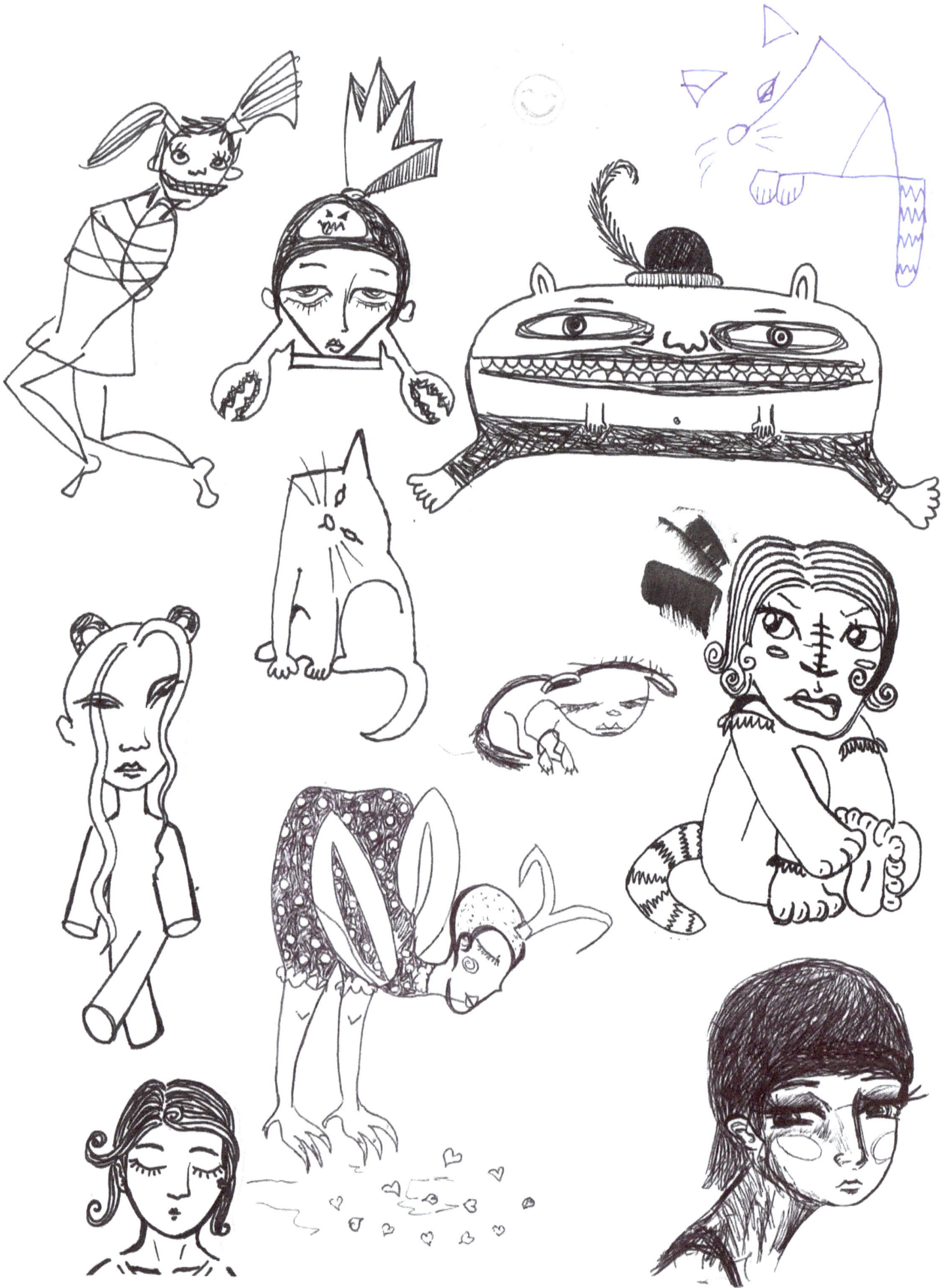

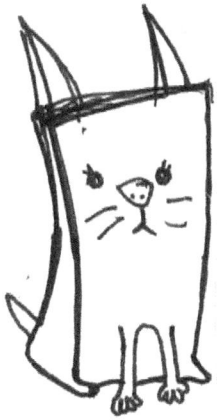
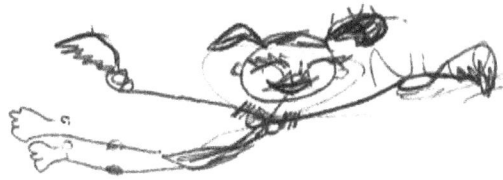
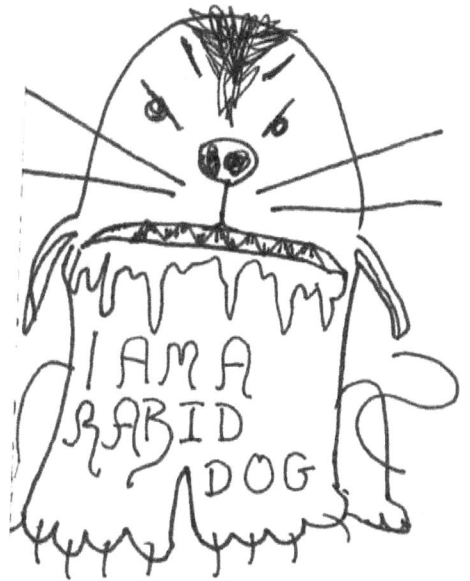

I AM A RABID DOG

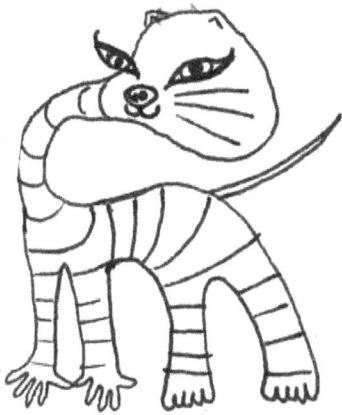
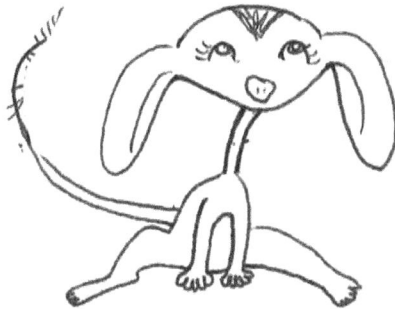
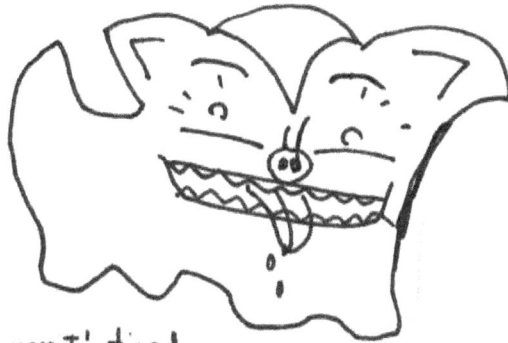
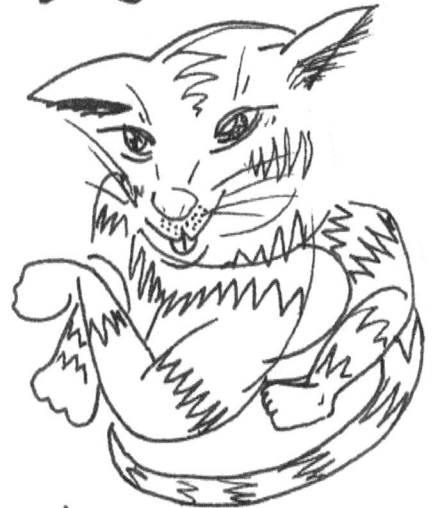

DamnImtired.

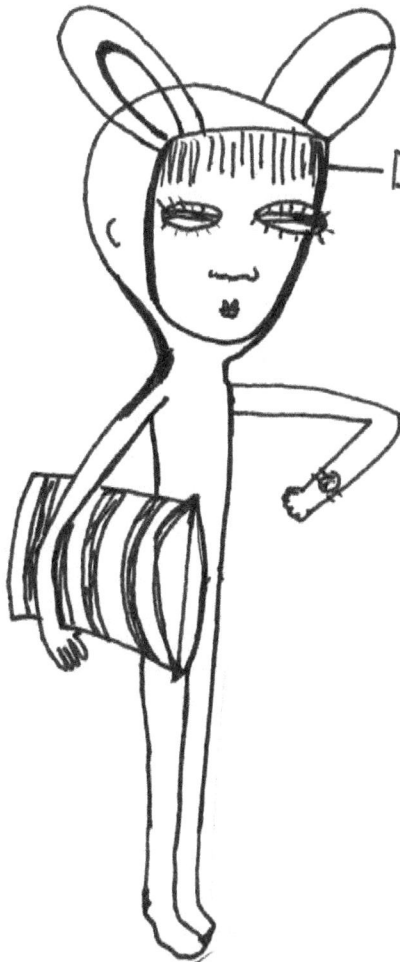
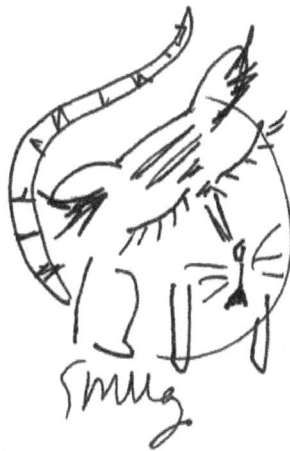
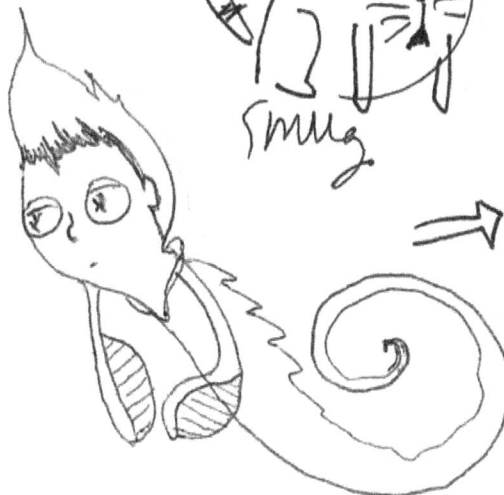
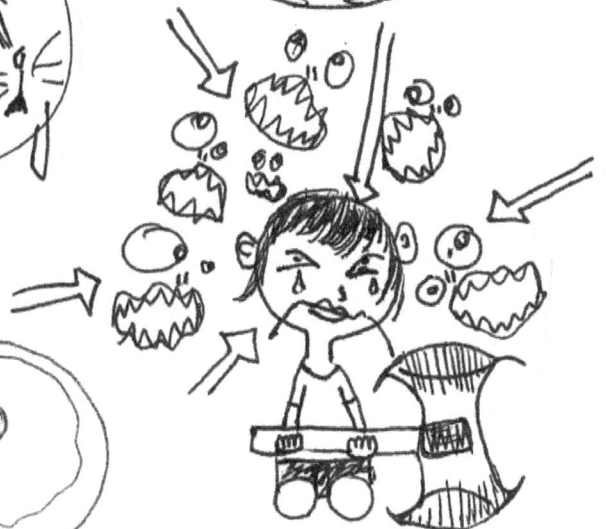

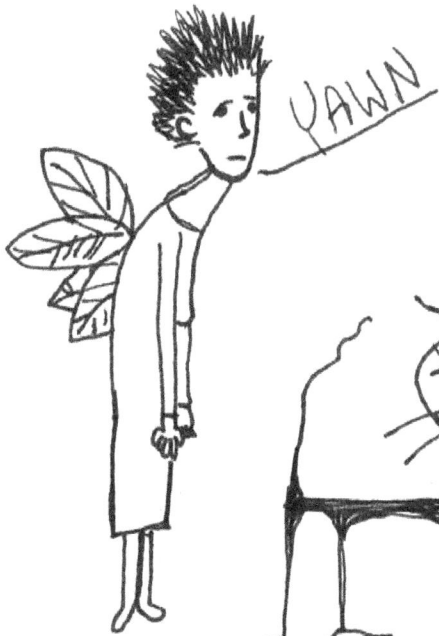
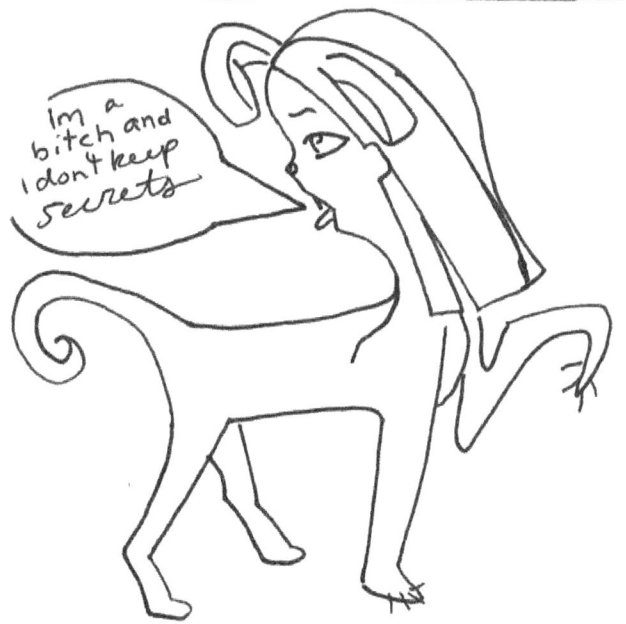
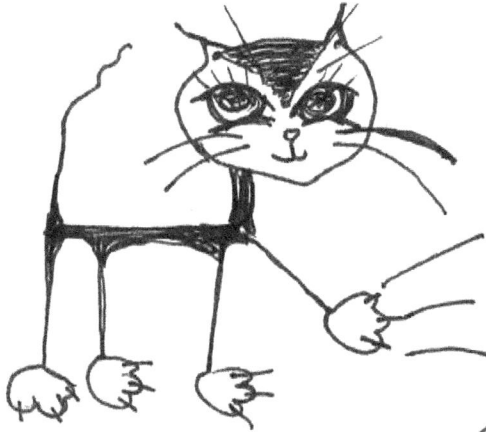
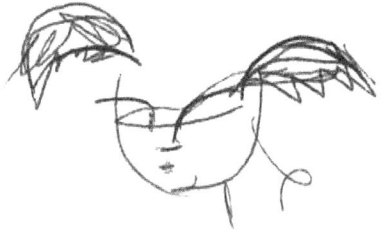
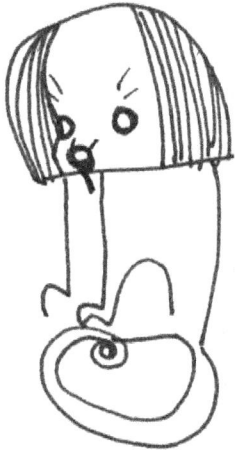
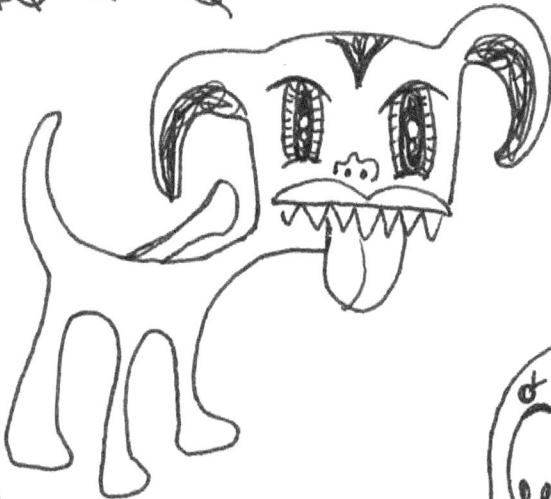
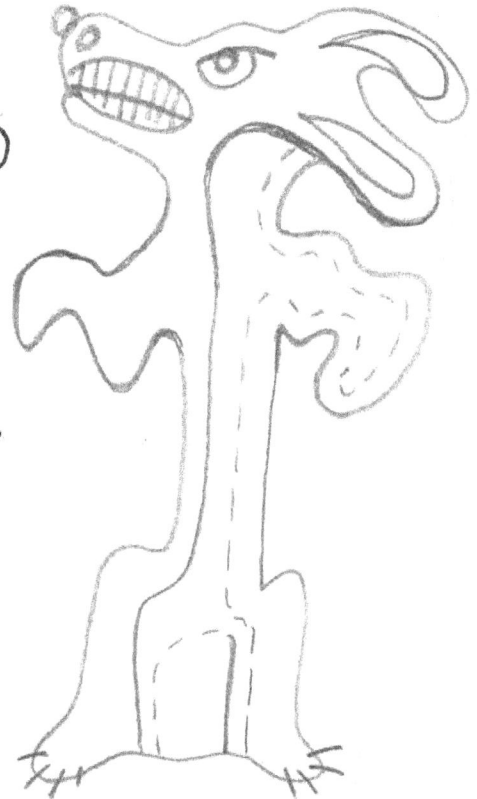
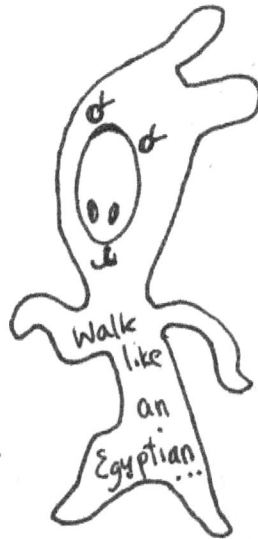
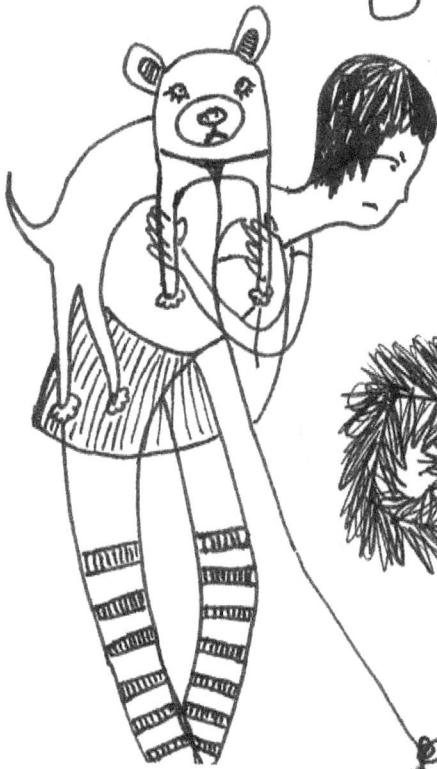
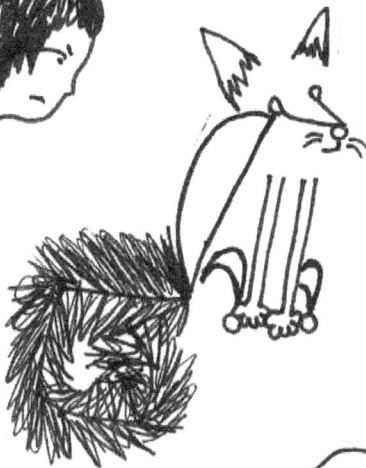
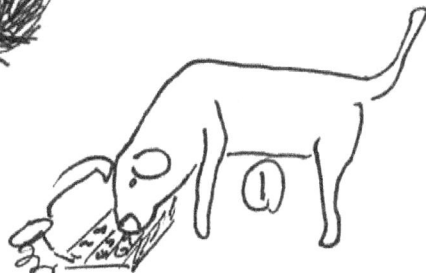
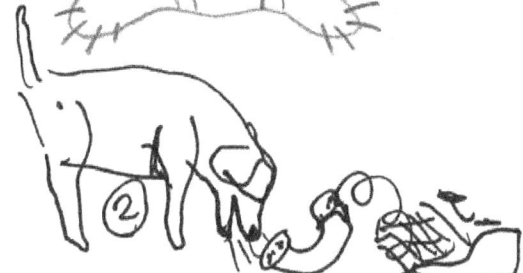

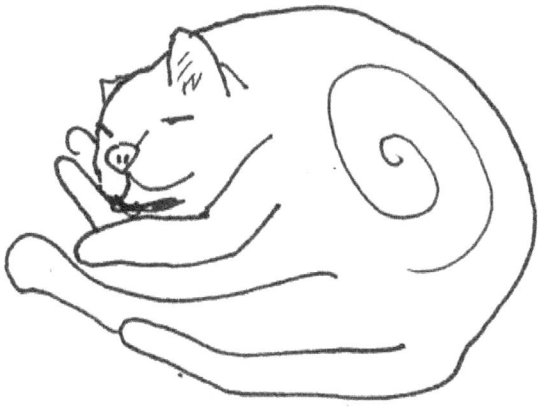
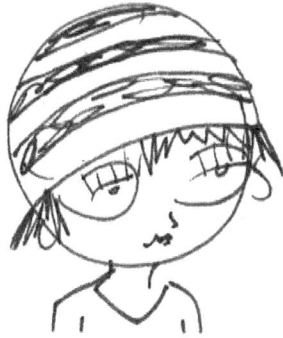
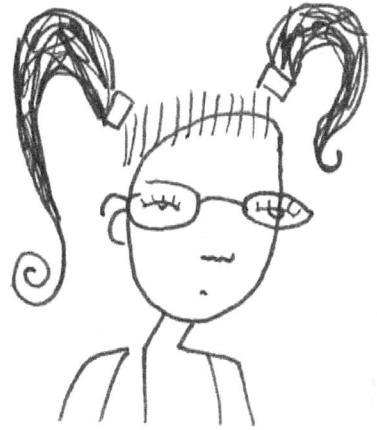
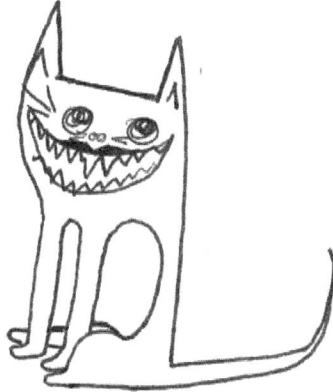
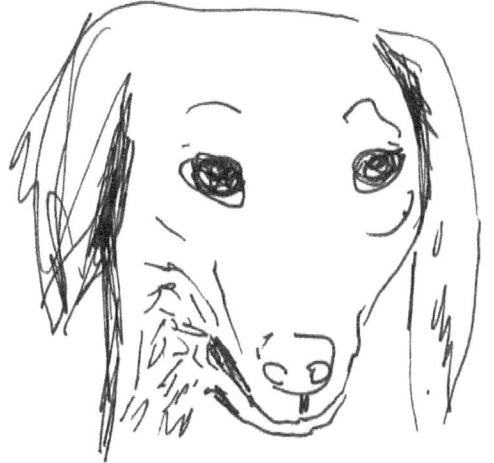

Lil
Roach

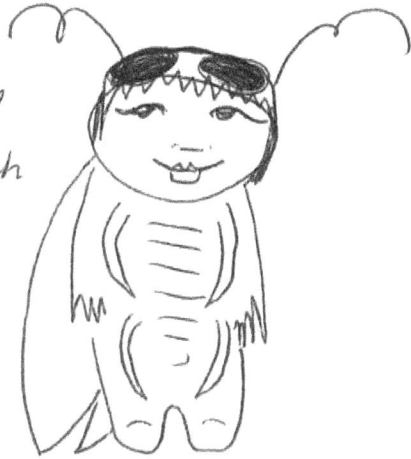
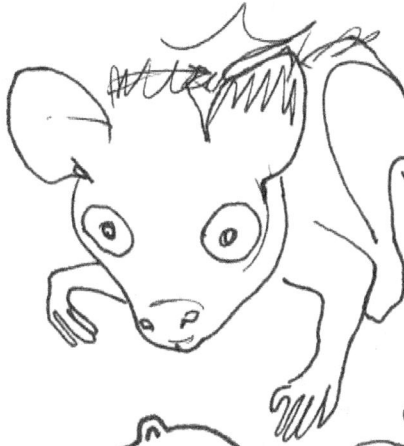

Rat
dog.

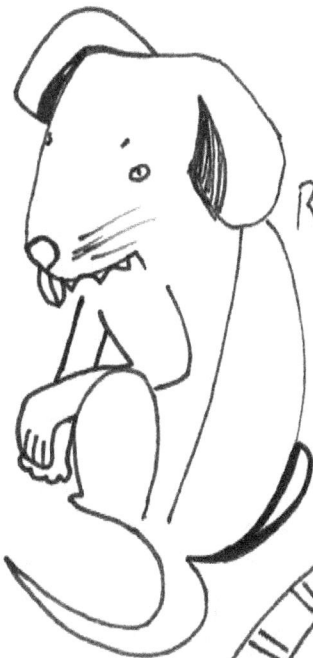

Fft!. Ffft!

Dah!

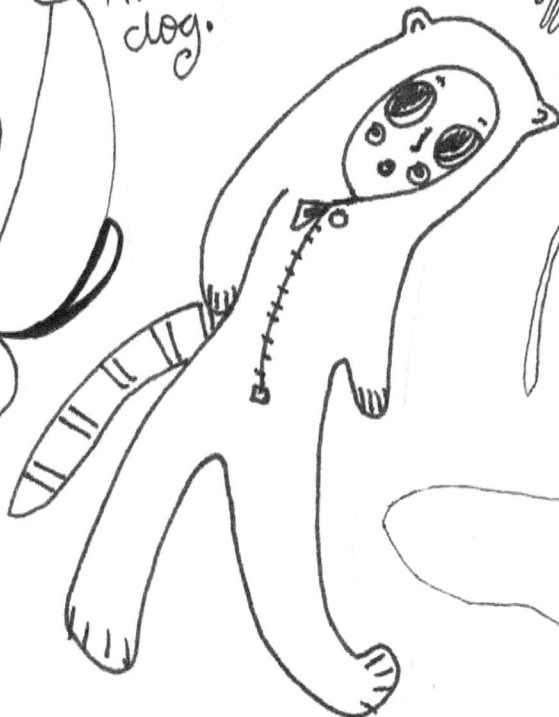
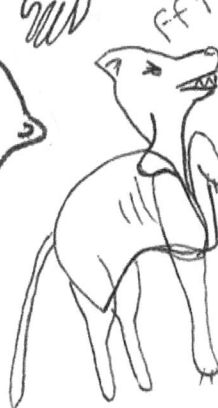
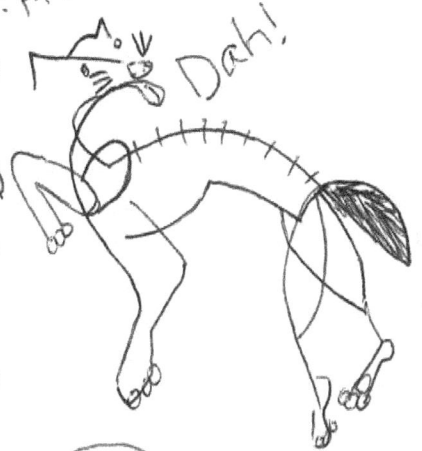
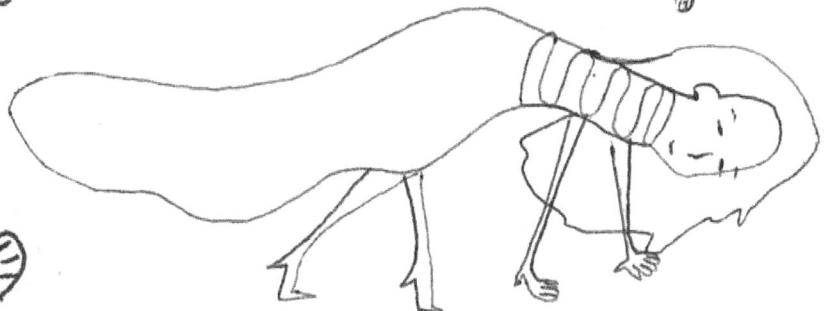

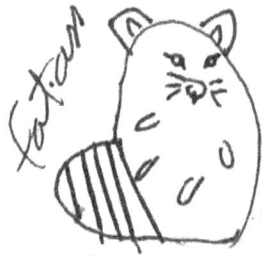

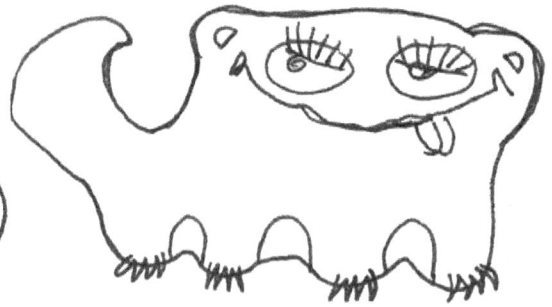

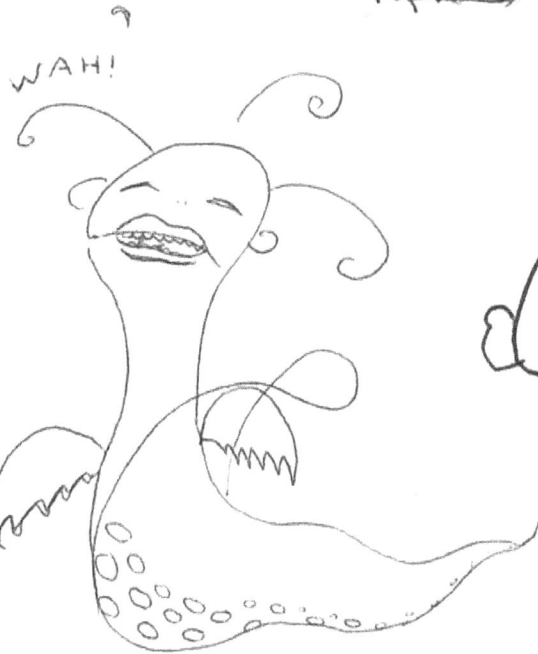

WAH!

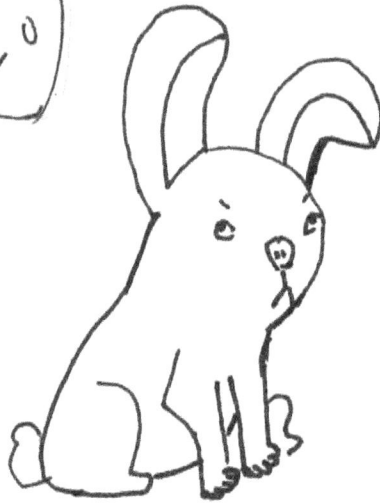

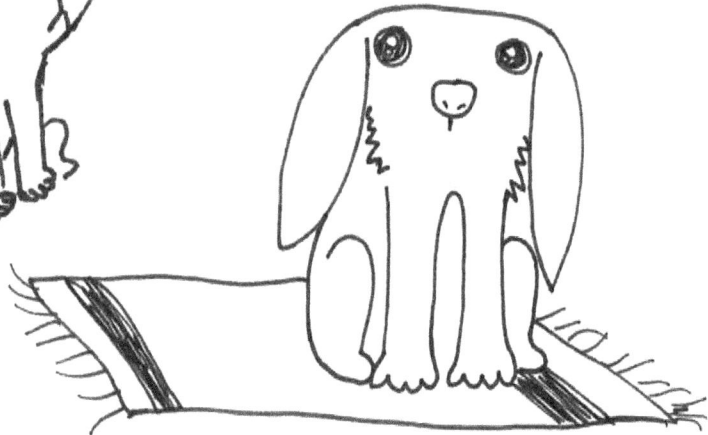

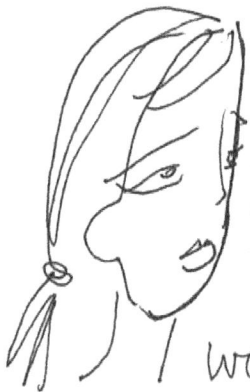

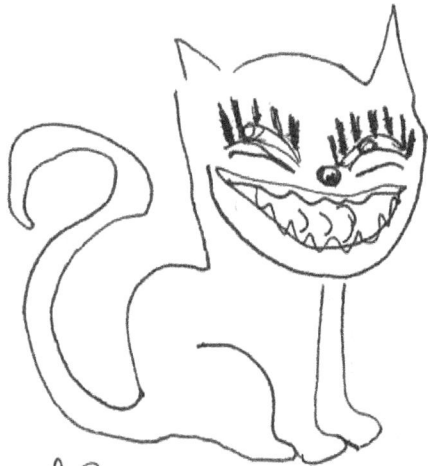

worried?

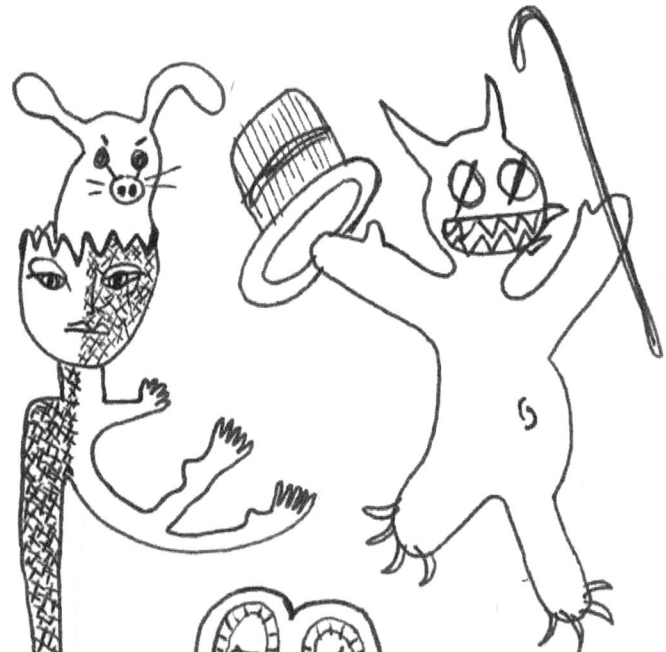

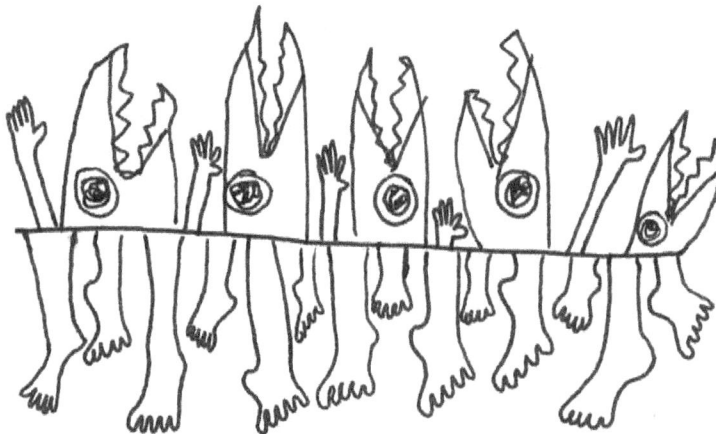

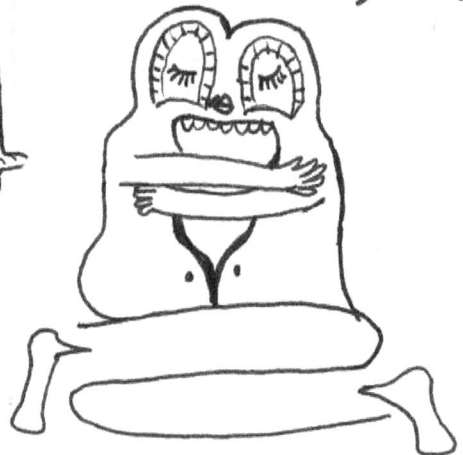

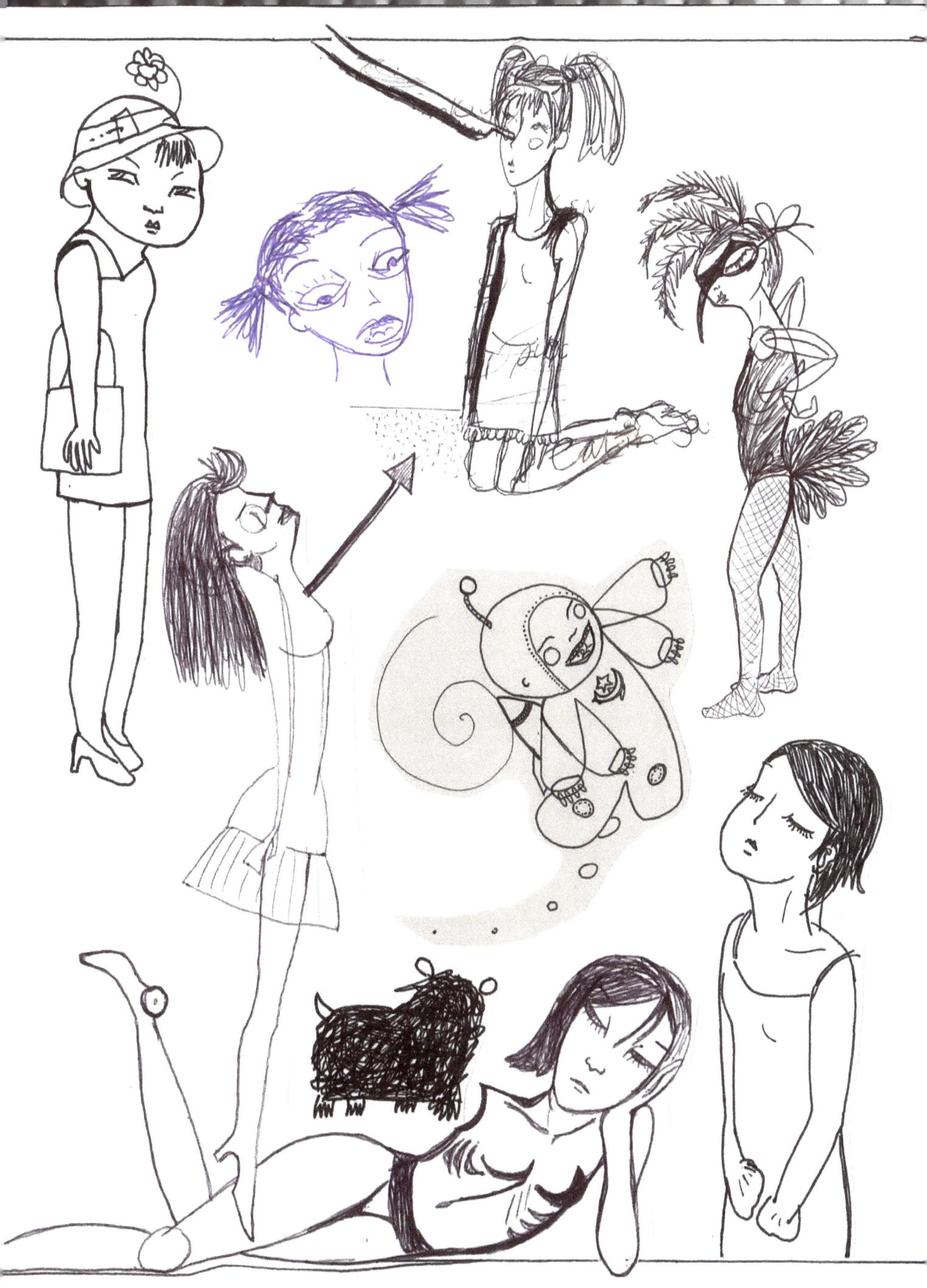

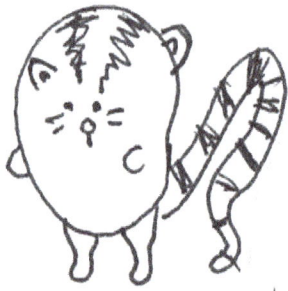

ouch ouch ouch
ouch ouch
ouch

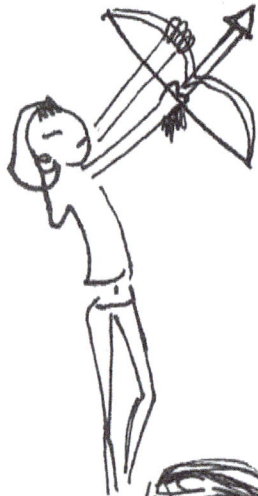

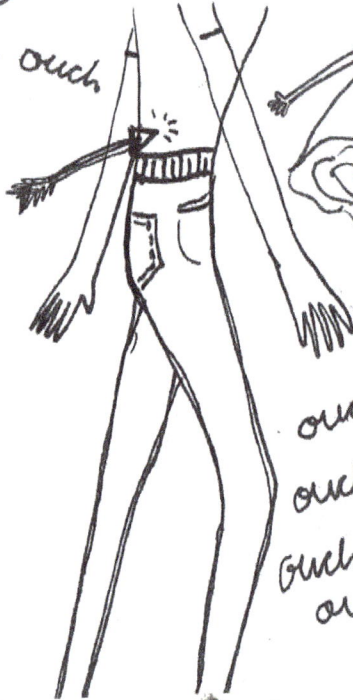

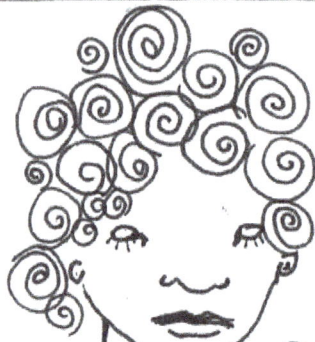

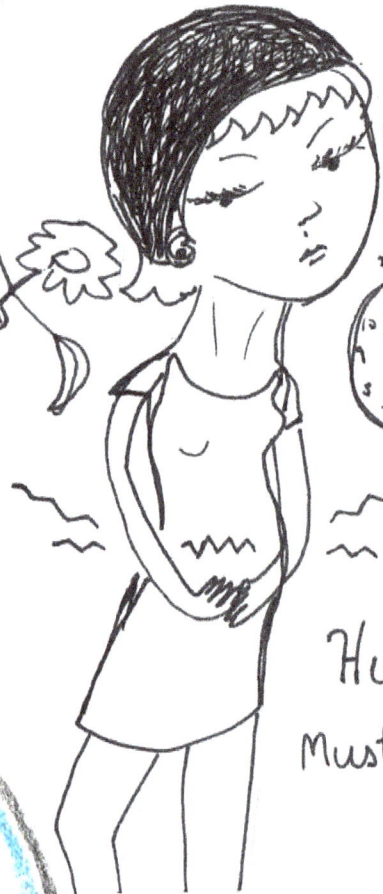

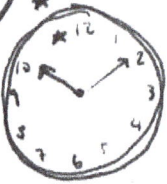

ouch
ouch ouch
ouch ouch
ouch

Hungry.
Must wait.

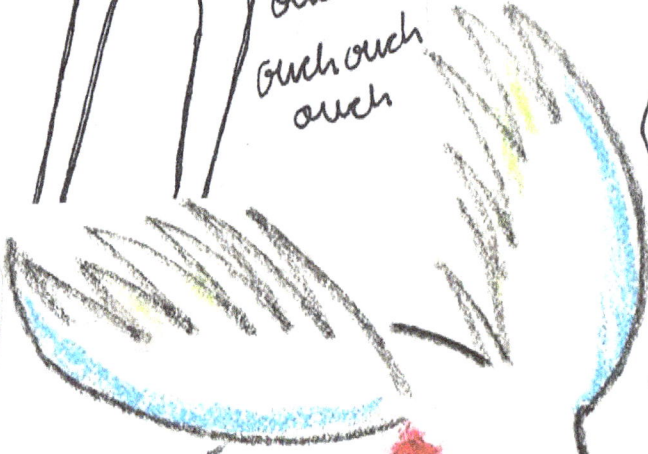

It is all
about
you.

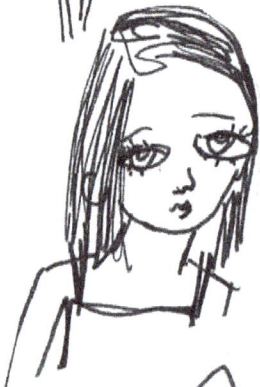

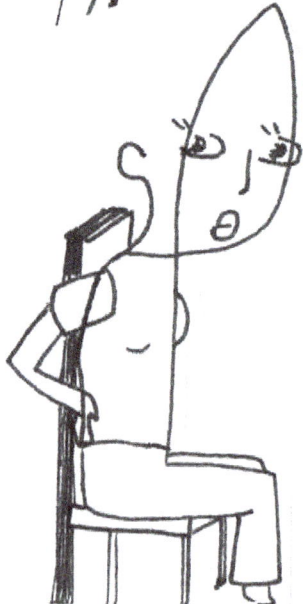

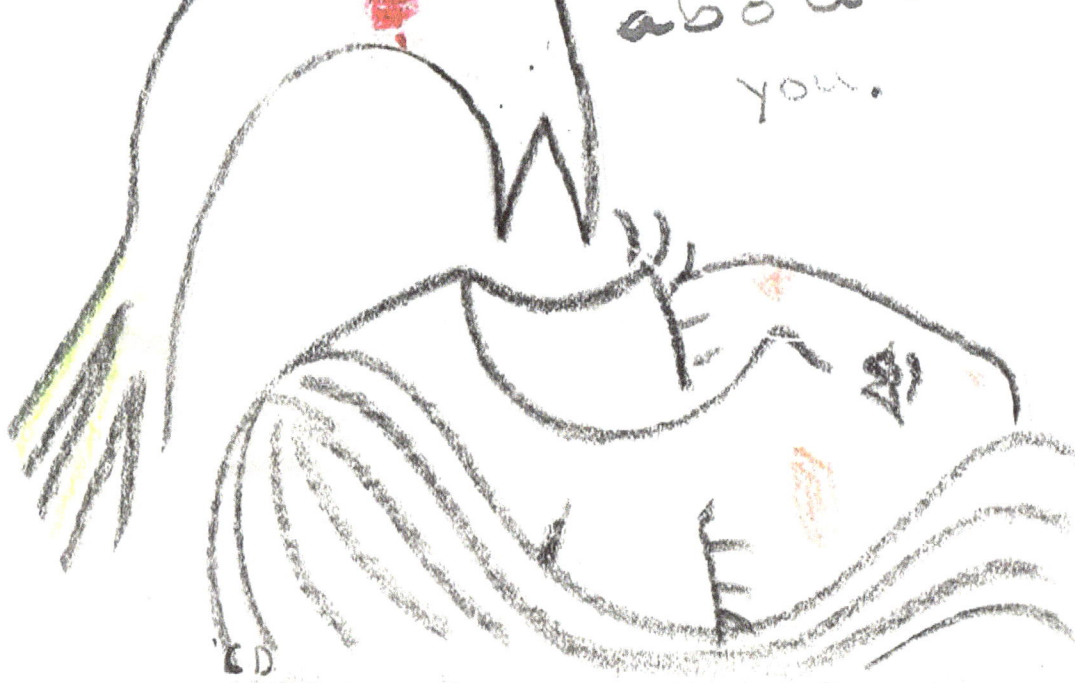

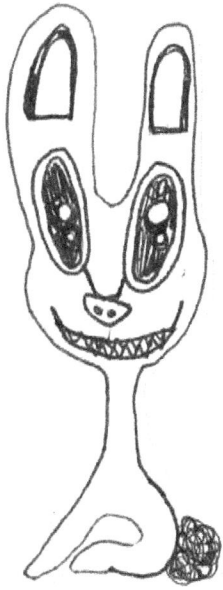
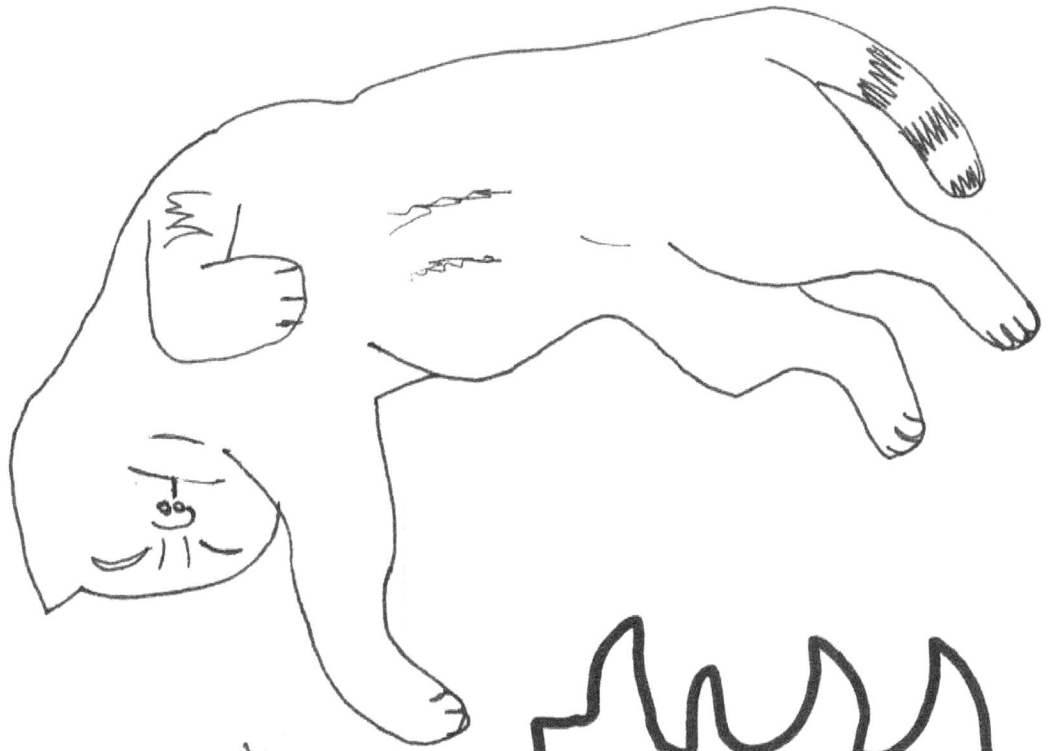
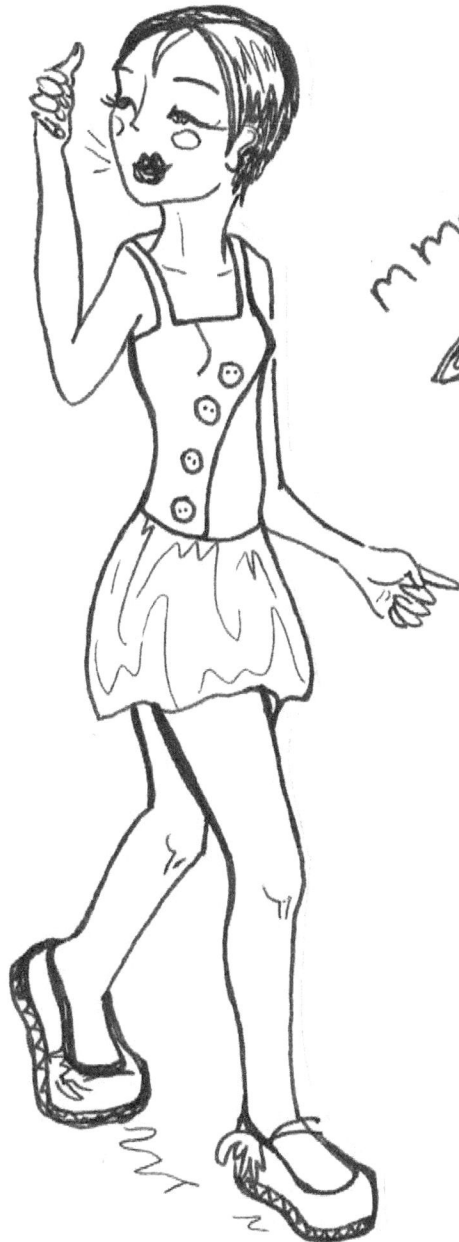

mmmoogh

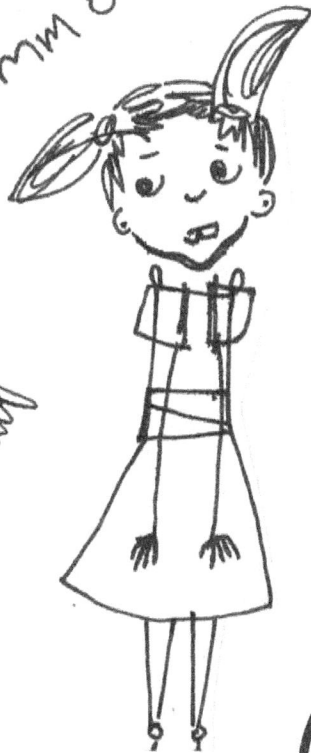
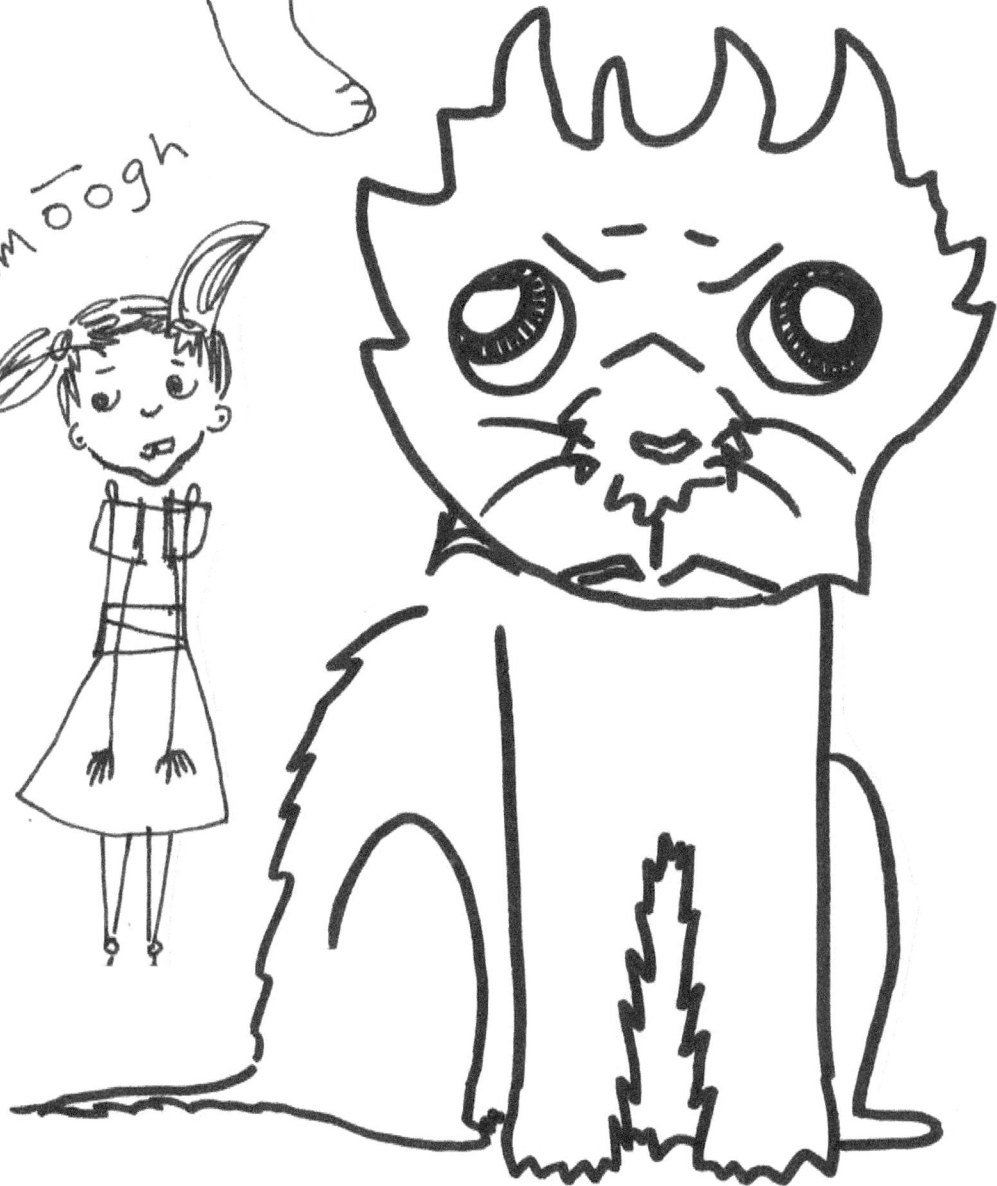

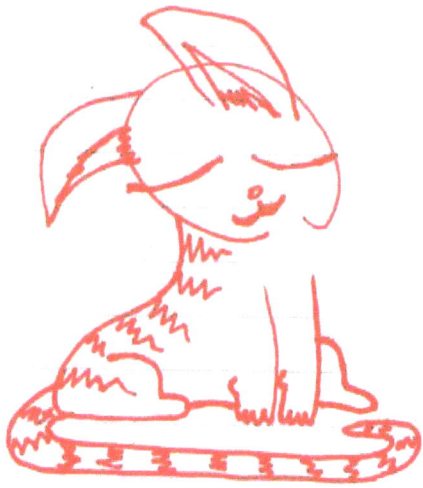
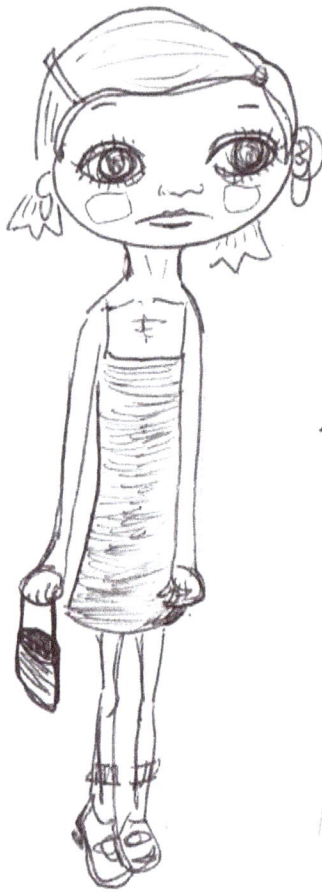
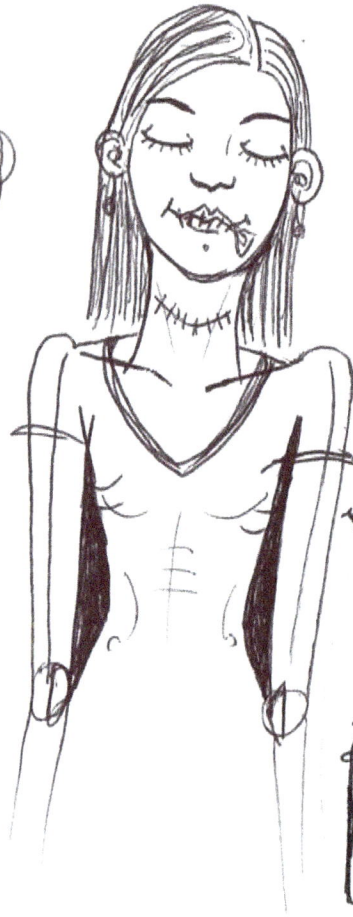
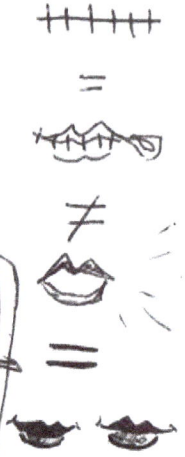
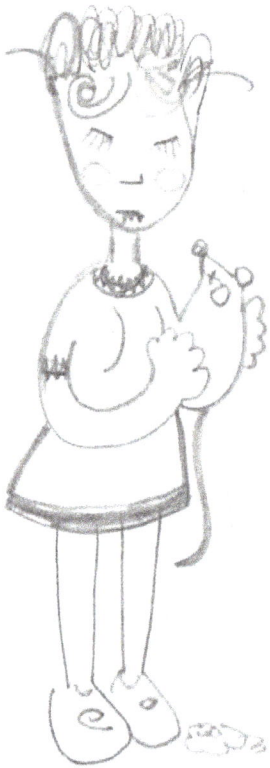
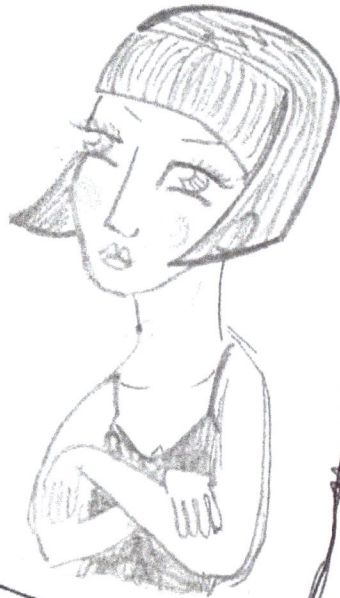
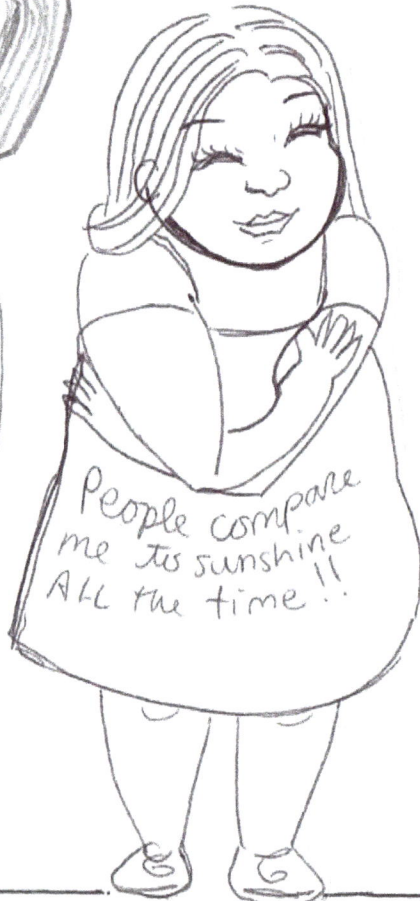
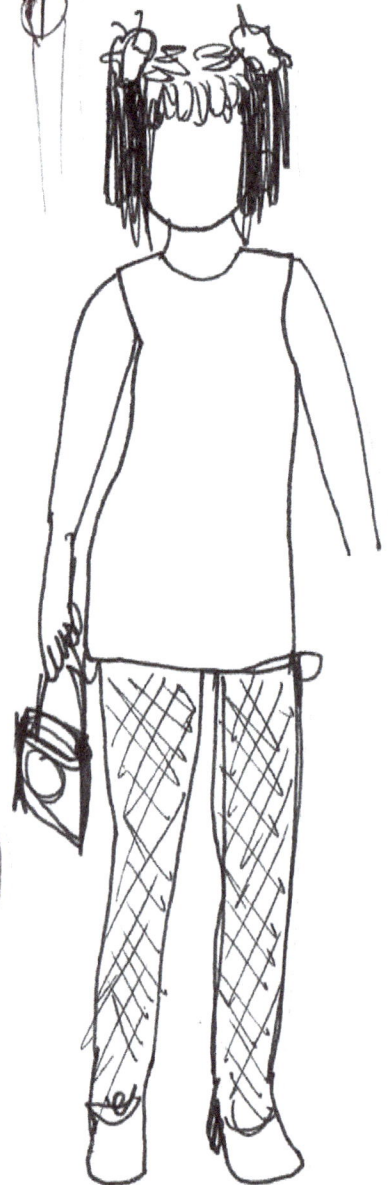
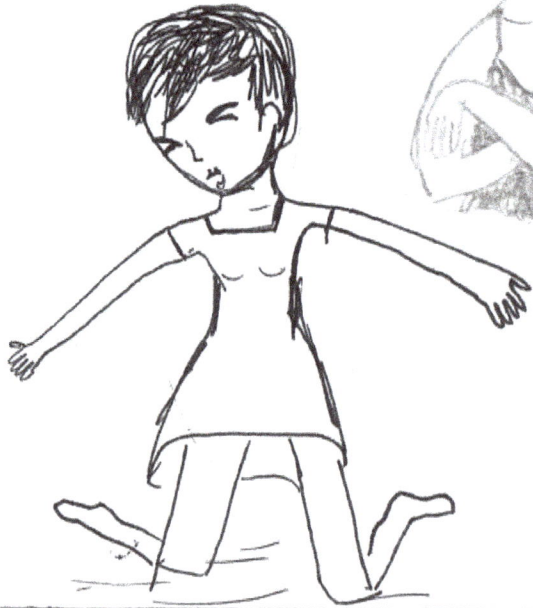

People compare
me to sunshine
All the time !!

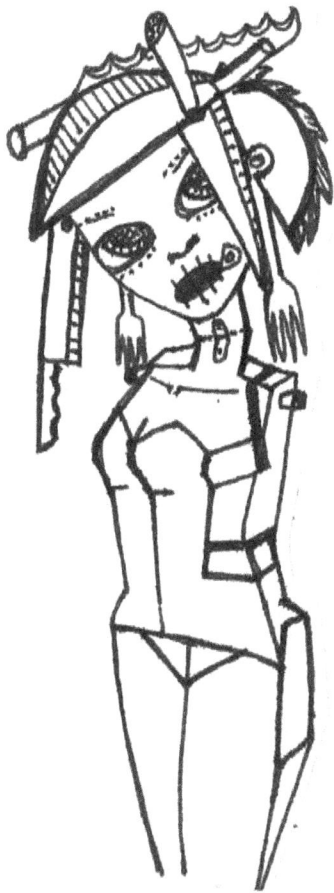

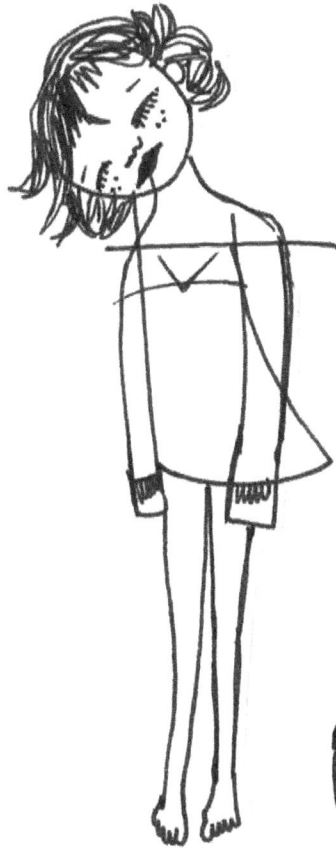

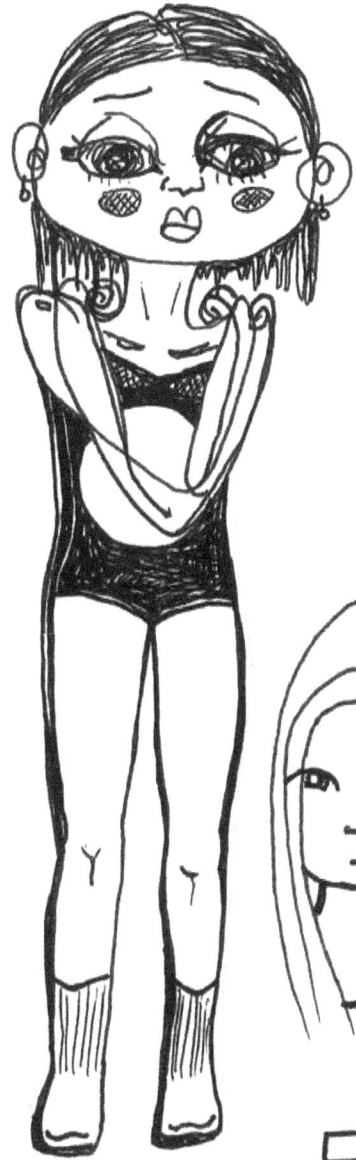

Why?
Why??
Why???

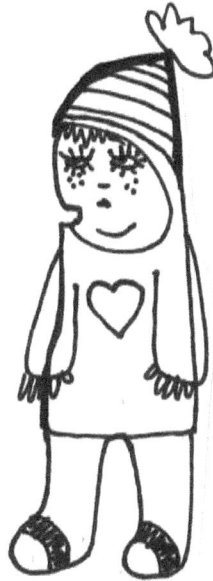

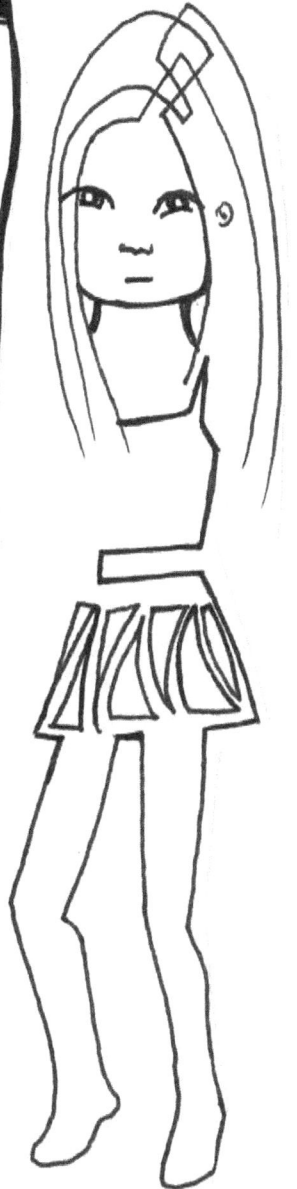

The overachiever always knows the ANSWER.

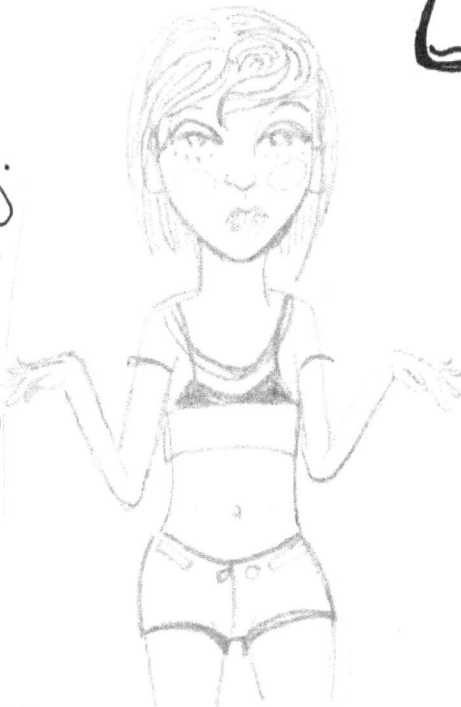

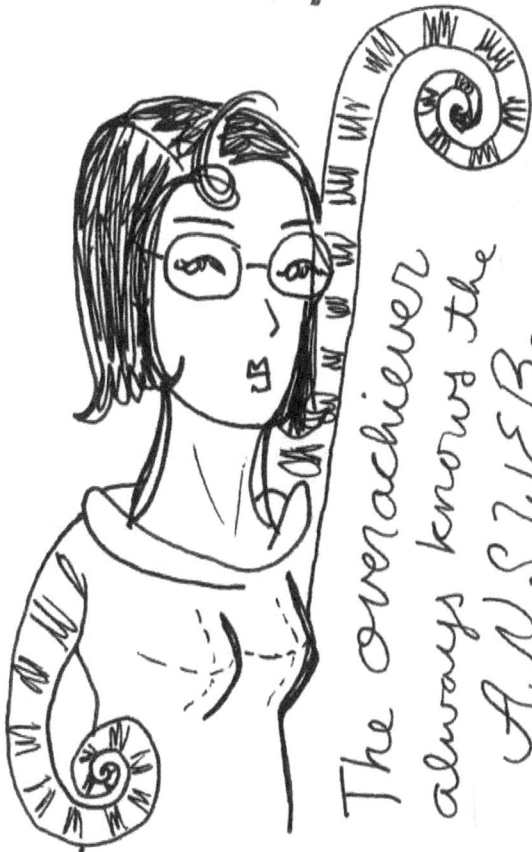

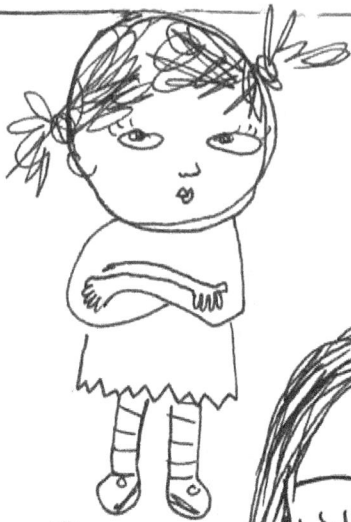

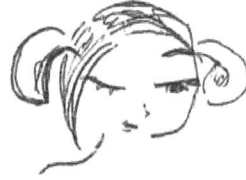

The sadness is back unexpected.

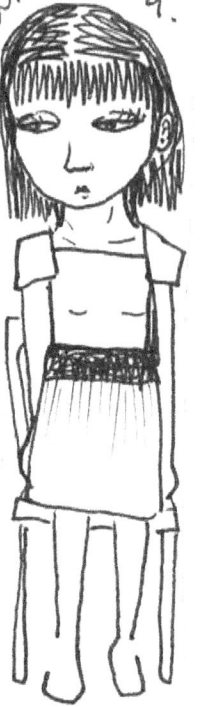

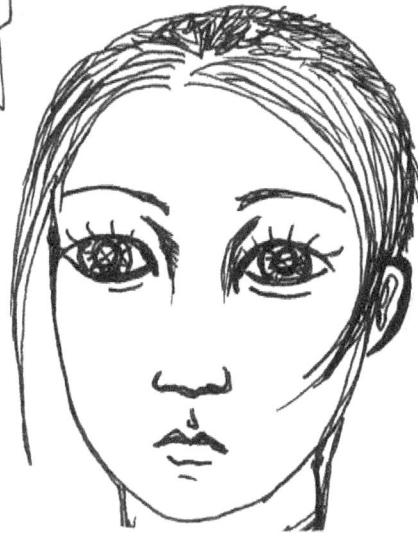

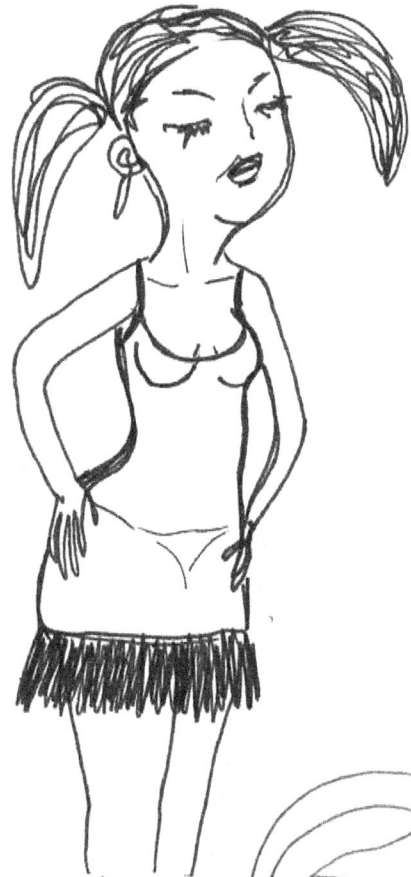

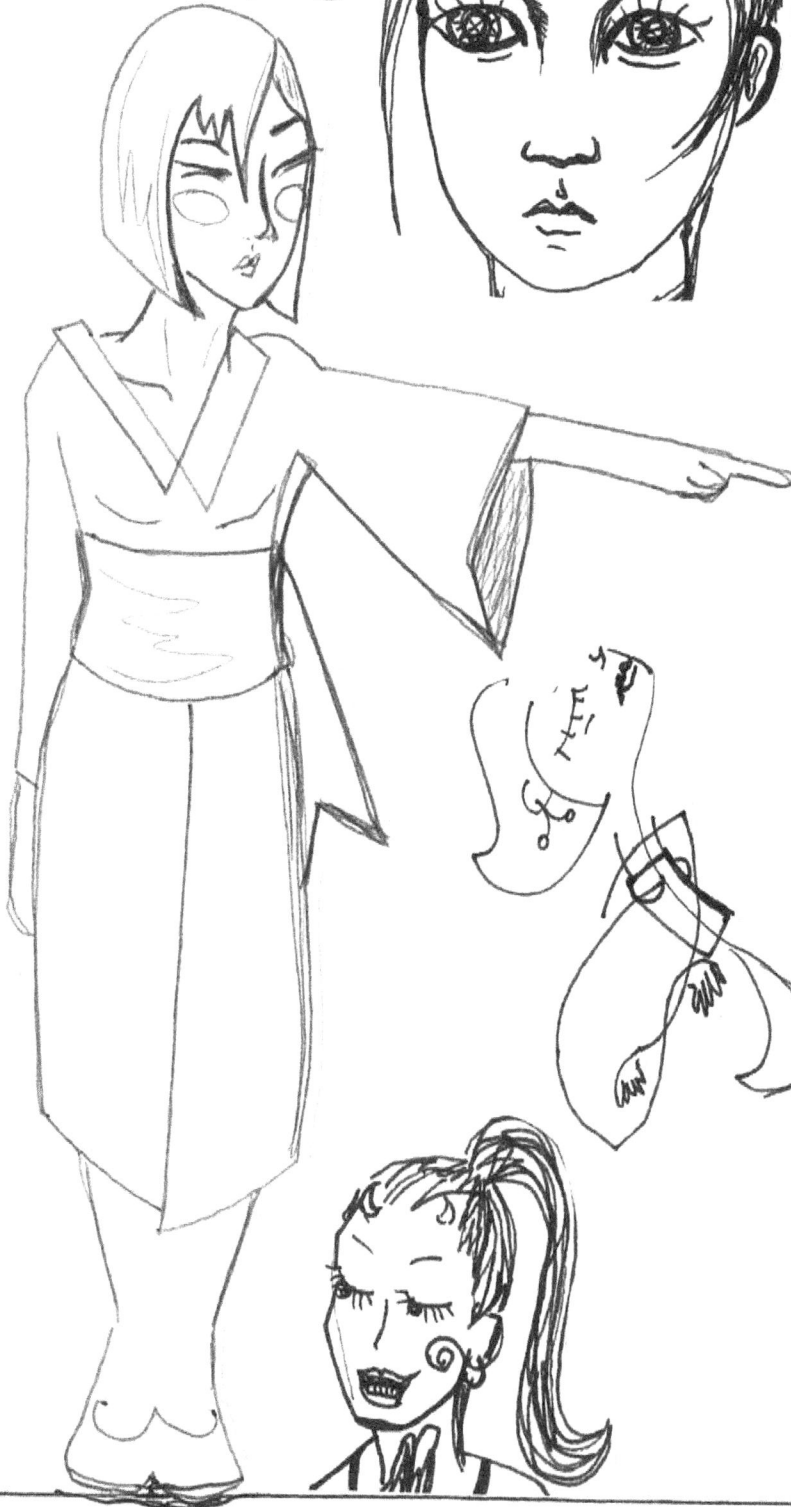

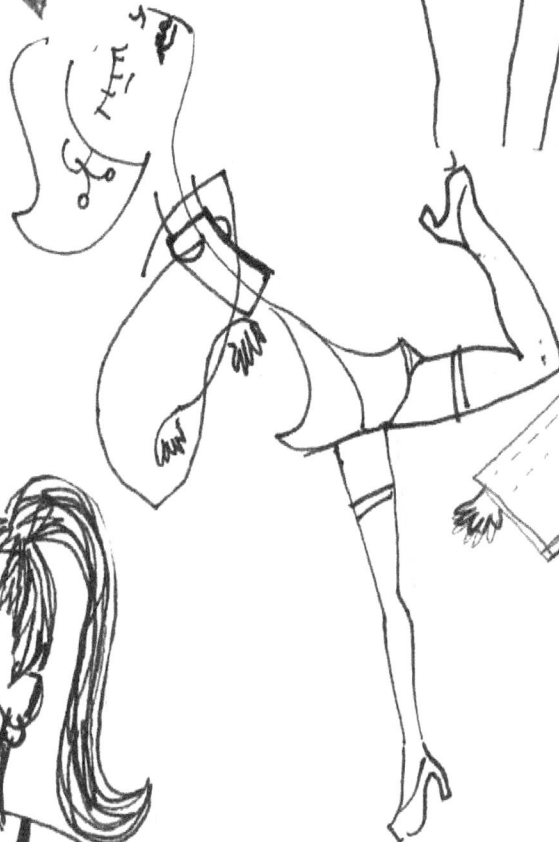

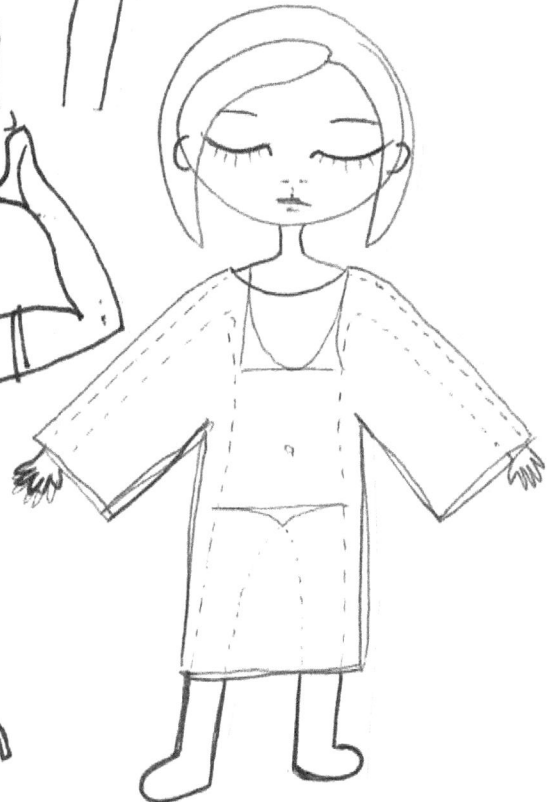

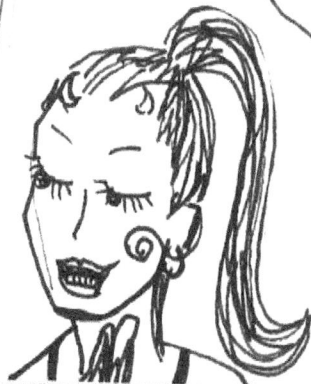

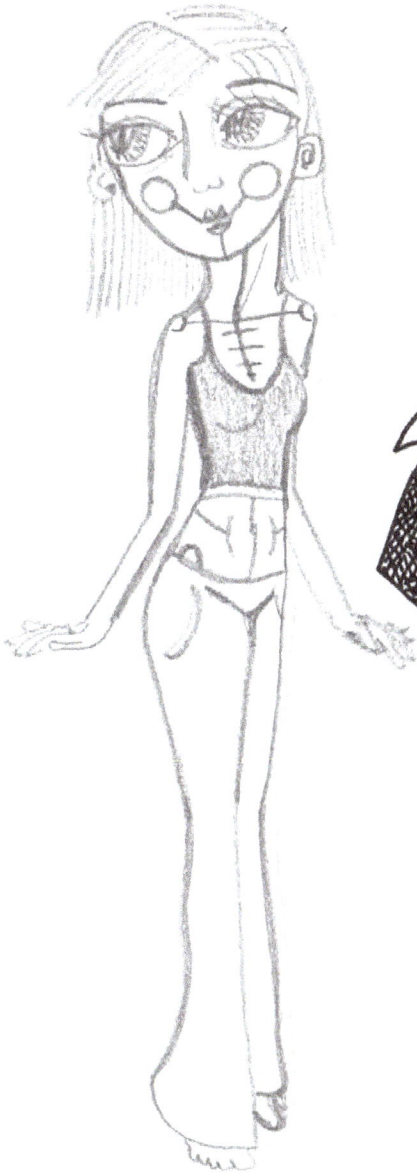
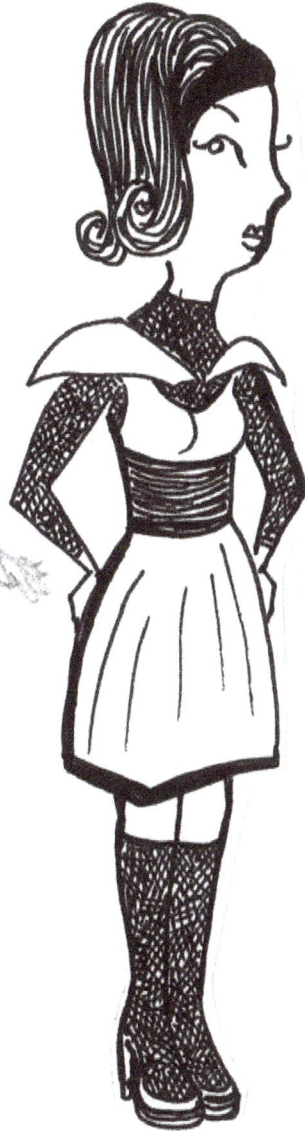
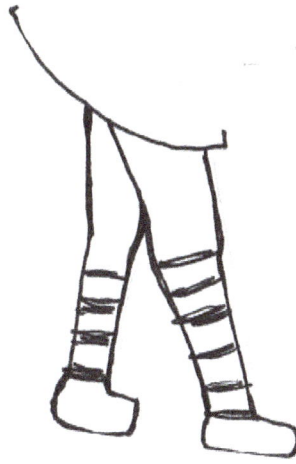
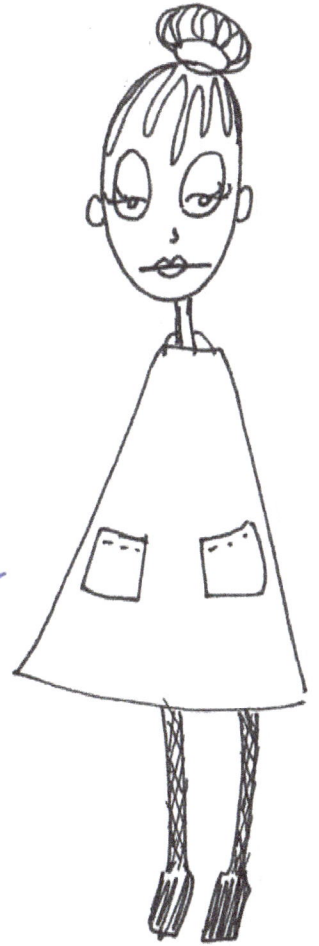
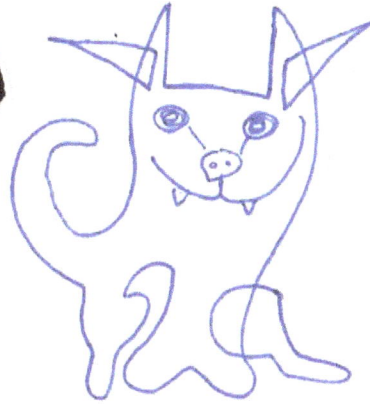
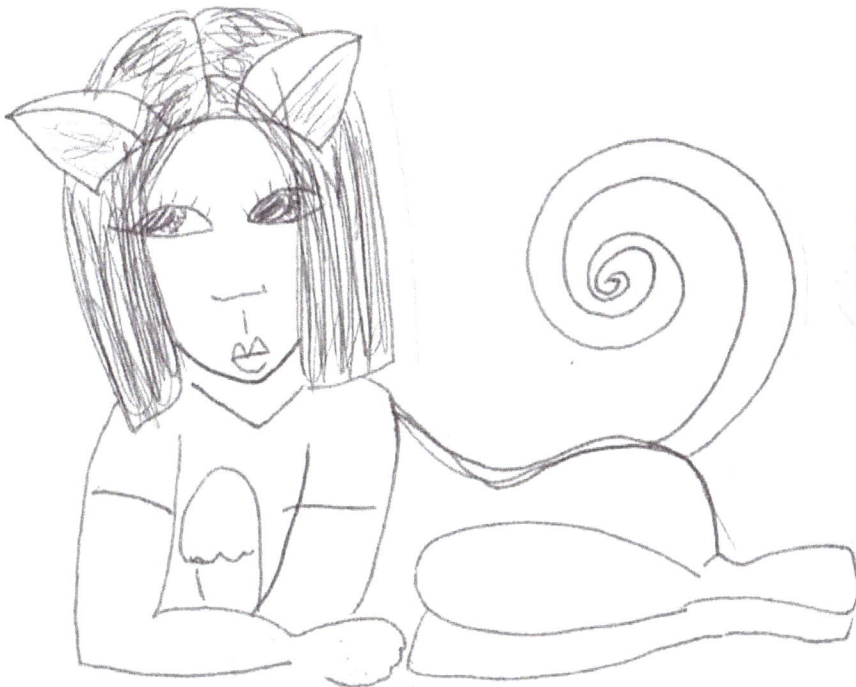
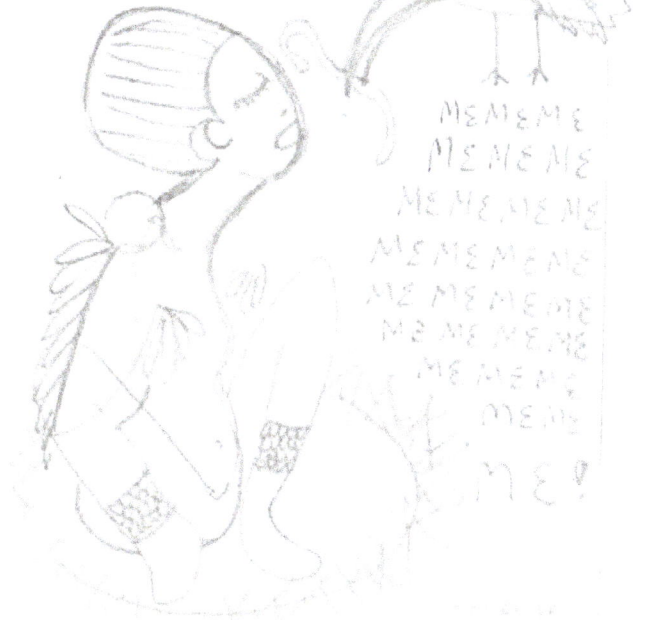

ME ME ME
ME ME ME
ME ME ME ME
ME ME ME ME
ME ME ME ME
ME ME ME ME
ME ME ME
ME ME
ME!

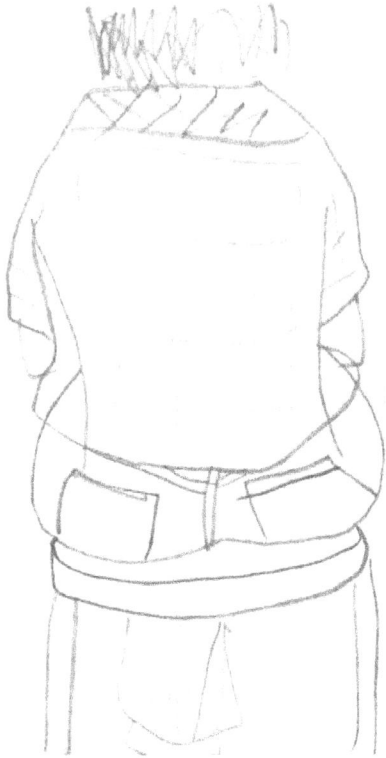

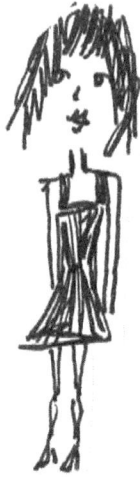

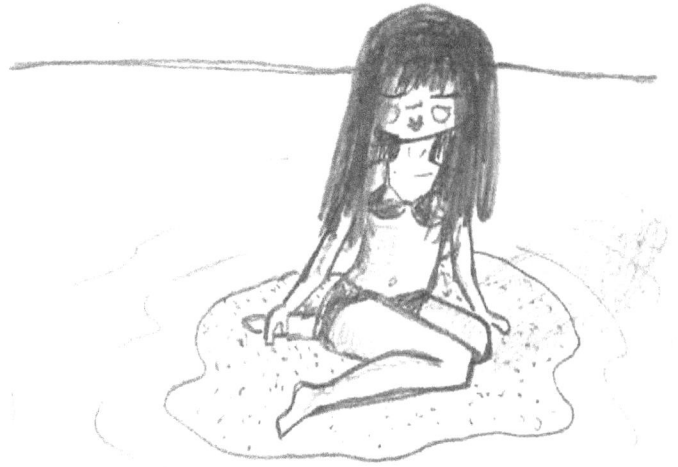

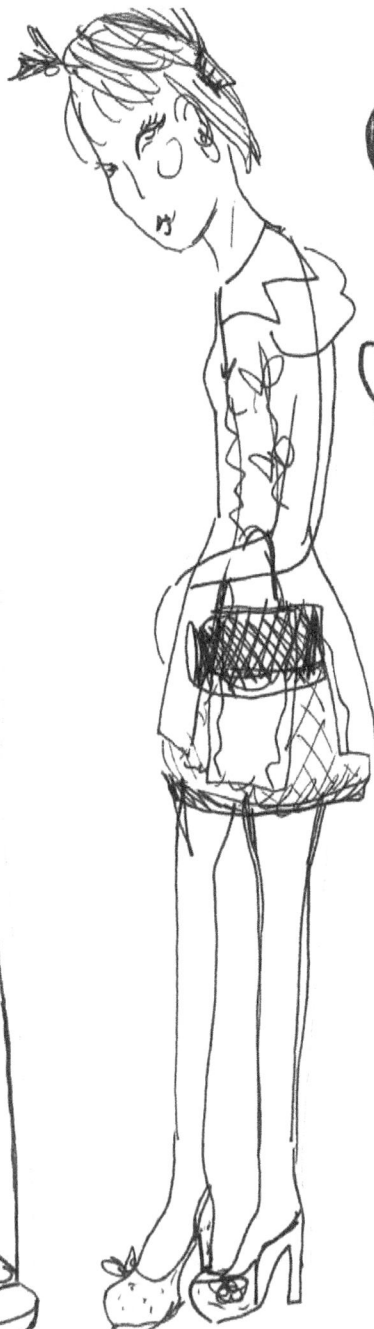

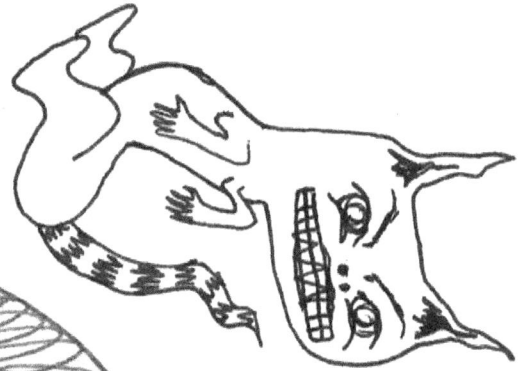

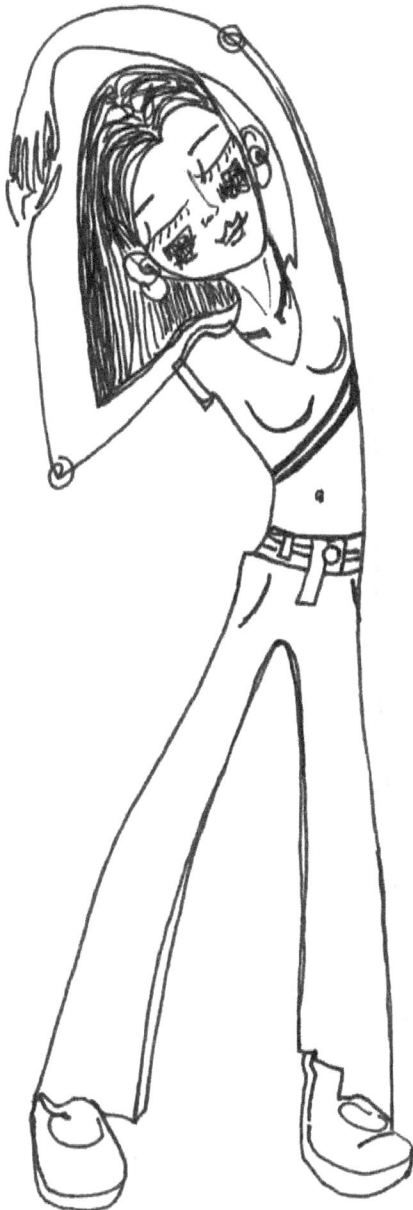

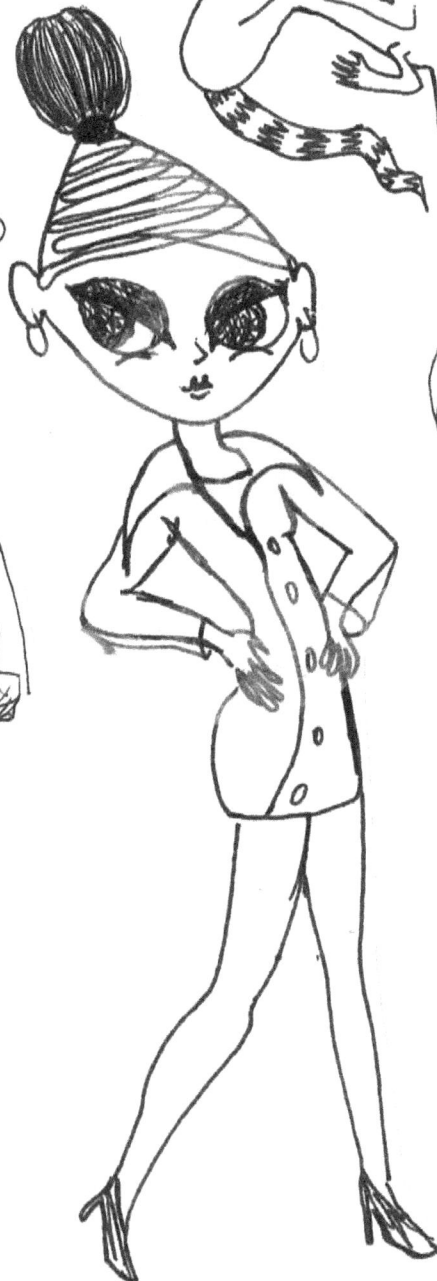

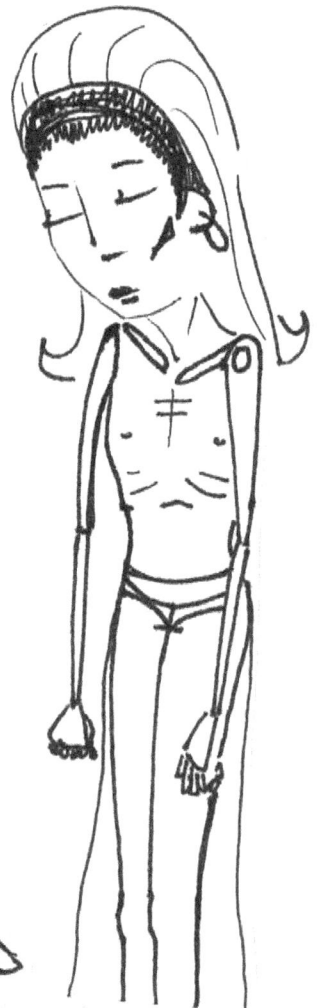

www.ingramcontent.com/pod-product-compliance
Lightning Source LLC
Chambersburg PA
CBHW061235270326
41929CB00031B/3494

* 9 7 8 0 5 7 8 2 7 5 5 6 7 *